Orthodontics: An Evidence-Based Approach

Orthodontics: An Evidence-Based Approach

Edited by Dave Clark

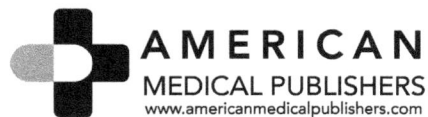

AMERICAN
MEDICAL PUBLISHERS
www.americanmedicalpublishers.com

American Medical Publishers,
41 Flatbush Avenue,
1st Floor, New York,
NY 11217, USA

Visit us on the World Wide Web at:
www.americanmedicalpublishers.com

ISBN: 978-1-63927-059-0

Cataloging-in-Publication Data

Orthodontics : an evidence-based approach / edited by Dave Clark.
    p. cm.
Includes bibliographical references and index.
ISBN 978-1-63927-059-0
1. Orthodontics. 2. Orthodontics--Diagnosis. I. Clark, Dave.
RK522 .O78 2022
617.643--dc23

Table of Contents

Preface

Every book is a source of knowledge and this one is no exception. The idea that led to the conceptualization of this book was the fact that the world is advancing rapidly; which makes it crucial to document the progress in every field. I am aware that a lot of data is already available, yet, there is a lot more to learn. Hence, I accepted the responsibility of editing this book and contributing my knowledge to the community.

Orthodontics is a branch of dentistry that focuses on the diagnosis, prevention and treatment of jaws and teeth that are malpositioned. Diagnosis and treatment in orthodontics include reorganization of the problem, defining the nature of the problem, designing a treatment based on the needs of the patient and present the treatment strategy to the patient. Diagnosis also includes an in-depth orthodontic assessment of the patient. Orthodontic treatment aims to promote good function and to produce stable results. The majority of orthodontic appliance therapy is done using fixed appliances and removable appliances. Active and functional appliances are the two main types of orthodontic appliances that are commonly used. The objective of this book is to give a general view of the different areas of orthodontics, and its applications. This book covers in detail some existent theories and innovative concepts revolving around this domain. This book is a vital tool for all researching and studying this field.

While editing this book, I had multiple visions for it. Then I finally narrowed down to make every chapter a sole standing text explaining a particular topic, so that they can be used independently. However, the umbrella subject sinews them into a common theme. This makes the book a unique platform of knowledge.

I would like to give the major credit of this book to the experts from every corner of the world, who took the time to share their expertise with us. Also, I owe the completion of this book to the never-ending support of my family, who supported me throughout the project.

Editor

Effects of rapid maxillary expansion in cleft patients resulting from the use of two different expanders

Daniel Santos Fonseca Figueiredo[1], Lucas Cardinal[1], Flávia Uchôa Costa Bartolomeo[1],
Juan Martin Palomo[2], Martinho Campolina Rebello Horta[3], Ildeu Andrade Jr[4], Dauro Douglas Oliveira[5]

Objective: The aim of this study was to evaluate the skeletal and dental effects of rapid maxillary expansion (RME) in cleft patients using two types of expanders. **Methods:** Twenty unilateral cleft lip and palate patients were randomly divided into two groups, according to the type of expander used: (I) modified Hyrax and (II) inverted Mini-Hyrax. A pretreatment cone-beam computed tomographic image (T_0) was taken as part of the initial orthodontic records and three months after RME, for bone graft planning (T_1). **Results:** In general, there was no significant difference among groups ($p > 0.05$). Both showed a significant transverse maxillary expansion ($p < 0.05$) and no significant forward and/or downward movement of the maxilla ($p > 0.05$). There was greater dental crown than apical expansion. Maxillary posterior expansion tended to be larger than anterior opening ($p < 0.05$). Cleft and non-cleft sides were symmetrically expanded and there was no difference in dental tipping between both sides ($p > 0.05$). **Conclusions:** The appliances tested are effective in the transverse expansion of the maxilla. However, these appliances should be better indicated to cleft cases also presenting posterior transverse discrepancy, since there was greater expansion in the posterior maxillary region than in the anterior one.

Keywords: Palatal expansion technique. Cleft palate. Cone-beam computed tomography.

[1] Former Orthodontic residents, Pontifícia Universidade Católica de Minas Gerais (PUC-MG), Belo Horizonte, Brazil.

[2] Associate Professor and Program Director, Case Western Reserve University, Department of Orthodontics, and Director of the Craniofacial Imaging Center, School of Dental Medicine, Cleveland, Ohio, USA.

[3] Associate Professor and Dean of Graduate Studies, Pontifícia Universidade Católica de Minas Gerais (PUC-MG), Belo Horizonte, Brazil.

[4] Associate Professor of Orthodontics, Pontifícia Universidade Católica de Minas Gerais (PUC-MG), Belo Horizonte, Brazil.

[5] Associate Professor and Program Director of Orthodontics, Pontifícia Universidade Católica de Minas Gerais (PUC-MG), Belo Horizonte, Brazil.

» The authors report no commercial, proprietary or financial interest in the products or companies described in this article.

Dauro Douglas Oliveira
Av. Dom José Gaspar, 500, prédio 46, sala 106
Belo Horizonte/MG – CEP: 30.535-610, Brazil
E-mail: dauro.bhe@gmail.com

INTRODUCTION

Cleft lip and palate (CLP) is a relatively common birth defect that affects the craniofacial complex.[1,2] During the first years of life, CLP patients are subjected to primary repair surgeries. As a consequence, the scar tissue compromises growth and development of the maxilla while frequently causing maxillary constriction. Therefore, rapid maxillary expansion (RME) is a therapy commonly used to correct this transverse deficiency.[3,4]

RME effects in non-cleft patients is well documented in the literature.[5-15] However, the biomechanical effects of RME in CLP patients seem to be different from those registered for patients without this craniofacial deformity, probably due to different anatomical structures.[16,17] This high anatomical variability in the maxillary arch has led to the development of maxillary expanders with alternative designs.[4,17,18,19] A recent study evaluated the effects of expanders designed to privilege anterior arch expansion: the fan-type and inverted mini-Hyrax (iMini) associated with a transpalatal arch (TPA).[17] However, the effects of the iMini without the TPA were not addressed. Therefore, the aim of the present study was to evaluate and compare the dentoskeletal effects of modified Hyrax and iMini supported on first permanent molars.

MATERIAL AND METHODS

The study sample consisted of 20 unilateral cleft lip and palate (UCLP) children (14 boys, 6 girls) who sought orthodontic treatment at the Center of Craniofacial Anomalies (CENTRARE), Department of Orthodontics, Pontifícia Universidade Católica de Minas Gerais. The selection criteria were: presence of UCLP, need for maxillary expansion treatment and age between 8 and 15 years. Exclusion criteria included: absence of maxillary first molars, periodontal disease, previous orthodontic treatment and presence of any syndrome. Cervical vertebral maturation revealed that all patients were before or during the pubertal growth spurt (cervical maturation between CS1 to CS4).[20] This study was approved by the local Ethics Committee, and an informed consent form was obtained from all patients' parents.

The sample was randomly allocated into two groups with 10 patients each: (1) modified Hyrax expander and (2) iMini supported on first permanent molars. Sex and age distributions are shown in Table 1 for all groups. The modified Hyrax is a tooth-borne appliance (Leone, Florence, Italy) with a jackscrew placed in the region of deciduous molars or premolars (Fig 1A). The iMini is a tooth-borne appliance (Dynaflex, Sait Ann, Missouri, USA) designed with a mini-screw positioned at the anterior region (Fig 1B). All expanders were made by the same technician, and the bands were placed only on maxillary first molars with wire extensions bonded to the adjacent teeth.

The methods were similar to those used in our previous study.[17] A pretreatment cone-beam computed tomographic image (CBCT) (T_0) was taken as part of the initial orthodontic records of all patients. The activation regimen was established at two turns/day until the tip of the lingual cusp of maxillary teeth touched the tip of the buccal cusp of mandibular teeth. The ap-

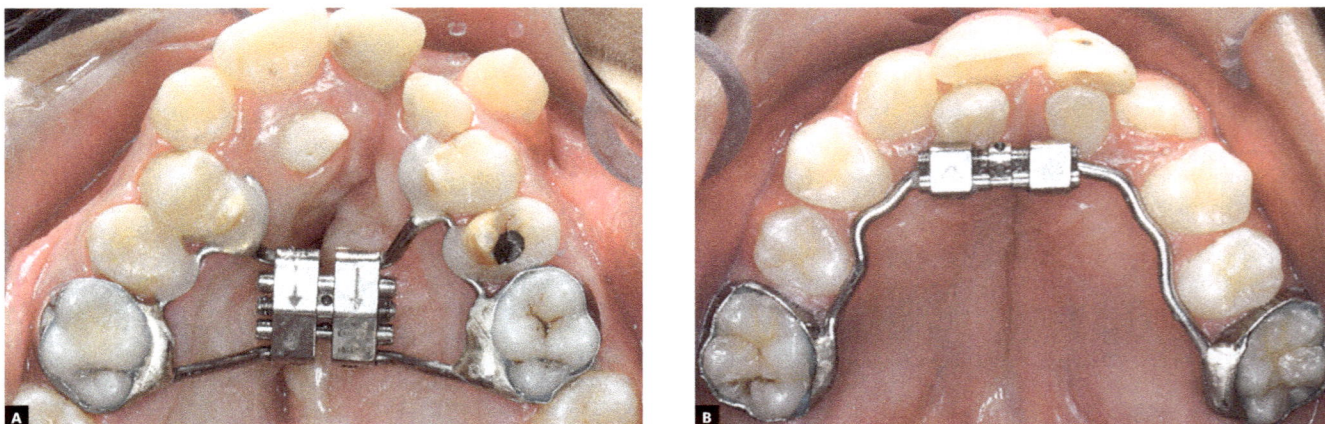

Figure 1 - Rapid maxillary expanders evaluated: **A)** modified Hyrax; **B)** inverted mini-Hyrax (iMini).

pliance was kept in place as a passive retainer for three months. After the retention period, the expander was removed and a post expansion CBCT image (T_1) was immediately taken. On the same day, a transpalatal bar with anterior extensions was inserted as a retainer. The T_1 CBCT was justified because of its valuable importance in bone graft planning. None of the patients received any brackets or wires in the maxillary arch until the second CBCT image was taken.

All scans were obtained by the same technician with an i-CAT machine (Imaging Sciences International, Hatfield, Pa, USA), performed at 120 kV, 8 mA, scan time of 40 seconds, and 0.3-mm voxel dimension. All CBTC images were oriented and standardized by means of Dolphin Imaging software (version 11.5, Dolphin Imaging & Management Solutions, Chatsworth, Calif, USA). Patient's head was oriented in the three planes of space for frontal, right lateral and top (facing down) views, as detailed previously.[17]

To examine the effects of RME, the measurements were evaluated at T_0 and T_1 in three planes of space: anteroposterior (AP), vertical and transversal. The AP plane was assessed in lateral cephalograms obtained through CBCT by the SNA measurement. The vertical plane was verified by means of CBCT sagittal slices, measuring the smaller distance between the Frankfort Horizontal Line and ANS (FH-ANS) (Fig 2).

Transverse changes were measured in the anterior and posterior regions of the maxilla. Transverse posterior maxillary measurements were taken at the level of the first permanent molars. Transverse anterior measurements were taken at the level of the most anterior appliance-supporting teeth. As described previously,[17] the following parameters were used to quantify the amount of transversal expansion (Figs 3A, 3B and 3C): dental crown width (DCW), maxillary basal width (MBW), dental apices width (DAW), nasal cavity width (NCW), and dental tipping (Tip).

To evaluate which maxillary segment was more expanded, a mid-sagittal line connecting the Crista Galli and Basion was defined as the reference line. In the axial slice, the smaller distance from this mid-sagittal line to the four MBW landmarks was measured (Fig 3D).

Statistical analysis

All measurements were performed by the same operator blinded to group status. In order to test in-

traexaminer reproducibility, 18 random images were remeasured by the same examiner, with at least one week between them, and compared to the original measurements. Intraexaminer reliability values were determined with the intraclass correlation coefficient. Chi-square test was performed to verify the distribution of the cleft-side as well as of patient's sex between groups. Paired t-test was used to evaluate whether the changes from T_0 to T_1 were significantly different in each group. Unpaired t-test was performed to statistically compare the patients' age between the two groups and to evaluate differences in the changes of each measurement between the different appliances. Data obtained from all measurements were processed with GraphPad Prism (version 5.01, GraphPad Software, San Diego, Calif, USA). The level of significance for all statistical tests was predetermined at 5%. Intraexaminer reproducibility test varied between 0.98 and 0.99, indicating high reproducibility among measurements.

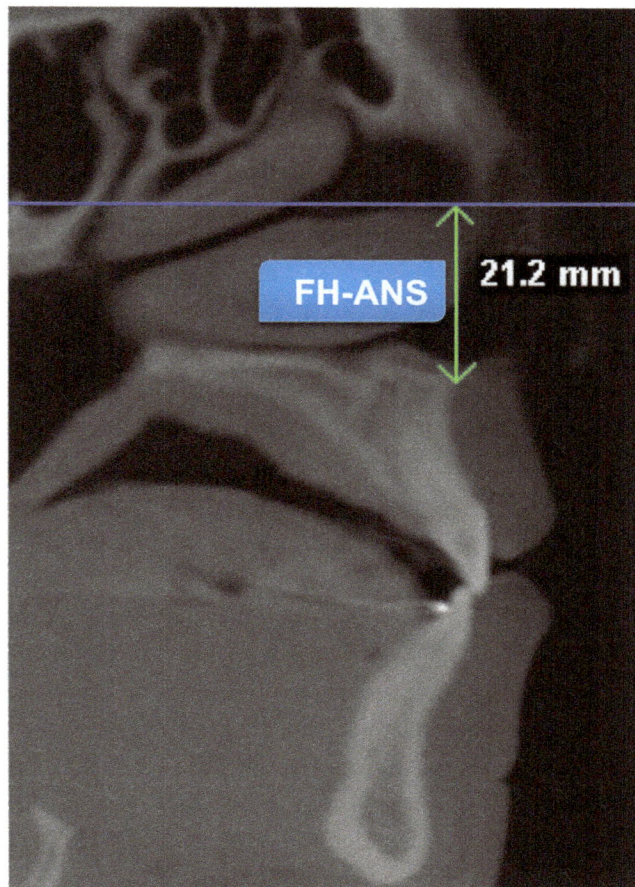

Figure 2 - Vertical measurement (FH-ANS).

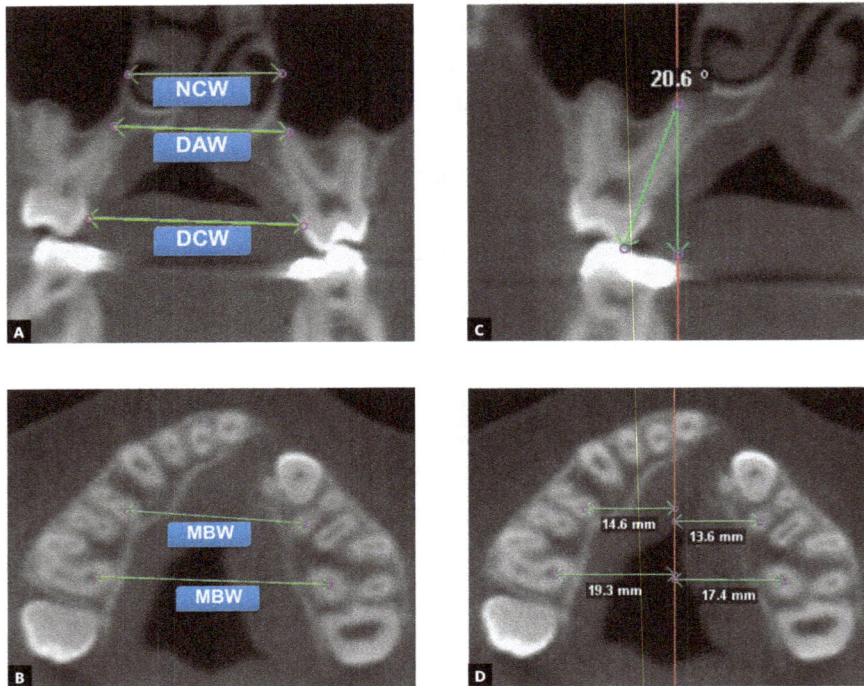

Figure 3 - Transversal measurements were performed in the anterior and posterior regions of the maxilla. **A)** Dental crown width (DCW), dental apices width (DAW), nasal cavity width (NCW) measurements. **B)** Anterior and posterior MBW measurements. **C)** Coronal slice showing dental tipping. **D)** Lateral displacement between cleft and non-cleft sides.

Table 1 - Distribution of age (years), sex and cleft-side.

Group	Age		Gender		Cleft-side	
	Mean	SD	M	F	R	L
Hyrax	11.3	2.4	7	3	4	6
iMini	10.4	2.4	7	3	3	7

Unpaired t-test showed no statistically difference between groups age (p=0.452); the chi-square test showed no statistically difference between groups for gender (p=1.000) and cleft-side (p=0.639) distribution.

RESULTS

There was no significant forward and/or downward movement of the maxilla in either one of the groups. As shown in Tables 2 and 3, there was no statistically significant maxillary movement in the vertical or anteroposterior planes ($p > 0.05$), and there was no difference between groups for this measurement ($p > 0.05$) (Table 4).

There was significant transverse maxillary expansion in both groups, and no significant difference was found between them. All linear parameters observed in the transverse maxillary dimensions demonstrated significant difference in both groups ($p < 0.05$), including NCW, as shown in Tables 2 and 3. In comparing both groups, there were no differences in any measurement studied ($p > 0.05$) (Table 4).

Both groups showed greater dental crown than apical expansion. Measurements (Tables 2 and 3) indicated

that the greatest widening occurred in the crown area, and that the widening effect of the device gradually decreased throughout the upper structures.

Maxillary posterior expansion tended to be larger than anterior opening in both groups. When comparing the means of difference between anterior and posterior regions within the same group, most variables showed greater posterior than anterior expansion ($p < 0.05$) (Table 5), except for NCW in both groups and for the variable DCW in the Hyrax group ($p > 0.05$).

There was no significant difference in dental tipping between appliances. There were no statistically significant differences in anterior or posterior dental tipping when the two appliances were compared ($p > 0.05$) (Table 4). Additionally, it was perceived that both groups demonstrated greater anterior than posterior dental tipping.

Table 2 - Comparison between T_0 and T_1 maxillary dimensions in the Hyrax group.

Measurements	T_0		T_1		Mean of difference	p-value
	Mean	SD	Mean	SD	(T_1-T_0)	
Antero-posterior						
SNA (degrees)	81.77	6.68	81.75	4.96	-0.02	0.981
Vertical						
FH-ANS (mm)	17.13	2.19	17.86	1.96	0.73	0.275
Transverse						
Anterior maxilla						
DCW (mm)	19.65	2.62	24.34	3.59	4.69	< 0.001*
MBW (mm)	25.95	2.35	29.80	3.05	3.85	< 0.001*
DAW (mm)	26.84	2.65	29.64	3.91	2.80	0.001*
NCW (mm)	25.15	3.17	26.74	2.87	1.59	< 0.001*
Dental Tip CS (degrees)	-3.73	14.88	0.21	14.19	3.94	0.250
Dental Tip NS (degrees)	3.99	9.12	12.50	8.17	8.51	0.005*
Posterior maxilla						
DCW (mm)	30.47	2.20	35.20	2.53	4.73	< 0.001*
MBW (mm)	38.15	2.59	42.49	2.63	4.34	< 0.001*
DAW (mm)	29.74	3.33	33.49	2.61	3.75	< 0.001*
NCW (mm)	29.41	2.85	31.28	2.67	1.87	0.003*
Dental Tip CS (degrees)	13.02	4.57	13.82	5.12	0.80	0.126
Dental Tip NS (degrees)	11.37	3.17	13.74	4.55	2.37	0.030*

p values were obtained by paired t-test; *statistically significant p value; SD = standard deviation; CS = cleft side; NS = non-cleft side.

Table 3 - Comparison between T_0 and T_1 maxillary dimensions in the iMini group.

Measurements	T_0		T_1		Mean of difference	p-value
	Mean	SD	Mean	SD	(T_1-T_0)	
Antero-posterior						
SNA (degrees)	80.68	5.18	80.44	5.45	-0.24	0.587
Vertical						
FH-ANS (mm)	1.56	0.32	1.63	0.27	0.07	0.132
Transverse						
Anterior maxilla						
DCW (mm)	20.41	2.61	25.17	3.15	4.76	< 0.001*
MBW (mm)	26.37	2.57	29.79	2.63	3.42	< 0.001*
DAW (mm)	27.18	3.67	29.28	3.51	2.10	< 0.001*
NCW (mm)	26.46	4.92	28.64	4.84	2.18	0.018*
Dental tip CS (degrees)	-9.18	14.26	0.59	17.71	9.77	0.046*
Dental Tip NS (degrees)	-1.4	10.78	7.81	12.02	9.21	0.013*
Posterior maxilla						
DCW (mm)	32.23	2.55	38.16	2.75	5.93	< 0.001*
MBW (mm)	39.78	2.56	45.10	2.85	5.32	< 0.001*
DAW (mm)	32.14	3.26	36.29	3.90	4.15	< 0.001*
NCW (mm)	30.33	3.43	33.07	3.65	2.74	0.007*
Dental Tip CS (degrees)	12.20	9.74	15.87	5.85	3.67	0.094
Dental Tip NS (degrees)	10.32	5.31	13.09	6.87	2.77	0.049*

p-values were obtained by paired t test; *statistically significant p-value; SD = standard deviation; CS = cleft side; NS = noncleft side.

Table 4 - Comparisons between the changes of both groups.

Measurements	Hyrax T_1-T_0			iMini T_1-T_0		p-value
	Mean	SD		Mean	SD	
Anteroposterior						
SNA (degrees)	-0.02	0.73		-0.24	1.31	0.813
Vertical						
FH-ANS (mm)	0.73	1.93		0.07	0.13	0.308
Transversal						
Anterior maxilla						
DCW (mm)	4.69	1.26		4.76	1.60	0.919
MBW (mm)	3.85	1.56		3.42	1.44	0.541
DAW (mm)	2.80	1.83		2.10	0.84	0.299
NCW (mm)	1.59	0.77		2.18	2.33	0.469
Dental Tip CS (degrees)	3.94	10.14		9.77	13.43	0.287
Dental Tip NS (degrees)	8.51	7.29		9.21	9.51	0.855
Posterior maxilla						
DCW (mm)	4.73	1.09		5.93	1.86	0.104
MBW (mm)	4.34	1.14		5.32	1.78	0.171
DAW (mm)	3.75	1.37		4.15	1.37	0.534
NCW (mm)	1.87	1.45		2.74	2.45	0.359
Dental Tip CS (degrees)	0.80	1.50		3.67	6.20	0.172
Dental Tip NS (degrees)	2.37	2.92		2.77	3.85	0.796

p-values were obtained by unpaired t test; *statistically significant p-value; SD = standard deviation; CS = cleft side; NS= noncleft side.

Table 5 - Transverse changes (mm) comparison between anterior and posterior region for each expander.

Groups	Variables	Anterior region		Posterior region		p-value
		Mean	SD	Mean	SD	
Hyrax	DCW	4.69	1.26	4.73	1.09	0.893
	MBW	3.85	1.56	4.34	1.14	0.048*
	DAW	2.80	1.83	3.75	1.37	0.014*
	NCW	1.59	0.77	1.87	1.45	0.480
iMini	DCW	4.76	1.60	5.93	1.86	0.028*
	MBW	3.42	1.44	5.32	1.78	< 0.001*
	DAW	2.10	0.84	4.15	1.37	0.002*
	NCW	2.18	2.33	2.74	2.45	0.371

p-values were obtained by paired t test; *statistically significant p-value; SD = standard deviation.

Cleft and non-cleft sides were symmetrically expanded and there was no difference in dental tipping between groups. There was no significant difference in the amount of expansion when cleft and non-cleft sides were compared in each group ($p > 0.05$) (Table 6). When the 20 patients were evaluated together, still there was no significant difference between cleft and non-cleft sides ($p > 0.05$) (Table 6). There was also no difference in dental tipping between the cleft side and the non-cleft side ($p > 0.05$) (Table 7).

DISCUSSION

Despite being a widely used procedure in patients with CLP, RME treatment-related structural changes in these patients have only been evaluated by a small number of studies.[17,21,22,23] A previous study in cleft patients using CBCT evaluated the effects of expanders developed to focus on expansion of the anterior region of the arch.[17] It was shown that fan-type and iMini expanders — both anchored in premolars associated with TPA — were effective in expanding the anterior region,

Table 6 - Dental tipping on cleft side and noncleft side.

Groups	Maxillary region	Dental Tip - CS Mean	Dental Tip - NS Mean	p-value
Hyrax (n=10)	Anterior	3.94°	8.51°	0.199
	Posterior	0.80°	2.37°	0.103
iMini (n=10)	Anterior	9.77°	9.21°	0.883
	Posterior	3.67°	2.77°	0.656
Both groups (n=20)	Anterior	6.85°	8.86°	0.431
	Posterior	2.23°	2.57°	0.759

p-values were obtained by paired t test; *statistically significant p-value; SD = standard deviation; CS = cleft side; NS = noncleft side.

Table 7 - Alveolar expansion (mm) on cleft side and noncleft side.

Groups	Maxillary region	CS expansion Mean	SD	NS expansion Mean	SD	Mean of differences (CS-NS)	p-value
Hyrax (n=10)	Anterior	2.00	1.43	1.83	1.25	0.17	0.809
	Posterior	2.87	2.80	1.83	0.87	1.04	0.370
iMini (n=10)	Anterior	1.86	1.72	1.56	1.25	0.30	0.724
	Posterior	2.83	1.25	2.33	1.12	0.50	0.344
Both groups (n=20)	Anterior	1.93	1.54	1.69	1.22	0.23	0.657
	Posterior	2.85	2.11	2.08	1.01	0.77	0.209

p-values were obtained by paired t test; *statistically significant p-value; SD = standard deviation; CS = cleft side; NS = noncleft side.

thus restricting the posterior expansion.[17,19] By using similar methods and evaluating the same variables, the objective of this study was to evaluate and compare the dentoskeletal effects of RME in cleft patients using the modified Hyrax expander and iMini anchored in first permanent molars without TPA.

The present study had some important features: it was a prospective study; patients were randomly divided between groups, and skeletal maturation was assessed. All sample subjects were treated when they were at the cervical maturation stage between CS1 and CS4. There was no untreated control group due to ethical concerns and short treatment time.

The iMini and modified Hyrax groups revealed no significant forward or downward movement of the maxilla. There were discordant results of studies with non-cleft patients which described significant forward[11,12,13,24] and downward[11,12,14,15,24] displacement. However, previous studies with CLP patients also showed no change in anteroposterior plane after RME.[17,23] Thus, these findings suggest that the differential anatomy in cleft patients, in comparison to non-cleft ones, can induce to a different behavior of the maxilla in the sagittal and vertical planes.[17]

All linear parameters observed in the transverse dimension presented significant changes for both appliances, indicating that both are effective in performing RME. As in previous RME studies,[7,9,10,14,25] the present findings indicated that the greatest widening occurred in the dentoalveolar area, and the widening effect of the device gradually decreased throughout the upper structures in a triangular pattern, indicating that dental overexpansion is necessary to gain the appropriate skeletal effect.

CLP patients most commonly present atresia in the anterior maxillary region.[3,4,26] Thus, posterior expansion may be undesirable in certain cases because the posterior limit of expansion can be reached before the desired anterior expansion is obtained. From this perspective, the present results showed a pattern of unfavorable opening when using both devices. Maxillary posterior expansion tended to be larger than anterior opening in both groups. There was a previous expectation that iMini would achieve greater expansion in the anterior maxilla because of the anterior location of the screw. The resultant force would be located more distant from the center of resistance of each maxillary half,[27] which would theoretically propitiate more expansion in the anterior region rather than in the posterior region. However, this expectation was not confirmed. Therefore, in order to prioritize expansion in the anterior region, it would be important to consider the association of a TPA with iMini or the use of a fan-type expander, as suggested by previous articles.[17,19] Thus, it is believed that some patients in this study would have more effective maxillary expansion if they were treated with these devices;[17,19] however, at the time they were treated, the effectiveness of these devices had not been evinced yet.

Considering dental tipping, both groups demonstrated greater anterior than posterior dental tipping. This would be expected, since posterior supporting teeth were banded and firmly attached to the appliance, whereas anterior supporting teeth were just connected by lingual wire extension. As the screw was activated, the bands provided resistance to tipping, which probably led to a greater bodily buccal movement of the banded teeth compared to non-banded teeth.[5]

Previous studies have shown an association between RME and various degrees of increase in nasal cavity dimension.[9,11,14,25] Ptresent data clearly showed that both groups demonstrated an increase at the posterior and anterior regions in nasal cavity width, and there was no significant difference when the two groups were compared.

Due to an asymmetrical anatomy of the maxilla, some studies have evaluated if the cleft and non-cleft sides of the maxilla are symmetrically expanded.[16,17,22] Our findings showed a symmetrical expansion in both groups, thereby confirming previous results.[17] When all 20 patients were evaluated together, still there were no significant differences between cleft and non-cleft sides. Furthermore, there was no significant difference in dental tipping in the cleft side when compared with the non-cleft side.

Despite showing similar dentoskeletal results, the Hyrax expander presents a greater size, volume and extent than iMini. Therefore, iMini, as described herein and in previous articles,[17,19] may be a good alternative expander to minimize the difficulty in maintaining appropriate oral hygiene during RME. Thus, the use of this more delicate expander may reduce the negative impact of orthodontic treatment in cleft patients. However, future studies evaluating the impact of these appliances on the quality of life of cleft patients are necessary to confirm this hypothesis.

CONCLUSIONS

Based on this clinical trial, the following conclusions can be drawn:

> » There was no significant anteroposterior or vertical movement of the maxilla with RME.
> » RME produced significant increases in all linear measurements of the maxillary transverse dimension for both groups, including nasal cavity.
> » The cleft side and the non-cleft side expanded symmetrically.
> » The tested appliances were effective in maxillary expansion. However, these appliances should be better indicated to cleft cases also presenting posterior transverse discrepancy, since there was greater expansion in the posterior maxillary region in comparison to the anterior region.

Author contributions

Conception/design of the study: IAJ, DDO; Data acquisition, analysis or interpretation: DSFF, FUCB, JMP, MCRH; Writing the article: DSFF, LC, DDO; Critical revision of the article: DSFF, IAJ, DDO; Final approval of the article: DSFF, LC, FUCB, JMP, MCRH, IAJ, DDO.

REFERENCES

1. Mossey PA, Shaw WC, Munger RG, Murray JC, Murthy J, Little J. Global oral health inequalities: challenges in the prevention and management of orofacial clefts and potential solutions. Adv Dent Res. 2011 May;23(2):247-58.

2. IPDTOC Working Group. Prevalence at birth of cleft lip with or without cleft palate: data from the International Perinatal Database of Typical Oral Clefts (IPDTOC). Cleft Palate Craniofac J. 2011 Jan;48(1):66-81.

3. Capelozza Filho L, De Almeida AM, Ursi WJ. Rapid maxillary expansion in cleft lip and palate patients. J Clin Orthod. 1994 Jan;28(1):34-9.

4. Townend PI. Technique of rapid expansion in patients with cleft lip and palate. Br J Orthod. 1980 Apr;7(2):65-7.

5. Garib DG, Henriques JF, Janson G, Freitas MR, Coelho RA. Rapid maxillary expansion—tooth tissue-borne versus toothborne expanders: a computed tomography evaluation of dentoskeletal effects. Angle Orthod. 2005 Jul;75(4):548-57.

6. Garrett BJ, Caruso JM, Rungcharassaeng K, Farrage JR, Kim JS, Taylor GD. Skeletal effects to the maxilla after rapid maxillary expansion assessed with cone-beam computed tomography. Am J Orthod Dentofacial Orthop. 2008 Jul;134(1):8-9.

7. Lione R, Ballanti F, Franchi L, Baccetti T, Cozza P. Treatment and posttreatment skeletal effects of rapid maxillary expansion studied with low-dose computed tomography in growing subjects. Am J Orthod Dentofacial Orthop. 2008 Sep;134(3):389-92.

8. Ballanti F, Lione R, Fanucci E, Franchi L, Baccetti T, Cozza P. Immediate and post-retention effects of rapid maxillary expansion investigated by computed tomography in growing patients. Angle Orthod. 2009 Jan;79(1):24-9.

9. Christie KF, Boucher N, Chung CH. Effects of bonded rapid palatal expansion on the transverse dimensions of the maxilla: a cone-beam computed tomography study. Am J Orthod Dentofacial Orthop. 2010 Apr;137(4 Suppl):S79-85.

10. Weissheimer A, Menezes LM, Mezomo M, Dias DM, Lima EM, Rizzatto SM. Immediate effects of rapid maxillary expansion with Haas-type and hyrax-type expanders: A randomized clinical trial. Am J Orthod Dentofacial Orthop. 2011 Sep;140(3):366-76.

11. Haas AJ. Rapid expansion of the maxillary dental arch and nasal cavity by opening the mid palatal suture. Angle Orthod. 1961 Apr;31(2):73-90.

12. Haas AJ. Palatal expansion: just the beginning of dentofacial orthopedics. Am J Orthod. 1970 Mar;57(3):219-55.

13. Chung CH, Font B. Skeletal and dental changes in the sagittal, vertical, and transverse dimensions after rapid palatal expansion. Am J Orthod Dentofacial Orthop. 2004 Nov;126(5):569-75.

14. Wertz RA. Skeletal and dental changes accompanying rapid midpalatal suture opening. Am J Orthod. 1970 Jul;58(1):41-66.

15. Silva Filho OG, Boas MC, Capelozza Filho L. Rapid maxillary expansion in the primary and mixed dentitions: a cephalometric evaluation. Am J Orthod Dentofacial Orthop. 1991 Aug;100(2):171-9.

16. Pan X, Qian Y, Yu J, Wang D, Tang Y, Shen G. Biomechanical effects of rapid palatal expansion on the craniofacial skeleton with cleft palate: a three-dimensional finite element analysis. Cleft Palate Craniofac J. 2007 Mar;44(2):149-54.

17. Figueiredo DS, Bartolomeo FU, Romualdo CR, Palomo JM, Horta MC, Andrade I Jr, Oliveira DD. Dentoskeletal effects of 3 maxillary expanders in patients with clefts: A cone-beam computed tomography study. Am J Orthod Dentofacial Orthop. 2014 Jul;146(1):73-81.

18. Levrini L, Filippi V. A fan shaped maxillary expander. J Clin Orthod. 1999 Nov;33(11):642-3.

19. Oliveira DD, Bartolomeo FU, Cardinal L, Figueiredo DS, Palomo JM, Andrade I Jr. An alternative clinical approach to achieve greater anterior than posterior maxillary expansion in cleft lip and palate patients. J Craniofac Surg. 2014 Nov;25(6):e523-6.

20. Baccetti T, Franchi L, McNamara JA. The cervical vertebrae maturation (CVM) method for the assessment of optimal treatment timing in dentofacial orthopedics. Semin Orthod. 2005 Sep;11(3):119-29.

21. Subtelny JD, Brodie AG. An analysis of orthodontic expansion in unilateral cleft lip and cleft palate patients. Am J Orthod. 1954 Sep;40(9):686-97.

22. Isaacson RJ, Murphy TM. Some effects of rapid maxillary expansion in cleft lip and palate patients. Angle Orthod 1964 Jul;34(4): 143-54.

23. Tindlund RS, Rygh P, Bøe OE. Intercanine widening and sagittal effect of maxillary transverse expansion in patients with cleft lip and palate during the deciduous and mixed dentitions. Cleft Palate Craniofac J. 1993 Mar;30(2):195-207.

24. Doruk C, Bicakci AA, Basciftci FA, Agar U, Babacan H. A comparison of the effects of rapid maxillary expansion and fan-type rapid maxillary expansion on dentofacial structures. Angle Orthod. 2004 Apr;74(2):184-94.

25. Silva Filho OG, Montes LA, Torelly LF. Rapid maxillary expansion in the deciduous and mixed dentition evaluated through posteroanterior cephalometric analysis. Am J Orthod Dentofacial Orthop. 1995 Mar;107(3):268-75.

26. Silva Filho OG, Ramos AL, Abdo RC. The influence of unilateral cleft lip and palate on maxillary dental arch morphology. Angle Orthod. 1992 Winter;62(4):283-90.

27. Braun S, Bottrel JA, Lee KG, Lunazzi JJ, Legan HL. The biomechanics of rapid maxillary sutural expansion. Am J Orthod Dentofacial Orthop. 2000 Sep;118(3):257-61.

28. Cozza P, De Toffol L, Mucedero M, Ballanti F. Use of a modified expander to increase anterior arch lenght. J Clin Orthod. 2003 Sep;37(9):490-5.

2

Relationship between mandibular symphysis dimensions and mandibular anterior alveolar bone thickness as assessed with cone-beam computed tomography

Pimchanok Foosiri[1], Korapin Mahatumarat[1], Soontra Panmekiate[2]

Objective: To determine the relationship between symphysis dimensions and alveolar bone thickness (ABT) of the mandibular anterior teeth. **Methods:** Cone-beam computed tomography images of 51 patients were collected and measured. The buccal and lingual ABT of the mandibular anterior teeth was measured at 3 and 6 mm apical to the cemento-enamel junction (CEJ) and at the root apices. The symphysis height and width were measured. The symphysis ratio was the ratio of symphysis height to symphysis width. Kendall's tau correlation coefficient was used to determine the relationships between the variables at a 0.05 significance level. **Results:** The mandibular anterior teeth lingual and apical ABT positively correlated with symphysis width ($p<0.05$). Moreover, these thicknesses negatively correlated with the symphysis ratio ($p<0.05$). Symphysis widths and ratios showed higher correlation coefficients with total and buccal apical ABT, compared with lingual ABT. Buccal ABT at 3 and 6 mm apical to the CEJ was not significantly correlated with most symphysis dimensions. The mean thickness of the buccal alveolar bone at the upper root half was only 0.2-0.6 mm, which was very thin, when compared with other regions. **Conclusion:** For mandibular anterior teeth, the apical alveolar bone and lingual alveolar bone tended to be thicker in patients with a wide and short symphysis, compared to those with a narrow and long symphysis. Buccal alveolar bone was, in general, very thin and did not show a significant relationship with most symphysis dimensions.

Keywords: Cone-beam computed tomography. Incisor. Chin. Mandible. Orthodontics.

[1] Chulalongkorn University, Department of Orthodontics (Bangkok, Thailand).
[2] Chulalongkorn University, Department of Radiology (Bangkok, Thailand).

» The authors report no commercial, proprietary or financial interest in the products or companies described in this article.

Pimchanok Foosiri
Resident, Department of Orthodontics, Chulalongkorn University
34 Henri-Dunant Rd, Patumwan, 10330, Bangkok, Thailand
E-mail: pimchanok.dentchula@gmail.com

INTRODUCTION

Orthodontic tooth movement (OTM) occurs from the biological response of alveolar bone to pressure and tension, i.e., resorption and apposition, respectively. Studies on secondary remodeling and tooth movement found decreased alveolar bone thickness and root perforations of the lingual cortical plates when anterior teeth were moved in an anteroposterior direction.[1-3] These results corresponded with those of Handelman,[4] which indicated that iatrogenic sequelae, such as root perforation, dehiscence or fenestration, may occur due to teeth moving beyond the dimensions of the alveolus. Proffit et al[5] proposed a theoretical model ("envelopes of discrepancy") that suggested that orthodontic movement without surgery or growth modification produced the least tooth movement due to anatomical limitations.

To determine the therapeutic limits of OTM, several studies examined alveolar bone thickness (ABT). Both buccal and lingual bone tended to be very thin in the mandibular incisor region, especially at the upper root half.[6,7] Additionally, bone dehiscence and fenestration prior to orthodontic treatment was commonly found in anterior regions, particularly in the mandibular incisor area, where thin alveolar bone support was seen.[8,9] Consequently, ABT, especially in the mandibular incisor area should be taken into consideration to avoid iatrogenic complications and minimize periodontal tissue and tooth structure damage during orthodontic treatment.

Prior studies demonstrated a relationship between vertical facial types and alveolar bone support at different tooth levels. Several studies concluded that long-face patients frequently showed thinner anterior alveolar bone at the root apex compared with normal-face and short-face patients[4,9-11] Furthermore, a thin anterior alveolus was typical in normal-face Class III patients due to the dentoalveolar compensatory mechanism,[4,10,12] and in patients with severe bimaxillary protrusion.[4] Although thin apical alveolar bone was more frequently found in long lower facial height patients, it could be encountered in any other skeletal types.[4]

Bone thickness measurements in most previous studies were limited to the root apex level.[4,7,9-11] Sarikaya et al[1] stated that both buccal and lingual marginal alveolar bone loss was inevitable during mandibular anterior teeth retraction. Accordingly, marginal and mid-root alveolar bone widths are as important as apical widths and should be taken into consideration when planning orthodontic treatment.[1] Hoang et al[13] concluded that the difference in bucco-lingual bone thickness at the alveolar crest was less pronounced than that at the root apex among the three vertical skeletal patterns.[13] Additionally, buccal and lingual ABT at the cervical and middle thirds of the root was similar for both hyperdivergent and hypodivergent vertical facial patterns.[14] Similarly, both buccal and lingual ABT at the middle root third demonstrated a weak correlation with vertical facial patterns.[15] Importantly, thin anterior alveolus could be found in any skeletal types.[4] Consequently, there may be other factors related to mandibular anterior bone support, especially in the upper root half, apart from vertical facial types. Wehrbein et al[16] showed that symphysis morphology might relate to alveolar bone support of the mandibular anterior teeth. Progressive alveolar support loss was found in an orthodontic patient with a narrow and long symphysis. However, the association between symphysis morphology and mandibular anterior alveolar bone support remains unsolved.

Lateral cephalometric radiography (LCR) has long been used to examine alveolar bone thickness. However, three-dimensional structures overlap in 2D images. Furthermore, 2D radiographs produce a magnification error due to X-ray beam divergence.[17] Thus, assessing mandibular ABT from LCR is unreliable due to overlapping in the incisor region. Cone-beam computed tomography (CBCT) provides three-dimensional data with higher accuracy and reliability, allowing for dimensional measurements that correspond to actual anatomical measurements.[18,19] This technique could be useful in assessing quantitative and qualitative alveolar bone morphology data.[19]

Currently, there are no reports using CBCT data to evaluate the correlation between mandibular symphysis dimensions and mandibular anterior ABT at various tooth levels, including coronal and mid-root. The aim of this study was to evaluate the relationship between symphysis dimensions and ABT of the mandibular anterior teeth using CBCT at the cervical, middle and apical root thirds, in a broad sample of patients.

MATERIALS AND METHODS

From 1,988 patients, whose CBCT images were acquired from January 2014 to March 2016, 51 consecutive subjects (21 males, mean age 26.19 years; 30 females, mean age 25.44 years) meeting the inclusion criteria were collected, resulting in a sample size of 306 mandibular anterior teeth. The inclusion criteria were subjects aged 18–35 years old, CBCT images displaying the entire mandibular symphysis and all mandibular anterior teeth regions, regardless of vertical skeletal pattern and type of occlusion. Subjects with prior orthodontic treatment, >3 mm of mandibular anterior crowding or blocked out teeth, periodontal disease, missing lower anterior teeth, or pathology that might affect the mandible and alveolar bone, were excluded. The data of the mandibular teeth were collected and separated into the following groups, divided into left and right sides: central incisors, lateral incisors, and canines. The CBCT images were acquired using 3D Accuitomo 170 machine (J. Morita, Kyoto, Japan) using 90 kV, 5 mA, 17.5 s exposure time, and a field of view of 8 x 8 or 10 x 10 cm, resulting in voxel sizes of 0.165 and 0.25 mm, respectively. Each CBCT scan was taken as part of treatment and diagnosis, including implant-site assessment and embedded tooth localization; therefore, no subjects received an unjustified radiation exposure. The study protocol was approved by the University Ethics Committee (HREC-DCU 2015-096).

I-Dixel One Volume Viewer Software (V. 2.0.0, J. Morita) was used for viewing and measuring images by a single operator who had been trained, and under the supervision of a certified oral and maxillofacial radiologist. A 1-mm slice thickness was used. For bone thickness measurements, the sagittal slice was positioned through the long axis of each tooth, perpendicular to the alveolar ridge curvature (Fig 1). Buccal and lingual ABT of the mandibular anterior teeth was measured from the root surface to the external limit of the mandibular buccal and lingual cortex, perpendicular to the long axis of each tooth, 3 and 6 mm apical to the cemento-enamel junction (CEJ) and at the root apices (Fig 2). FDI tooth numbering system was used to identify each tooth. For the symphysis dimension measurements, a sagittal slice was placed along the

mandibular midline (Fig 3). The symphysis height was measured from midpoint of anterior alveolus (Idm) to Menton (Me). The buccal symphysis width was measured from the buccal pogonion (Pog) to the external limit of the lingual cortex, perpendicular to the symphysis height. The lingual symphysis width was measured from the lingual pogonion (Pogl) to the external limit of the buccal cortex,

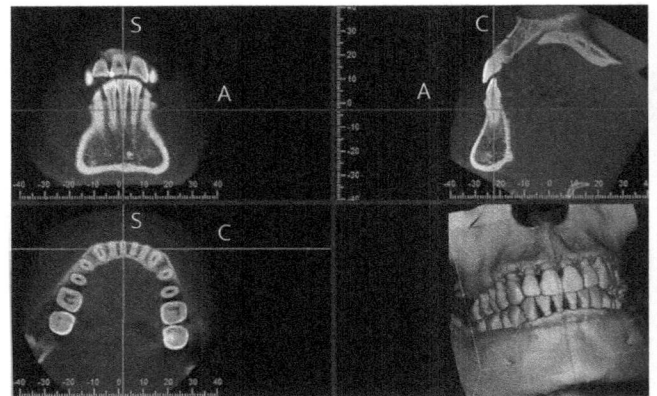

Figure 1 - Lower anterior tooth sagittal cross-section construction using I-Dixel Software. The sagittal slice was positioned through the long axis of each lower anterior tooth, perpendicular to the curvature of the alveolar ridge. The sagittal cross-section (upper right image) was used to measure alveolar bone thickness. A, C, and S represent the lines corresponding to the axial, coronal, and sagittal planes, respectively.

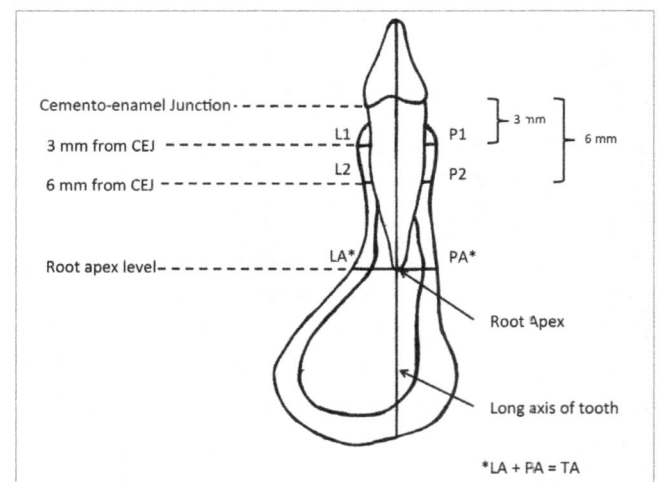

Figure 2 - Sagittal cross-section of the lower anterior tooth. Bone thickness was measured perpendicular to the long axis of the tooth. Variables: L1, buccal bone thickness 3 mm apical to the CEJ; L2, buccal bone thickness 6 mm apical to the CEJ; LA, buccal bone thickness at the root apex; P1, lingual bone thickness 3 mm apical to the CEJ; P2, lingual bone thickness 6 mm apical to the CEJ; PA, lingual bone thickness at the root apex; TA, total apical bone thickness, LA+PA, sum of the buccal and lingual bone thickness at the root apex.

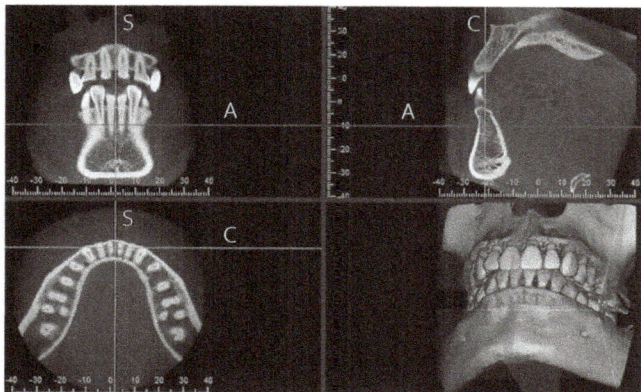

Figure 3 - Mandibular symphysis sagittal cross-section construction using I-Dixel software. The sagittal slice was positioned through the mandibular midline. The sagittal cross-section (upper right image) was used for symphysis dimensions measurements. A, C, and S represent the lines corresponding to the axial, coronal, and sagittal planes, respectively.

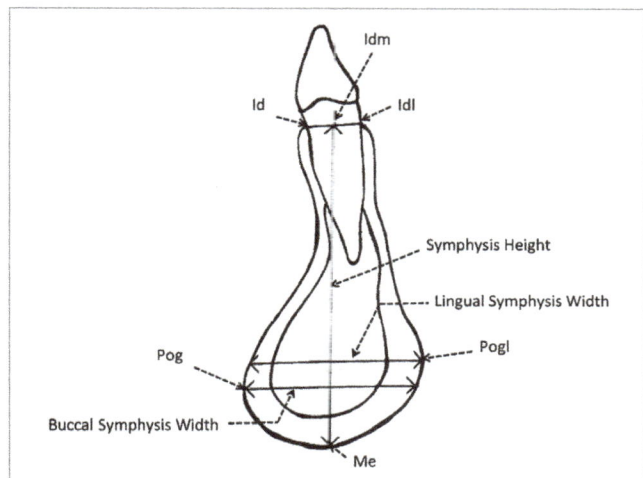

Figure 4 - Sagittal cross-section of the mandibular symphysis displaying symphysis region landmarks and variables.

perpendicular to the symphysis height (Fig 4, Table 1). The buccal symphysis ratio was calculated by dividing the symphysis height by the buccal symphysis width. The lingual symphysis ratio was calculated by dividing symphysis height by the lingual symphysis width. One month after the first measurement, 20% of the subjects were selected at random and all variables were measured again. An intraclass correlation coefficient of 0.91–0.99 was found, showing excellent intra-rater reliability.

Statistical analysis

The Mann-Whitney U test was used to analyze the difference between the male and female subjects' variables. The variables of the same tooth were compared between the right and left sides by the Wilcoxon Signed-Rank test. The Kolmogorov-Smirnoff test was used to determine the normality of the data, which were not normally distributed. Therefore, Kendall's tau correlation coefficient was used to determine the relationship between the symphysis dimensions and ABT of the mandibular anterior teeth. A $p < 0.05$ was considered significant for all tests. The statistical analyses were performed with SPSS software package (IBM SPSS Statistics for Windows, version 22.0. Armonk, NY: IBM Corp.).

Table 1 - Landmarks and variables of symphysis region.

Abbreviation	Name	Definition
Id	Infradentale	The most superior anterior point on mandibular alveolar process between central incisors
Idl	Lingual point of infradentale	The most superior posterior point on mandibular alveolar process of tooth between central incisors
Me	Menton	The most inferior point of mandibular symphysis
Pog	Buccal Pogonion	The most anterior point of mandibular symphysis
Pogl	Lingual Pogonion	The most convex point of lingual curvature of symphysis
Idm*	Midpoint of anterior alveolus	Midpoint of line drawn from Id to Idl
-	Buccal symphysis width	Total width of mandibular symphysis measured from buccal pogonion to the external limit of lingual cortex perpendicular to symphysis height
-	Lingual symphysis width	Total width of mandibular symphysis measured from lingual pogonion to the external limit of buccal cortex perpendicular to symphysis height
-	Symphysis height	Linear distance from Idm to Me
-	Buccal symphysis ratio	Ratio of symphysis height to buccal symphysis width
-	Lingual symphysis ratio	Ratio of symphysis height to lingual symphysis width

*Based on Suri et al.[20]

RESULTS

No significant difference was found between the male and female variables; therefore, the data were combined for subsequent analysis. The ABT measurements between the left and right sides were not significantly different, with the exception of the following: (1) lingual alveolar bone at the mandibular central incisor root apex (PAx31 and PAx41), (2) lingual alveolar bone 6 mm from the CEJ of the mandibular lateral incisors (P2x32 and P2x42), (3) lingual alveolar bone 3 mm from the CEJ of the mandibular canines (P1x33 and P1x43). Consequently, the measurements of these three pairs were analyzed separately as left and right values. The other pairs were combined (Table 2). Symphysis dimensions of the subjects are illustrated in Table 3.

Symphysis width and height

Buccal symphysis width showed a positive correlation with the buccal, lingual and total ABT at the root apices of all mandibular anterior teeth. Buccal symphysis width also positively correlated with lingual ABT 6 mm apical to the CEJ of all teeth, and lingual ABT 3 mm apical to the CEJ for canines (P1xCanine). Lingual symphysis width demonstrated a similar relationship, with a weaker correlation compared with the buccal symphysis width, except for the lingual ABT 3 mm apical to CEJ for the lower right canine (P1x43). In contrast, the symphysis height was not significantly correlated with most ABT measurements. No significant relationship was found between most symphysis dimensions and buccal ABT 3 mm or 6 mm apical to the CEJ (Tables 4, 5 and 6).

Symphysis ratio

The buccal and lingual symphysis ratios (ratio of height/width) negatively correlated with the buccal, lingual and total ABT at the root apices for almost all teeth, except for the lingual ABT at the canine root apices (PAxCanine). Both ratios also negatively correlated with lingual ABT 3 and 6 mm apical to the CEJ for all teeth. Buccal symphysis ratio mostly showed a higher correlation compared with the lingual symphysis ratio. There was no significant relationship between buccal or lingual symphysis ratios and buccal ABT 3 mm or 6 mm apical to the CEJ (Tables 4, 5 and 6).

Table 2 - Mean alveolar bone thickness for lower anterior teeth

Variables*	Mean	Std. Deviation
L1xCentral	0.56	0.27
L2xCentral	0.36	0.17
LAxCentral	3.63	1.22
P1xCentral	0.38	0.22
P2xCentral	0.80	0.55
PAx31	4.44	1.27
PAx41	4.24	1.14
TAxCentral	7.97	1.91
L1xLateral	0.58	0.33
L2xLateral	0.27	0.15
LAxLateral	3.99	1.39
P1xLateral	0.49	0.30
P2x32	1.28	0.83
P2x42	1.08	0.70
PAxLateral	4.39	1.18
TAxLateral	8.38	2.02
L1xCanine	0.40	0.23
L2xCanine	0.25	0.10
LAxCanine	4.49	1.56
P1x33	1.33	0.90
P1x43	1.09	0.68
P2xCanine	2.25	1.06
PAxCanine	5.53	1.44
TAxCanine	10.02	2.00

*L1, L2, LA, P1, P2, PA, TA: see these sites in Figure 2.
*Central, Lateral, Canine: means mandibular central incisors, lateral incisors and canines, respectively.
*31, 32, 33, 41, 42, 43: refer to the teeth according to the FDI tooth numbering system.

Table 3 - Mean and standard deviation of symphysis dimensions.

Variables	Mean	Std. Deviation
Buccal symphysis width	13.54	1.71
Lingual symphysis width	14.24	1.88
Symphysis height	32.13	2.55
Buccal symphysis ratio	2.41	0.33
Lingual symphysis ratio	2.29	0.34

Table 4 - Correlation between buccal symphysis/ lingual symphysis and mandibular central incisor alveolar bone thickness.

		L1xCentral	L2xCentral	LAxCentral	P1xCentral	P2xCentral	PAx31	PAx41	TAxCentral
Buccal symphysis width	Correlation Coefficient	0.028	0.03	0.365**	0.094	0.298**	0.352**	0.352**	0.475**
	Sig. (2-tailed)	0.776	0.763	0.000	0.333	0.002	0.000	0.000	0.000
Lingual symphysis width	Correlation Coefficient	0.090	0.123	0.234*	0.157	0.263**	0.291**	0.270**	0.339**
	Sig. (2-tailed)	0.358	0.212	0.016	0.107	0.007	0.003	0.006	0.000
Symphysis height	Correlation Coefficient	0.133	0.203*	-0.227*	-0.088	-0.133	0.057	0.052	-0.075
	Sig. (2-tailed)	0.174	0.039	0.019	0.367	0.170	0.558	0.592	0.440
Buccal symphysis ratio	Correlation Coefficient	0.037	0.058	-0.478**	-0.207*	-0.360**	-.303**	-0.296**	-0.501**
	Sig. (2-tailed)	0.708	0.557	0.000	0.033	0.000	0.002	0.002	0.000
Lingual symphysis ratio	Correlation Coefficient	-0.002	-0.035	-0.390**	-0.220*	-0.331**	-0.232*	-0.217*	-0.405**
	Sig. (2-tailed)	0.987	0.720	0.000	0.024	0.001	0.017	0.025	0.000

** Correlation is significant at the 0.01 level (2-tailed).
* Correlation is significant at the 0.05 level (2-tailed).
See Table 2 legend for abbreviation explanation.

Table 5 - Correlation between buccal symphysis/ lingual symphysis and mandibular lateral incisor alveolar bone thickness.

		L1xLateral	L2xLateral	LAxLateral	P1xLateral	P2x32	P2x42	PAxLateral	TAxLateral
Buccal symphysis width	Correlation Coefficient	0.056	0.027	0.361**	0.150	0.298**	0.216*	0.383**	0.518**
	Sig. (2-tailed)	0.564	0.788	0.000	0.124	0.002	0.027	0.000	0.000
Lingual symphysis width	Correlation Coefficient	0.086	0.103	0.225*	0.155	0.263**	0.193*	0.322**	0.377**
	Sig. (2-tailed)	0.380	0.297	0.021	0.113	0.007	0.049	0.001	0.000
Symphysis height	Correlation Coefficient	0.146	0.098	-0.322**	-0.178	-0.097	-0.066	0.214*	-0.074
	Sig. (2-tailed)	0.135	0.320	0.001	0.067	0.317	0.500	0.027	0.445
Buccal symphysis ratio	Correlation Coefficient	0.029	0.030	-0.509**	-0.264**	-0.330**	-0.247*	-0.238*	-0.522**
	Sig. (2-tailed)	0.764	0.763	0.000	0.007	0.001	0.011	0.014	0.000
Lingual symphysis ratio	Correlation Coefficient	0.012	-0.039	-0.413**	-0.292**	-0.317**	-0.251*	-0.194*	-0.431**
	Sig. (2-tailed)	0.903	0.690	0.000	0.003	0.001	0.010	0.045	0.000

** Correlation is significant at the 0.01 level (2-tailed).
* Correlation is significant at the 0.05 level (2-tailed).
See Table 2 legend for abbreviation explanation.

Table 6 - Correlation between buccal symphysis/ lingual symphysis and mandibular canine alveolar bone thickness.

		L1xCanine	L2xCanine	LAxCanine	P1x33	P1x43	P2xCanine	PAxCanine	TAxCanine
Buccal symphysis width	Correlation Coefficient	0.086	0.140	0.380**	0.280**	0.212*	0.307**	0.264**	0.497**
	Sig. (2-tailed)	0.375	0.158	0.000	0.004	0.030	0.002	0.006	0.000
Lingual symphysis width	Correlation Coefficient	0.128	0.261**	0.285**	0.215*	0.162	0.235*	0.269**	0.424**
	Sig. (2-tailed)	0.190	0.009	0.003	0.028	0.099	0.016	0.006	0.000
Symphysis height	Correlation Coefficient	0.067	0.059	-0.214*	-0.113	-0.070	0.006	0.235*	-0.025
	Sig. (2-tailed)	0.490	0.552	0.027	0.248	0.474	0.955	0.015	0.795
Buccal symphysis ratio	Correlation Coefficient	-0.087	-0.079	-0.480**	-0.339**	-0.263**	-0.272**	-0.126	-0.453**
	Sig. (2-tailed)	0.371	0.424	0.000	0.001	0.007	0.005	0.194	0.000
Lingual symphysis ratio	Correlation Coefficient	-0.095	-0.203*	-0.395**	-0.310**	-0.233*	-0.247*	-0.135	-0.400**
	Sig. (2-tailed)	0.329	0.040	0.000	0.001	0.017	0.011	0.162	0.000

** Correlation is significant at the 0.01 level (2-tailed).
* Correlation is significant at the 0.05 level (2-tailed).
See Table 2 legend for abbreviation explanation.

DISCUSSION

The results of the present study demonstrated a positive correlation between symphysis widths and apical ABT, as well as lingual ABT at the middle root third. Moreover, apical ABT and lingual ABT at the cervical and middle thirds of the roots negatively correlated with symphysis ratios. The wider the symphysis, the thicker the apical and lingual alveolar bone tended to be. The smaller the symphysis ratio, which represents a short and wide symphysis, the thicker the apical and lingual alveolar bone tended to be. These findings partially conformed to a study demonstrating that mandible with a long and narrow symphysis underwent progressive loss of both buccal and lingual bone due to thinner alveolar bone support.[16]

Lingual symphysis width and ratio showed a weaker correlation with ABT, compared with their buccal counterparts. The buccal symphysis ratio significantly correlated with the lingual ABT 3 and 6mm apical to the CEJ for all teeth, while the buccal symphysis width showed a significant relationship with the lingual ABT 6mm apical to the CEJ for all teeth and lingual ABT 3mm apical to the CEJ for canines only. Consequently, the parameters that showed the strongest relationships with ABT were the buccal symphysis ratio and buccal symphysis width, respectively.

In the present study, the buccal symphysis ratio tended to have a stronger relationship with the buccal and total ABT at root apices, compared with the lingual ABT at every level. The significant correlation coefficients between the buccal symphysis ratio and lingual ABT at 3mm and 6mm apical to the CEJ, and at the root apices ranged from 0.207 to 0.360. The correlation coefficients between the buccal symphysis ratio and total apical ABT, as well as buccal apical ABT, ranged from 0.453 to 0.522 and 0.478 to 0.509, respectively. This suggests that patients with a wide and short symphysis tended to have thicker apical and lingual alveolar bone than those with a narrow and long symphysis. Evaluating symphysis morphology before initiating orthodontic treatment might help orthodontists to estimate the mandibular anterior teeth bony support and design an appropriate treatment plan. Patients with a wide and short symphysis might allow more lingual tooth movement within the anatomical limits than those with a narrow and long symphysis. The possibility of estimating total and buccal apical ABT might be stronger than for lingual ABT, because the former presented a stronger relationship with the buccal symphysis ratio. However, the present results showed only a tendency for the correlations. Orthodontists should keep in mind that the correlation coefficients between the symphysis dimensions and ABT in this study were not high enough to accurately predict alveolar bone support based only on symphysis dimensions.

No significant relationships were found between most buccal ABT at 3 and 6 mm apical to the CEJ and symphysis dimensions. However, mean buccal ABT at 3 and 6 mm apical to CEJ tended to be thin (0.4-0.6 and 0.2-0.4 mm, respectively). These results corresponded with those of several studies that documented thin buccal alveolar bone at the mandibular anterior region, especially at the upper root half.[6-8] Similarly, dehiscence was also found, primarily at the cervical third of the buccal alveolar bone of the mandibular anterior region.[21] The majority of fenestrations were observed at the upper part of the buccal bone plates of mandibular incisors.[22] Therefore, orthodontic buccal movement of the mandibular anterior teeth should be performed with great care, irrespective of symphysis dimensions.

According to a study of postnatal mandibular growth patterns, the mental protuberance of the chin, together with the lingual cortex of the anterior mandible, showed accumulative periosteal bone deposition.[23] The buccal cortex superior to the mental protuberance exhibited variable degrees of periosteal bone resorption, ranging from restricted resorption at the interdental area to an entirely resorbed periosteal surface. This study showed comparable bone remodelling activity between the anterior mandibular lingual cortical bone and the mental protuberance. This might explain the positive association we found between the lingual ABT and the symphysis width. The fact that the buccal ABT at the upper root half did not show a significant relationship with most symphysis dimensions might be due to the differences in bone remodelling between these areas and a variable degree of periosteal bone resorption at the buccal cortex superior to the mental protuberance.

Some studies investigated symphysis width by measuring ABT at the root apices of the mandibular central incisors.[7,10,13] The measurements at the root apex level generally presented smaller widths, compared with the measurements at the mental protuberance, and were influenced by the variation in mandibular incisor root length. A prior study demonstrated that mandibular central incisor root length ranged from 9.13 to 17.24 mm.[24] In the present study, symphysis width was measured at the pogonion level, while the ABT at the root apices was defined as total apical ABT. Prior studies determined average symphysis width at the pogonion using CBCT and LCR. Beaty and Le[25] demonstrated mean symphysis width using CT images of the head and neck region of 14.03±1.53 mm and 13.21±1.46 mm for men and women, respectively. Another study found that the mean symphysis width of Caucasian Brazilian adults with a well-balanced face and normal occlusion measured from LCR was 15.61 mm, with no significant difference between sexes.[26] Compared with the present findings, the wider symphysis thickness measured in that study might result from LCR image magnification, different ethnic origin, and measuring methodology. They measured the distance from the buccal to the lingual pogonion, whereas the buccal symphysis width in the present study was derived from the perpendicular distance from the buccal pogonion to its counterpart, which might not be the most posterior point of the lingual curvature.

Numerous studies have investigated the relationships between vertical facial patterns and mandibular anterior ABT at the root apices.[4,7,9-11,13] Some studies showed that ABT, particularly in the upper root half, might not related to vertical facial patterns[13-15], and thin anterior alveolus could be found in other skeletal types, apart from hyperdivergent faces.[4] Thus, the present study evaluated other factors that might correlated with ABT at various tooth levels. The main objective was to examine whether the relationships existed between symphysis dimensions and mandibular anterior ABT, which had not yet been reported. It was found a significant correlation between certain symphysis dimensions and ABT at the cervical, middle and apical root thirds, in a broad sample of consecutive subjects. To expand the understanding of these relationships, further studies with larger sample sizes are indicated to investigate the correlations in subjects with different skeletal patterns.

CONCLUSION

The symphysis widths of the mandibular anterior teeth positively correlated with total, buccal and lingual ABT at the root apices and lingual ABT at the middle root third. Symphysis ratios, which are ratios of symphysis height to symphysis width, negatively correlated with total, buccal and lingual ABT at the root apices and lingual ABT at the cervical and middle root thirds. Therefore, apical alveolar bone and lingual alveolar bone tended to be thicker in patients with a wide and short symphysis compared with those with a narrow and long symphysis. Buccal alveolar bone at the cervical and middle thirds of the roots was, in general, thin and showed no significant correlation with most symphysis dimensions.

REFERENCES

1. Sarikaya S, Haydar B, Ciger S, Ariyurek M. Changes in alveolar bone thickness due to retraction of anterior teeth. Am J Orthod Dentofacial Orthop. 2002;122:15-26.

2. Wainwright WM. Faciolingual tooth movement: its influence on the root and cortical plate. Am J Orthod. 1973;64:278-302.

3. Vardimon AD, Oren E, Ben-Bassat Y. Cortical bone remodeling/tooth movement ratio during maxillary incisor retraction with tip versus torque movements. Am J Orthod Dentofacial Orthop. 1998;114:520-529.

4. Handelman CS. The anterior alveolus: its importance in limiting orthodontic treatment and its influence on the occurrence of iatrogenic sequalae. Angle Orthod. 1996;66(2):95-109.

5. Proffit WR, Fields HW, Sarver DM. Contemporary Orthodontics. 4th ed. St Louis, Mo: Mosby Elsevie; 2007.

6. Garib DG, Yatabe MS, Ozawa TO, Silva Filho OG. Alveolar bone morphology under the perspective of the computed tomography: Defining the biological limits of tooth movement. Dental Press J Orthod. 2010;15(5):192-205.

7. Gracco A, Luca L, Bongiorno MC, Siciliani G. Computed tomography evaluation of mandibular incisor bony support in untreated patients. Am J Orthod Dentofacial Orthop. 2010;138:179-87.

8. Evangelista K, Vasconcelos KF, Bumann A, Hirsch E, Nitka M, Silva MAG. Dehiscence and fenestration in patients with Class I and Class II Division 1 malocclusion assessed with cone-beam computed tomography. Am J Orthod Dentofacial Orthop. 2010;138:133.e1-133.e7.

9. Baysal A, Ucar FI, Buyuk SK, Ozer T, Uysal T. Alveolar bone thickness and lower incisor position in skeletal Class I and Class II malocclusions assessed with cone-beam computed tomography. Korean J Orthod. 2013; 43(3):134-140.

10. Molina-Berlanga N, Llopis-Perez J, Flores-Mir C, Puigdollers A. Lower incisor dentoalveolar compensation and symphysis dimensions among Class I and III malocclusion patients with different facial vertical skeletal patterns. Angle Orthod. 2013;83:948-55.

11. Ponraj RR, Korath VA, Nagachandran et al. Relationship of anterior alveolar dimensions with mandibular divergence in Class I malocclusion – a cephalometric study. J Clin Diagn Res. 2016;10(5):ZC29-33.

12. Al-masri MMN, Ajaj MA, Hajeer MY, Al-Eed MS. Evaluation of bone thickness and density in the lower incisors' region in adults with different types of skeletal malocclusion using cone-beam computed tomography. J Contemp Dent Pract 2015;16(8):630-7.

13. Hoang N, Nelson G, Hatcher D, Oberoi S. Evaluation of mandibular anterior alveolus in different skeletal patterns. Prog Orthod. 2016;17:22.

14. Ferreira MC, Garib DG, Cotrim-Ferreira F. Padronização de um método para mensuração das tábuas ósseas vestibular e lingual dos maxilares na tomografia computadorizada de feixe cônico (cone beam). Dental Press J Orthod. 2010;15:49e1-49e7.

15. Gama A, Vedovello S, Vedovello-Filho M, Lucato AS, Junior MS. Evaluation of the alveolar process of mandibular incisor in Class I, II and III individuals with different facial patterns. UNOPAR Cient Ciênc Biol Saúde. 2012;14(2):95-8.

16. Wehrbein H, Bauer W, Diedrich P. Mandibular incisors, alveolar bone, and symphysis after orthodontic treatment. A retrospective study. Am J Orthod Dentofacial Orthop. 1996;110:239-246.

17. Adams GL, Gansky SA, Miller AJ, Harrell WE Jr, Hatcher DC. Comparison between traditional 2-dimensional cephalometry and a 3-dimensional approach on human dry skulls. Am J Orthod Dentofacial Orthop. 2004;126(4):397-409.

18. Lagravère MO, Carey J, Toogood RW, Major PW. Three-dimensional accuracy of measurements made with software on cone-beam computed tomography images. Am J Orthod Dentofacial Orthop. 2008;134:112-116.

19. Timock AM, Cook V, McDonald T, Leo MC, Crowe J, Benninger BL, Covell DA Jr. Accuracy and reliability of buccal bone height and thickness measurements from cone-beam computed tomography imaging. Am J Orthod Dentofacial Orthop. 2011;140(5):734-44.

20. Suri, S, Ross RB, Tompson BD. Mandibular morphology and growth with and without hypodontia in subjects with Pierre Robin sequence. Am J Orthod Dentofacial Orthop. 2006;130:37-46.

21. Enhos S, Uysal T, Yagci A, Veli I, Ucar FI, Ozer T. Dehiscence and fenestration in patients with different vertical growth patterns assessed with cone-beam computed tomography. Angle Orthod. 2012;82:868-874.

22. Nauert K, Berg R. Evaluation of labio-lingual bony support of lower incisors in orthodontically untreated adults with the help of computed tomography. J Orofac Orthop. 1999;60(5):321-334.

23. Enlow DH, Haris DB. A study of the postnatal growth of human mandible. Am J Orthod Dentofacial Orthop. 1964;50(1):25-50.

24. Alves N. Morphometric study of the dental roots of permanent lower anterior teeth in Brazilian individuals. Int J Morphol. 2015;33(1):210-212.

25. Beaty NB, Le TT. Mandibular thickness measurements in young dentate adults. Arch Otolaryngol Head Neck Surg. 2009;135:920-923.

26. Arruda KEM, Neto JV, Almeida GA. Assessment of the mandibular symphysis of Caucasian Brazilian adults with well-balanced faces and normal occlusion: the influence of gender and facial type. Dental Press J Orthod. 2012;17(3):40-50.

3

Cephalometric norms and esthetic profile preference for the Japanese

Caroline Nemetz Bronfman[1], Guilherme Janson[2], Arnaldo Pinzan[3], Thais Lima Rocha[4]

Objective: To determine the cephalometric parameters and esthetic preferences of a pleasant face for the Japanese population. **Methods:** For the present study, the following databases were accessed: PubMed, Embase, Scopus and Web of Science. Initial inclusion criteria comprised studies written in English and quoting cephalometric norms and/or facial attractiveness in Japanese adults. No time period of publication was determined. The quality features evaluated were sample description, variables analyzed and how cephalometric standards or facial profile were evaluated. **Results:** Initially, 60 articles were retrieved. From the selected studies, 13 abstracts met the initial inclusion criteria. They were divided into two groups; seven articles were included in Group I and six articles in Group II, according to the criteria of evaluation: cephalometric or facial analyses. **Conclusion:** Japanese are characterized by having a less convex skeletal profile, bilabial protrusion, less prominent nose, more retruded chin and protruded mandibular incisor. Despite living in a society with homogeneous patterns, they seem to get an esthetic preference for white-like features. Therefore, in addition to ethnic normative values, patient's preferences to establish individual treatment plans should always be considered.
Keywords: Japan. Face. Dental radiography. Review.

[1] PhD resident in Orthodontics, Universidade de São Paulo (USP), School of Dentistry, Bauru, São Paulo, Brazil.
[2] Full professor, Universidade de São Paulo (USP), School of Dentistry, Department of Orthodontics, Bauru, São Paulo, Brazil.
[3] Associate professor, Universidade de São Paulo (USP), School of Dentistry, Department of Orthodontics, Bauru, São Paulo, Brazil.
[4] PhD resident in Orthodontics, Universidade de São Paulo (USP), School of Dentistry, Bauru, São Paulo, Brazil.

» The authors report no commercial, proprietary or financial interest in the products or companies described in this article.

Caroline Nemetz Bronfman
Alameda Dr. Octávio Pinheiro Brisolla, 9-75
Bairro Vila Universitária - CEP: 17012-901, Bauru / SP - Brazil
E-mail: carolbronfman@yahoo.com.br

INTRODUCTION

Anatomists and physical anthropologists generally classify men into various racial groups based on their cephalometric features.[1]

Currently, metropolitan areas have a more diverse population, emphasizing the need to recognize that a single standard of facial esthetics may not be appropriate when making diagnostic and treatment planning decisions for patients with diverse racial and ethnic backgrounds.[2]

The Japanese population is a well-defined and homogeneous group with features that are proper even when compared with other Asian groups. Japanese subjects have more proclined incisors, thicker soft tissues, a more projected midface and a flat facial profile.[3] Nowadays, an increasing number of Japanese are looking for orthognathic and orthodontic treatment and plastic surgery. Therefore, it has become important to determine the cephalometric parameters of hard and soft tissues for this ethnic group.[4] Furthermore, orthodontists and surgeons should recognize these differences when interpreting measurements.[3]

The purpose of orthodontic treatment is to achieve a proper and functional occlusion combined with a well-balanced and esthetically pleasing facial appearance. Consensus is comparatively easy to achieve regarding occlusion. One way of expressing that consensus is known as "the six keys for normal occlusion", as proposed by Andrews.[5] However, it is sometimes hard to define the treatment goal based on esthetic profile because no single facial type is believed to be attractive by all. Facial attractiveness might be related to several factors: ethnic group, age, sex, region and professional background. In particular, ethnic and racial differences play a major role in judging facial esthetics. Such judgments might be affected by differences in skeletal pattern among various ethnic groups. Thus, it is important to know the facial preferences of each ethnic group before orthodontic treatment.[6]

There are many studies about cephalometric norms and well-balanced faces in the Japanese population,[1,2,4,6-16] but up to date, none of these studies have compared the interrelationship between the bone pattern displayed by this ethnic group and its esthetic preferences for a pleasant face. People who are potential candidates for orthodontic treatment are likely to be profoundly influenced by the media, including the Internet, magazines, television and newspapers. Worldwide communication provides daily reinforcement for facial stereotypes and these are the major reasons why the perception of beauty might be changing to a more internationally pleasing one, thereby unifying preferences. This systematic review aims to determine the cephalometric parameters and esthetic preferences of a pleasant face for the Japanese population.

MATERIAL AND METHODS

Using "cephalometric", "Japanese", "norms", and "profile" as keywords, research was conducted until February 2014 in the following electronic databases: PubMed, Embase, Scopus and Web of Science. To ensure that the research would encompass all studies related to the topic, the keywords were used, as follows: cephalometric AND Japanese AND (norms OR profile). Cochrane database was investigated for a systematic review on the subject and no data were found.

To identify potential articles, the initial research was performed by title. Initial inclusion criteria were studies written in English and quoting cephalometric norms and/or facial attractiveness in Japanese adults No limitation on the year of publication of the studies was imposed. This selection process was independently conducted by two researchers. Thereafter, the articles from the selected titles were evaluated by abstract and independently valued by the examiners. Interexaminer conflicts were solved by discussion on each article, so as to reach a consensus regarding which articles fulfilled the main selection criteria.

The ultimately selected articles were then classified based on the following quality features: sample description, description of the analyzed variables and description of how the cephalometric standards or facial profiles were evaluated.

Sample description was considered adequate when the author clearly established the evaluated sample. The inclusion criteria were: adult Japanese, with an ANB angle between 2° and 5°, good facial symmetry, normal occlusion with minor or no crowding, all teeth present except third molars, no previous orthodontic treatment and no prosthetic replacement of teeth.

The analyzed variables were adequate when the article showed which angular and linear variables were evaluated and from which cephalometric analysis they were from.

The study was considered appropriate when the author described with which ethnic group the Japanese were compared to, and when their profiles were evaluated, in addition to examiners description.

Afterwards, the articles were divided into two groups: Group I (studies on cephalometric norms) and Group II (studies on facial profile). Then, qualification features were created to classify the articles based on the scientific weight.[17] Articles with most of the qualification features, earning 5 to 6 points, were classified as with high quality; articles with some of them, earning 3 to 4 points, as average; and those with few characteristics, earning 2 points or less, were classified as with low quality.

RESULTS

After database search, 60 articles were found from PubMed, 37 from Embase, 36 from Scopus and 52 from Web of Science, but some of them were repeated. From hand search, 12 studies were identified. The entire search strategy, excluding the repeated articles, resulted in 22 abstracts (Fig 1 and Table 1). Studies retrieved from 1965 up to the present demonstrate that the interest in different racial groups still attracts a number of orthodontists.

Thirteen articles met the initial inclusion criteria: cephalometric norms and facial profile. They were divided into two groups. The division in groups and their respective qualification features are shown in Tables 2 and 3. After quality feature analysis, all articles were classified as high-quality level in Group I; and four articles were classified as high-level, and two as average-quality level in Group II.

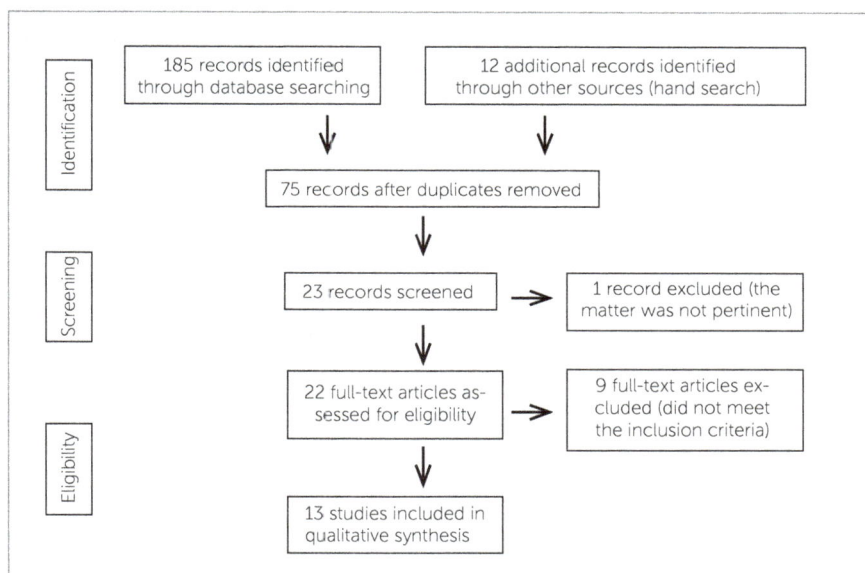

Figure 1 - Flow diagram of information through the different phases of article selection.

Table 1 - Search terms and number of articles processed in each selection phase.

Database	Keywords	Results	Selected	% of total selected abstracts
PubMed	Cephalometric, Japanese, norms or profile	60	7	5
Embase	Cephalometric, Japanese, norms or profile	37	8	5
Scopus	Cephalometric, Japanese, norms or profile	36	11	6
Web of Science	Cephalometric, Japanese, norms or profile	52	11	9
Cochrane	Cephalometric, norms, Japanese	0	0	0
Hand search		12	6	6
Total		23*	22*	13*

* The final sum corresponds to the total references without repetition.

Table 2 - Group I: quality features analyzed from studies on cephalometric norms.

Article	Year of publication	Quality feature					
		Ethnic group compared	Sample size	Balanced sample of man and woman	Provides table with measurements	Measures soft and hard tissues	Inclusion criteria of sample
Reitz et al[13]	1973	X	X	X	X	X	X
Miyajima et al[2]	1996	X	X	X		X	X
Alcade et al[4]	1998	X	X	X	X	X	X
Alcade et al[7]	2000	X	X	X	X		X
Scavone et al[15]	2006	X	X	X	X		X
Ioi et al[9]	2007	X	X	X	X	X	X
Shindoi et al[3]	2013	X	X		X	X	X

Table 3 - Group II: quality features analyzed from studies on facial profile.

Article	Year of publication	Quality feature					
		Kind of raters	Sample size	Balanced sample of man and woman	Elimination of distracting variables	Measures soft and hard tissues	Inclusion criteria of sample
Mantzikos T.[11]	1998	X	X	X	X		
Ioi et al[8]	2005	X	X	X	X	X	X
Ioi et al[10]	2008	X	X	X	X	X	X
Nomura et al[12]	2009		X	X	X	X	X
Kuroda et al[6]	2009	X	X			X	X
Shimomura et al[16]	2011	X	X	X	X	X	X

Comparison of cephalometric norms

In Group I, cephalometric parameters of adult Japanese with normal occlusion and well-balanced faces were evaluated in seven studies. In these studies, cephalometric values were obtained from lateral cephalometric radiographs of different ethnic groups and compared with each other. Only one article used facial-profile photographs to set landmarks and measure soft tissue profile variables.[15]

Each article used a specific cephalometric analysis to compare the Japanese with another racial group. Angular and linear measurements used in these studies derived from different cephalometric analyses.

In all selected articles, cephalometric radiograph tracings were made by hand, traced and digitized by a single author in order to eliminate interexaminer variability.

Table 4 shows the cephalometric analyses used and the ethnic groups compared to the Japanese.

Data extracted from the articles were separated according to individuals' sex and grouped according to skeletal or dental relationships as well as soft tissue analysis, as shown in Tables 5 and 6.

The differences found in Japanese when compared with white standards are:

» In anteroposterior dimension: the Japanese showed a more retruded mandibular position, retrognathic maxilla, more protruded mandibular incisors and lip position, and reduced nasal projection.

» In vertical dimension: the Japanese showed reduced midfaces and larger lower facial height.

Table 4 - Characterization of cephalometric analysis and ethnic group compared.

Article	Year of publication	Cephalometric landmarks	Ethnic group compared with the Japanese
Reitz et al[13]	1973	The authors describe lines and planes to create 17 angular measurements.	Caucasian – American
Miyajima et al[2]	1996	McNamara	European – American
Alcade et al[4]	1998	Burstone and Leagan	White American
Alcade et al[7]	2000	Ricketts Epker et al Legan and Burstone Holdaway	White
Scavone et al[15]	2006	Arnett et al	White American
Ioi et al[9]	2007	Riolo et al McNamara Miyajima et al Legan and Burstone Bishara Burstone and Marcotte	Caucasian
Shindoi et al[3]	2013	Arnett et al	White

Table 5 - Comparison of cephalometric norms between Japanese and Caucasian men.

Japanese men		Reitz et al,[13] 1973	Miyajima et al,[2] 1996	Alcalde et al,[4] 1998	Alcalde et al,[7] 2000	Scavone et al,[15] 2006	Ioi et al,[9] 2007	Shindoi et al,[3] 2013
Skeletal relationship	More retruded mandibular A-P position						X	
	Shorter maxilla in A-P dimension			X	X			X
	Reduced midfaces		X					
	Smaller facial axis angle		X					
	Larger Frankfort to mandibular plane angle						X	
Soft tissue	Bilabial protrusion	X	X	X	X	X	X	X
	Smaller nasolabial angle		X				X	
	Less prominent nose	X			X	X		
	Retruded chin				X			X
	Larger labiomental sulcus						X	
	Smaller Z-angle						X	
Dental relationship	More protruded lower incisor		X				X	X

Comparison of facial profile

In Group II, six articles evaluated the components of a well-balanced Japanese facial profile. The studies assessed the most favored or most well-balanced profile selected by different methods. Japanese silhouettes as well as profile photographs were based on Japanese adults with a harmonious facial profile, and the images were modified creating profiles with more or less protruded lips, or by horizontally altering middle and lower facial thirds. To avoid subjective considerations, four articles used facial silhouettes,[8,10,12,16] whereas the other two[6,11] used facial profile photographs in which distracting variables, such as hairstyle and make-up, were eliminated.

Table 6 - Comparison of cephalometric norms between Japanese and Caucasian women.

Japanese women		Reitz et al,[13] 1973	Miyajima et al,[2] 1996	Alcalde et al,[4] 1998	Alcalde et al,[7] 2000	Scavone et al,[15] 2006	Ioi et al,[9] 2007	Shindoi et al,[3] 2013
Skeletal relationship	More retruded mandibular A-P position						X	
	Shorter maxilla in A-P dimension			X	X			X
	Reduced midfaces		X					
	Larger lower facial height						X	X
	Steeper mandibular plane angle		X					
Soft tissue	Bilabial protrusion	X	X	X	X	X	X	X
	Smaller nasolabial angle		X					
	Less prominent nose	X			X	X		
	Retruded chin				X	X		
Dental relationship	More protruded lower incisor		X				X	X

Table 7 - Methods, examiners and results of evaluation of Japanese profiles.

Article	Year of publication	Methods to evaluate the profiles	Examiners	Results
Mantzikos et al[11]	1998	Five facial profile types were computer-generated to represent distinct facial types.	Japanese cultural and educational background that have immigrated from Japan within the past 5 years.	The profiles preferred were (in descending order): orthognatic, bimaxillary dentoalveolar retrusion, bimaxillary dentoalveolar protrusion, mandibular retrognathism and mandibular prognathism.
Ioi et al[8]	2005	Series of facial silhouettes with varying anteroposterior lip position.	Japanese orthodontists and young adult Japanese dental students.	Both orthodontists and students preferred a profile with slightly retruded lips.
Ioi et al[10]	2008	Series of facial silhouettes with varying anteroposterior lip position.	Young Korean and Japanese adults.	Both the Korean and Japanese tended to prefer slightly more retruded lip position.
Nomura et al[12]	2009	Silhouette profiles with various distances from lip to E-line.	Lay judges of European American, Hispanic American, Japanese and African.	All judges preferred lips located posterior to the E-line.
Kuroda et al[6]	2009	Profile images with point B and Menton anteriorly or distally moved by software.	Male and female Japanese laypeople.	Moderate mandibular retrusion was the most favored profile. A slight mandibular retrusion is more favorable than the mean image, and mandibular protrusion is less attractive.
Shimomura et al[16]	2011	Series of facial silhouettes with varying anteroposterior lip position.	Male and female orthodontic Japanese patients.	Patients tended to prefer a lip position that was slightly retruded compared with the average facial profile for both men and women.

Table 7 shows the methods used to evaluate profiles, the types of examiners and the results.

According to the results, the Japanese preferred a retruded profile with moderate mandibular and lip retrusion.

DISCUSSION
Group I

Cephalometric norms for the Japanese have been studied and extensively used for research and clinical purposes. In order to determine the differences in skeletal relationship, dental relationship and soft tissue analysis, seven articles were used in this systematic review. All selected studies compared a group of non growing Japanese (males and females) to white samples.

The Japanese showed a less convex skeletal profile due to the retruded position of the maxilla and mandible. They presented a significantly less prominent nose[7] and the upper and lower lips anteriorly positioned in all studies, which agreed with the concept of bilabial protrusion.[2,3,4,7,9,13,15]

Two articles[7,13] analyzed and compared soft tissue measurements while one compared hard tissue measurements.[13] Males and females adults were included in the samples, but data were not segregated according to sex. These articles showed that Japanese subjects have a less convex skeletal profile, less proeminent nose, anteriorly positioned upper and lower lips and a retruded chin, thereby increasing the H-angle. The H-angle is the angle between the H-line (soft tissue pogonion - upper lip) and soft tissue facial line (soft tissue nasion to soft tissue pogonion).

Five articles[2,3,4,9,15] grouped data according to sex and are discussed as follows.

Japanese males

Skeletally, Japanese males showed a vertically larger middle third as well as larger posterior dental height.[4] The maxilla was shorter in the anteroposterior dimension,[2,7] with a more retruded chin and mandible.[9] They also had a steeper Frankfort-to-mandibular-plane angle.[9]

Regarding soft tissues, Japanese males exhibited bilabial protrusion,[2,4,9,15] smaller noses,[15] less proeminent chin,[4] as well as posteriorly positioned maxilla and mandible in relation to the glabella, leading to less convex facial form.[4] They also presented a smaller nasolabial angle,[2,3,9,15] larger labiomental

sulcus,[9] smaller Z-angle[9] and a thinner base of the upper lip.[9]

Regarding dental relationships, there was greater protrusion of mandibular incisors.[2,9]

Japanese females

Skeletally, Japanese females showed anteroposteriorly shorter maxilla, greater anterior middle third of the face[4] and significantly larger lower facial height.[9] The midface and the facial axis angle were smaller,[2,9] and the Frankfort to mandibular plane angle was larger,[9] with a more retruded mandible and chin.[9]

Regarding soft tissues, Japanese females exhibited bilabial protrusion[2,4,9,15] and a less proeminent chin.[4] The nasolabial angle was more acute,[2] with a smaller nasal projection.[15] There was no difference in the Z-angle between Japanese and Caucasian females,[9] and racial differences in the cant of the upper lip were less obvious in women than in men.[2]

Regarding dental relationships, there was greater protrusion of mandibular incisors.[2,3,9] The distance of mandibular incisors and molars to the mandibular plane was significantly larger than in Caucasian subjects. These differences might be attributed to longer lower face height in Japanese females.[9]

Sexual dimorphism

Sexual dimorphism was found in Japanese adults, with Japanese males showing longer anteroposterior cranial base length and longer vertical skeletal and dental values than the female group. Longer maxillary and mandibular measurements and larger gonial angle were found in Japanese men. Japanese women had a more obtuse angle between occlusal and mandibular planes,[4] and had a more projected midface and convex profile .[3] Despite sexual differences in some dentoskeletal variables, there were no sexual differences regarding soft-tissue variables.[15]

Group II

The average anteroposterior lip position in Japanese adults is regarded to be more protrusive than that of white people. Because one of the goals of orthodontic treatment is to create an esthetic profile, it is important to study the Japanese esthetic preferences because different racial groups have different perceptions of attractiveness.

In Group II, the studies were conducted with various types of examiners, such as: Japanese laypeople,[6,11] Japanese orthodontic patients,[16] lay judges from different ethnicities,[10,12] Japanese orthodontists and dental students,[8] representing a wide variety of esthetic preferences of a particular population. These data suggest that the Japanese prefer a retruded or a straight profile, even though Japanese profiles have been characterized as being more protrusive due to typically protruded incisors. Thus, orthodontic treatment should consider patient's opinion to establish individual treatment plans.

Some studies were performed to determine how sex, age or different ethnicity influences the perception of beauty.

Sex

Orthodontists and dental students examiners preferred a slightly more retruded profile for both men and women; but for Japanese females, even a more retruded lip position is preferable.[8]

Age

There was no age difference regarding the preference for male profile. However, examiners over 30 years old preferred a more retruded lip position than those aged between 15 to 19 and 20 to 29 years old for the female profile.[16]

Ethnicity

Examiners' race had significant influence on preference judgement of lip profile. American, Japanese and African preferred lip position posterior to the E-line, but American and Japanese examiners preferred a more retruded lip profile than did the African.[12]

Korean and Japanese people have similar cultural backgrounds and both tended to prefer slightly more retruded lip positions.[10]

According to the profile

According to Mantzikos,[11] an orthognathic profile was most preferred and mandibular protrusion was the least favored off all profiles in the Japanese population. Mandibular retrusion was generally more favored than mandibular protrusion, but the Japanese's favorite profile depends much more on lip position than on chin position.[6]

CONCLUSION

» Japanese adults are characterized by having a less convex skeletal profile, bilabial protrusion, less proeminent nose, more retruded chin and protruded mandibular incisors, when compared to a white population.

» Although anteroposterior lip position in Japanese adults is more protrusive, they prefer a more retruded profile.

» Orthodontists should always consider, in addition to ethnic normative values, patient's preferences before establishing individual treatment plans.

REFERENCES

1. Altemus LA. Cephalofacial relationships. Angle Orthod. 1968;38(3):175-84.

2. Miyajima K, McNamara JA Jr, Kimura T, Murata S, Iizuka T. Craniofacial structure of Japanese and European-American adults with normal occlusions and well-balanced faces. Am J Orthod Dentofacial Orthop. 1996 Oct;110(4):431-8.

3. Shindoi JM, Matsumoto Y, Sato Y, Ono T, Harada K. Soft tissue cephalometric norms for orthognathic and cosmetic surgery. J Oral Maxillofac Surg. 2013 Jan;71(1):e24-30.

4. Alcalde RE, Jinno T, Pogrel MA, Matsumura T. Cephalometric norms in Japanese adults. J Oral Maxillofac Surg. 1998 Feb;56(2):129-34.

5. Andrews L. The straight-wire appliance, origin, controversy, commentary. J Clin Orthod. 1976 Feb;10(2):99-114.

6. Kuroda S, Sugahara T, Takabatake S, Taketa H, Ando R, Takano-Yamamoto T. Influence of anteroposterior mandibular positions on facial attractiveness in Japanese adults. Am J Orthod Dentofacial Orthop. 2009 Jan;135(1):73-8.

7. Alcalde RE, Jinno T, Orsini MG, Sasaki A, Sugiyama RM, Matsumura T. Soft tissue cephalometric norms in Japanese adults. Am J Orthod Dentofacial Orthop. 2000 Jul;118(1):84-9.

8. Ioi H, Nakata S, Nakasima A, Counts AL. Anteroposterior lip positions of the most-favored Japanese facial profiles. Am J Orthod Dentofacial Orthop. 2005 Aug;128(2):206-11.

9. Ioi H, Nakata S, Nakasima A, Counts AL. Comparison of cephalometric norms between Japanese and Caucasian adults in anteroposterior and vertical dimension. Eur J Orthod. 2007;29(5):493-9.

10. Ioi H, Shimomura T, Nakata S, Nakasima A, Counts AL. Comparison of anteroposterior lip positions of the most-favored facial profiles of Korean and Japanese people. Am J Orthod Dentofacial Orthop. 2008;134(4):490-5.

11. Mantzikos T. Esthetic soft tissue profile preferences among the Japanese population. Am J Orthod Dentofacial Orthop. 1998;114(1):1-7.

12. Nomura M, Motegi E, Hatch JP, Gakunga PT, Ng'ang'a PM, Rugh JD, et al. Esthetic preferences of European American, Hispanic American, Japanese, and African judges for soft-tissue profiles. Am J Orthod Dentofacial Orthop. 2009 Apr;135(4 Suppl):S87-95.

13. Reitz PV, Aoki H, Yoshioka M, Uehara J, Kubota Y. A cephalometric study of tooth position as related to facial structure in profiles of human beings: a comparison of Japanese (Oriental) and American (Caucasian) adults. J Prosthet Dent 1973;29(21):157-66.

14. Nakahara C, Nakahara R. A study on craniofacial morphology of Japanese subjects with normal occlusion and esthetic profile. Odontology. 2007 Jul;95(1):44-56.

15. Scavone H Jr, Trevisan H Jr, Garib DG, Ferreira FV. Facial profile evaluation in Japanese-Brazilian adults with normal occlusions and well-balanced faces. Am J Orthod Dentofacial Orthop. 2006 Jun;129(6):721.e1-5.

16. Shimomura T, Ioi H, Nakata S, Counts AL. Evaluation of well-balanced lip position by Japanese orthodontic patients. Am J Orthod Dentofacial Orthop. 2011 Apr;139(4):e291-7

17. Janson G, Branco NC, Fernandes TM, Sathler R, Garib D, Lauris JR. Influence of orthodontic treatment, midline position, buccal corridor and smile arc on smile attractiveness. Angle Orthod. 2011 Jan;81(1):153-61.

4

Evaluation of the reliability of measurements in cephalograms generated from cone beam computed tomography

Maurício Barbosa Guerra da Silva[1], Bruno Cabús Gois[2], Eduardo Franzotti Sant'Anna[3]

Objective: The purpose was to compare angular and linear measurements generated in digital cephalometric radiographs and cephalograms synthesized from three-dimensional images. **Methods:** Twenty-six individuals (12 men and 14 women) with mean age of 26.3 years were selected. Digital cephalometric radiographs and CBCTs were taken on the same day. The images were imported and analyzed on Dolphin Imaging V.10.5 software, which synthesized cephalograms in perspective projection and magnification of 9.7%. A single observer marked the points and repeated the procedure with an interval of time of ten days to evaluate intraexaminer error. In the statistical analysis paired Student's t test was used to establish the correlation between the measurements. **Results:** The angular measurements GoGn.SN and IMPA, which involved the Gonial point (Go) and the linear measurements that involved the lips presented significant difference ($p < 0.05$). The other measurements presented good correlation. **Conclusion:** The measurements in the synthesized cephalograms proved to be reliable.

Keywords: Cone beam computed tomography. Digital dental radiography. Interventional radiography.

[1] MSc in Orthodontics.
[2] Specialist in Radiology, APCD. MSc in Dentistry, UNESP.
[3] Assistant Professor of Orthodontics, Federal University of Rio de Janeiro (UFRJ).

» The authors report no commercial, proprietary or financial interest in the products or companies described in this article.

Eduardo Franzotti Sant'Anna
Av. Professor Rodolpho Paulo Rocco, 325 – Cidade Universitária – Ilha do Fundão
CEP: 21941-590 – Rio de Janeiro/RJ, Brazil
E-mail: eduardo.franzotti@gmail.com

INTRODUCTION

The cephalometric radiograph is an essential tool for orthodontic practice and research, providing valuable information to elaborate the diagnosis and treatment plan for growth prediction, evaluation of results and post-treatment stability and surgical evaluation.[1-4] For over fifty years, the cephalograms have been used to analyze the dental and skeletal relations in orthodontics.[5] However, the radiographs represent three-dimensional structures through two-dimensional images and for this reason, present inherent characteristics such as superposition, distortion and magnification of structures of the craniofacial complex, limiting the diagnostic value.[1,6]

Attempting to overcome such limits, the use of medical computed tomography (CT) was introduced in some dental specialties.[6,7] However, high cost, high exposition to radiation and presence of artefacts produced by metallic brackets, damaging the quality of the obtained image, compromised the use for orthodontic purposes.[1,8,9]

A new generation of tomographs was developed specifically to obtain images of head and neck, the cone beam computed tomography(CBCT). Since the introduction of the first equipment, the use of CBCT has increased significantly, specifically in orthodontics.[10,11,12]

The CBCT has been described as the 3D method of choice for obtaining craniofacial images, because of the following characteristics: Dose of radiation around 10 times lower than the medical tomographs, similarity to radiographic exams as panoramic radiograph and full periapical,[13] reduced cost, high spatial resolution for facial bones and teeth, and possibility of obtaining all traditional orthodontic images in a single exposition.[9,14]

However, despite all advantages offered by the CBCT, we must be careful in relation to this new technique in this period of transition, since many points still need to be clarified in relation to the acuity of the measures obtained through radiographs from CBCT.

Thus, it was the objective of this work to determine if the cephalograms generated from radiographs simulated through CBCT reproduce with the same accuracy the measures from the conventional cephalogram.

MATERIAL AND METHODS

The sample had 26 individuals, 12 men and 14 women, with mean age of 26.3 years, from the records of the dental database in Maceió/AL, Brazil. A cephalometric radiograph and a cone beam computed tomograph, obtained on the same day by the same operator should be available in the file. Individuals presenting full permanent dentition, and that signed the Free and Clarified Consent Term allowing the use of the images, were included in this research. The present study was approved by the Board of Ethics of the Federal University of Rio de Janeiro, with number 90/2008. Patients that presented absence of teeth and/or presence of osseointegrated implants or fixed orthodontic retainers were not included.

The x-ray device that was used to obtain the radiographs was the Cranex D (Soredex, Tuusula, Finland) with a digital system that uses CCD sensor (charge-coupled device) as image captivator, eliminating the necessity of radiographic films and/or scanning. The images were generated with resolution of 300 dpi and automatically sent to the work station. The regulation of the Kv was done automatically by the device according to the size of the patient's head, positioned with Frankfurt's horizontal plane parallel to the ground.

All digital radiographs included the image of a milimetric ruler on the right upper quadrant, present on the x-ray device, necessary to perform the adjustment of the image's size.

The CBCTs were obtained through the NewTom 3G tomograph (AFP Imaging, Elmsford, New York, USA). The individuals were positioned in the tomograph lying with their head in natural position, so that the Frankfurt's horizontal plane was perpendicular to the ground.

A 12-in field of view was used, necessary to visualize all structures that compose the cephalometric tracing. The images were exported by the tomograph in DICOM format (Digital Imaging and Communication in Medicine) and the thickness of the slices was of 0.3 mm generating voxels with 0.3 x 0.3 x 0.3 mm of resolution.

All images were imported by the software Dolphin Imaging Version 10.5.02.65 Premium (Dolphin Imaging & Management Solutions) for analysis.

The digital cephalometric images were positioned with Frankfurt's horizontal plane parallel to the lower border of the monitor, for posterior analysis.

The first step to simulate the cephalometric image from the tomogram, was to standardize the orientation of the three-dimensional models. Using the coronal view, the midsagittal plane was vertically oriented passing through nasion and through the anterior nasal spine; the right sagittal view was used as reference to determine the Frankfurt plane, horizontally oriented; the right and left sagittal visualizations were used to make the coronal plane touch the anterior walls of the right and left poria (Fig 1).[9]

After the standardization for the volume positioning was performed, adjusting the image segmentation was done for better contrast between structures of the soft tissue and the skull.

Using the 3D module of the Dolphin software, the perspective radiographs were generated using a 9.7% magnification at the sagittal plane, following orientations from the software, and the right and left sides of the image were present, so that the comparison with the digital radiograph could be established.

The center of the X-ray projection on perspective radiographs was determined on the porion of each three-dimensional image, so that it was the closest to the incidence of rays on the conventional or digital device, which pass at the ear rods.

When generating the simulated cephalometric images, a 100 mm ruler was virtually added to the right side of all images, so that during the cephalometric tracing, the images could be resized.

The 2D image analyses were performed using the module Ceph Tracing of the Dolphin Software. In this research 13 common cephalometric measures were compared, 9 being angular and 4 linear (Table 1), based on 14 cephalometric references: Lateral and on the midsagittal plane.

The projection magnification could be corrected by the computer at the beginning of the tracing, marking two points on the ruler present in the 2D image, so that the program could adequate it to its real size.

The craniofacial structures were automatically drawn by the program as the cephalometric points were being marked. After all markings, the cephalogram and the results from the measurements were automatically provided.

The porion point was considered the most superior point of the external auditory canal, since on the tomographic image there is no similar reference to the mechanical porion, present on the digital radiograph.

On a second step, 10 days after making the cephalograms, 6 exams were randomly selected and analyzed again, to perform the reliability study.

During the marking of points, image tools were used for better visualization of the structures, allowing alterations on the level of contrast, saturation and brightness. On the digital image, the possibility of inversion of colors allowed better visualization of bone structures (Fig 2).

On the simulated radiograph, there was the possibility of navigation among several filters pre-defined by the software. Each filter texture facilitates the visualization of bone structures, soft profile or teeth (Fig 3).

RESULTS

The descriptive statistical analysis including mean, median and standard deviation, was calculated for each cephalometric measure of the digital and simulated radiographs (Table 2).

Table 1 - Measurements used in this study.

Angular	Linear
SNA	Upper Lip – Line E
SNB	Lower Lip – Line E
ANB	1-NA
FMA	1-NB
Ocl.SN	
GoGn.SN	
IMPA	
1.SN	
Y axis	

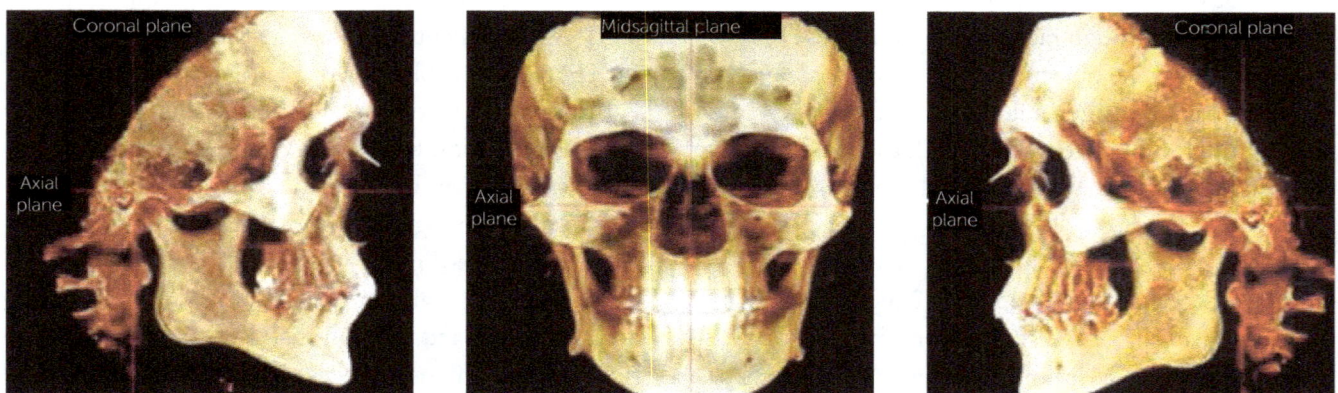

Figure 1 - Image showing the auxiliary reference lines on the positioning of three-dimensional volumes.

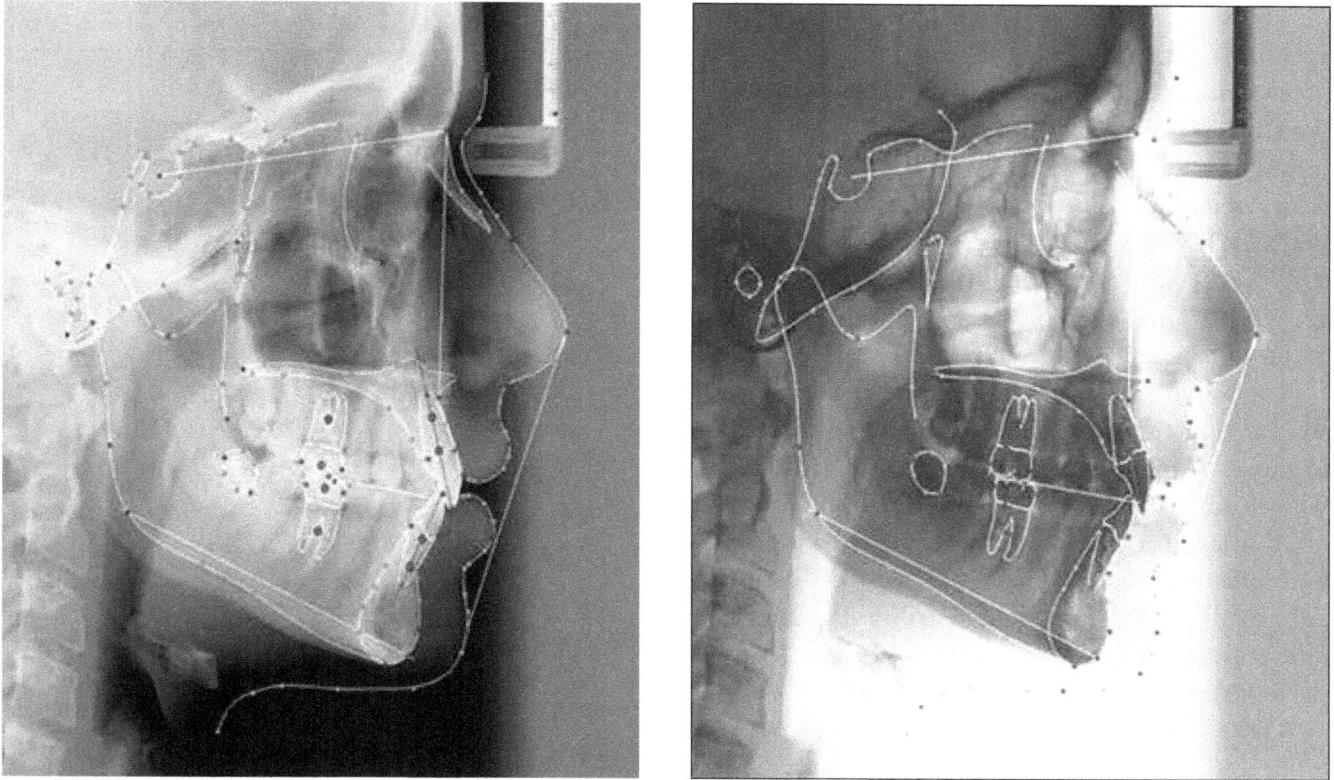

Figure 2 - Difference between original and modified images (inversion of colors).

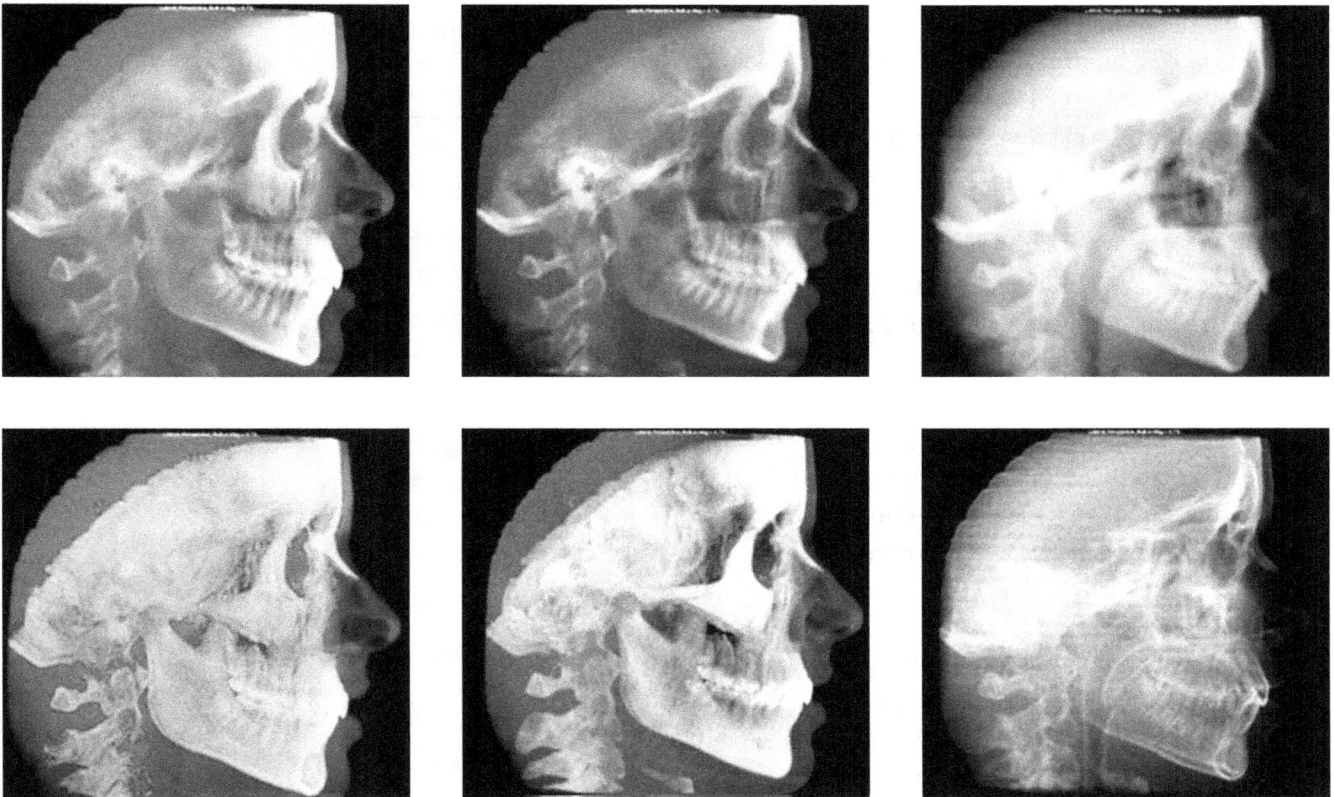

Figure 3 - Several image filters that are provided by Dolphin 3D.

The reliability study on the image capturing was determined by the repetition of six tracings (23%) randomly selected, performed in two different periods by the same examiner. The same point, lines, planes and measures were traced again after a 10 day interval. The values obtained were compared by Intraclass Correlation Coefficient (ICC) and were between 0.969 and 0.999 with statistical significance of $p < 0.05$. Thus, the correlation was shown to be high, indicating reliability on the obtainment of measures.

The paired Student's t test was used on the comparison between the means of values found on the cephalometric tracings of digital and simulated radiographs, with a confidence interval of 95%.

Most angular measures (78%) presented an irrelevant difference between the means (0.07° - 0.56°), and only two measures presented a statistically significant difference ($p < 0.05$), GoGn.SN and IMPA, however the difference was 1.8° and 1.5° respectively.

The linear measurements presented two measures using teeth as reference that showed minimum difference (0.28 mm and 0.30 mm, respectively) and two measures that used the lip as reference presenting differences of up to 1.81 mm ($p < 0.05$) (Table 3).

The Intraclass Correlation Coefficient between the two modalities of images in all the measurements in this work presented an index over 0.927, indicating a strong correlation, as can be seen on Table 4.

The statistical analysis was performed through the software SPSS 16.0 (SPSS Inc.,Chicago, Illinois).

DISCUSSION

The first reports about computed tomography for dentistry occurred in the late 90s.[15] With the appearance of specific softwares, the possibility of simulating radiographs used in the orthodontic diagnosis such as panoramic, lateral and frontal cephalometric became promising especially because of the advantage of taking only one exam.

The validation of extracting two-dimensional images from three-dimensional images becomes extremely important in this transition period or change of paradigm from the 2D to the 3D diagnosis, so that the clinician can continue to use the same cephalometric analysis, until three-dimensional analysis be established in the orthodontic literature and become available for the daily practice.[14] At first sight, the reconstruction of a 3D model and subsequent return to a 2D image seems paradoxical,

Table 2 - Descriptive analysis of linear and angular measurements, including mean, median and standard deviation, of each cephalometric measurement.

Measurement		Mean	Median	S.D.
Angular measurements (degrees)				
SNA	Digital	82.71	82.70	3.65
	3D	82.40	81.75	3.60
SNB	Digital	80.06	79.75	3.56
	3D	79.83	79.30	3.44
ANB	Digital	2.66	2.40	2.27
	3D	2.58	2.70	2.08
FMA	Digital	24.13	24.70	5.97
	3D	24.58	25.10	5.27
Ocl.SN	Digital	14.16	14.85	4.56
	3D	14.09	14.45	5.02
GoGn.SN	Digital	29.72	30.35	7.03
	3D	31.22	32.30	6.17
IMPA	Digital	94.68	93.30	8.47
	3D	92.88	91.70	7.58
1.SN	Digital	104.77	103.75	8.77
	3D	104.21	102.95	8.43
Y axis	Digital	58.33	57.60	3.73
	3D	58.65	58.80	3.65
Linear measurements (mm)				
UL-Line E	Digital	-3.41	-3.55	2.35
	3D	-5.23	-5.20	2.08
LL-Line E	Digital	-0.46	-0.15	2.97
	3D	-1.50	-1.90	2.78
1-NA	Digital	5.40	5.25	3.25
	3D	5.70	4.80	3.01
1-NB	Digital	5.76	5.60	3.17
	3D	6.05	6.05	3.17

Table 3 - Difference between mean and standard deviation of angular and linear cephalometric measurements, carried on digital radiographs simulated from CBCT.

Measurement	Mean	S.D.	p
Angular measurements (degrees)			
SNA	0.31	0.69	0.081
SNB	0.22	0.74	0.142
ANB	0.07	0.66	0.583
FMA	-0.45	2.46	0.361
Ocl.SN	0.07	2.50	0.883
GoGn.SN	-1.50	1.63	0.009*
IMPA	1.80	1.92	0.006*
1.SN	0.56	1.54	0.074
Y axis	-0.31	1.92	0.410
Linear measurements (mm)			
UL-Line E	1.81	0.88	0.002*
LL-Line E	1.03	0.80	0.007*
1-NA	-0.30	1.01	0.146
1-NB	-0.28	0.67	0.040

* $p < 0.05$. Result statistically significant.

Table 4 - Intraclass correlation coefficient between measurements carried on digital radiographs simulated from CBCT (n = 26).

Measurement	ICC
Angular measurements (degrees)	
SNA	0.991
SNB	0.988
ANB	0.976
FMA	0.950
Ocl.SN	0.927
GoGn.SN	0.985
IMPA	0.986
1.SN	0.992
Y axis	0.928
Linear measurements (mm)	
UL-Line E	0.958
LL-Line E	0.980
1-NA	0.973
1-NB	0.990

but this can make the progressive introduction of CBCT easier to the practice of the orthodontist and research.

Before the employment of cephalometric radiographs simulated from computed tomography, the evaluation of the reliability of the data of the new images is necessary, and this was the objective of the present study.

Some cephalometric points as Gonion and Porion that are used to define the mandibular plane and the Frankfurt horizontal plane, respectively, are located in curved surfaces, which can make the identification more difficult. For this reason, such points have considerable margin of error when marked.[16-20]

The results of comparison between the modalities of images showed statistically significant difference (p < 0.05) in two angular measures (IMPA and GoGn.SN) and in two linear measures (UL-Line E and LL-Line E). These 4 measures presented differences of ± 1.8 mm or 1.8°. These differences are probably clinically irrelevant.

The two angular measures that presented statistical difference used the mandibular plane as reference and the difference between mandibular contours on the two modalities of images can be noticed, which probably contributed to the difference between the two measurements (Fig 4).

In a similar work, the angular measure that presented differences was the FMA (-4.36°) that also uses the mandibular plane as one of the cephalometric references. However, when the anatomic porion could not be determined, the most superior part of the image of the auricular positioner (mechanical porion) was used as reference;[9] on the present study all markings were performed on the anatomic porion.

The linear measures that had statistical difference involved lips and E Line (nose tip, soft pogonion). Some hypotheses must be considered in this regard: First, it cannot be assured that the positioning of the lips was exactly the same in both exams; then, the tomography is not the most recommended exam to reproduce soft tissues with high accuracy; and last but not least, the gravity working on soft tissues, when medical or cone beam tomographs are taken with the patient lying dorsally, and the same method used in the present work.

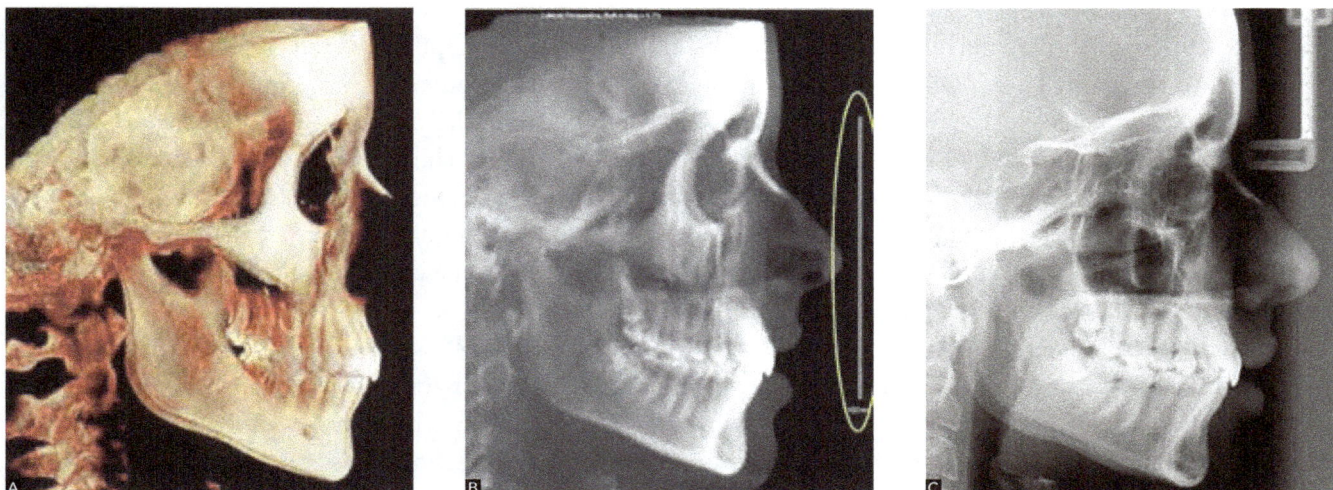

Figure 4 - Illustration of images: **A)** 3D image in a right profile visualization; **B)** perspective simulated cephalometric radiograph, with 100 mm ruler on the right; **C)** digital cephalometric radiograph.

The stability of the points is affected by several factors. On the lateral radiograph, when the head is deviated from the exact profile position, the sagittal points experience the minimum degree of displacement, while the structures located outside the midsagittal plane change position significantly. In this case, structures in opposite sides of the head move in opposite directions.[21]

The questioning about the validity of the two-dimensional cephalometry in orthodontics is due to four aspects: First, the limitation of the 2D technique in representing a three-dimensional object. When a three-dimensional object is represented in two dimensions, the structures are vertical and horizontally displaced proportionally to the distance to the film or record plane; then, symmetry on the right and left side is very rare, which makes it difficult to evaluate patients with craniofacial anomalies and facial asymmetries; third, the problems inherent to obtaining the image; and fourth, the operational error on the elaboration of the cephalogram and on the process of cephalometric analysis. Despite the amount of variables that compete to make the cephalometric analysis liable, it remains widely used by orthodontist from all around the world and, in many cases, it is essential for the diagnosis and treatment of patients.

Cephalometric analysis is still the only practical quantitative method that allows the investigation and evaluation of the relations between skull, dental and soft-tissue structures.[22-25]

The conventional radiography, as well as the perspective simulated image, show a superimposition of bilateral structures that does not correspond to reality. It is taught that the structures on the left must be traced for being closer to the film and consequently experience lower magnification than those on the right. Probably this error was repeated numerous times until the advent of the tomography. Figure 4 shows one patient from the sample, that clinically did not present any remarkable facial asymmetry and after positioning the exams on the Dolphin software, it was noticed that the left side showed to be larger. However, as the magnification on the right side (closer to the frame) is larger, what is observed is an almost complete overlap of the mandibular planes on both sides, suggesting symmetry. It would be necessary, however, three-dimensional visualization to be sure on which side is larger or smaller in cases of evident asymmetry.

The positioning of the patient is considered a critical factor for cephalometric analysis.[26,27] When the conventional exam is performed, the technician uses reference lines on the tissue, which can complicate the reproducibility. On CBCT, there is the advantage of visualizing only bone structures that can be used to reorient the patient on a better position with greater reproducibility.

Since the research was about a comparison to digital radiographs, that had divergence on X-ray beam and consequently, magnification of the image size, the radiographs from tomographies, were also simulated with divergence on X-rays and magnification. The magnification factor is the amount of magnification of the image on the midsagittal plane and it was defined in 9.7% following orientation from the manufacturer of the Dolphin software. Some researchers used magnification factor of 7.5% justified by the relation between distance object-film and distance x-ray source-object.[1,9] However this calculation cannot be surely used, since some patients who take radiographs in two different x-ray devices have radiographs with different size structures, but the distances from the focus to the object and from the object to the film are similar.

Considering the values related to radiation that the patient absorbs,[28] the substitution of panoramic radiograph for CBCT would not be justified, panoramic radiographs solely could be appropriate for the diagnosis. But, in the case of orthodontic diagnosis, the substitution of panoramic, lateral and frontal cephalometric radiographs for the CBCT can be done, so that the dosage of NewTom 3G with a 12-in FOV, for example, it is approximately two times the dosage of conventional expositions, except for the full periapical exam.

Although some authors propose three-dimensional cephalometric analysis[23,29,30] it is believed that the 3D analysis, in clinical practice, is a lot more qualitative, with spatial visualization and relation between the structures, than quantitative, with preestablished measures; this last one is preferred for the research field.

CONCLUSION

After analysis of results, it can be concluded that the cephalometric measures obtained by cephalograms generated from simulated radiographs through CBCT reproduce with significant accuracy the conventional cephalogram measures.

REFERENCES

1. Kumar V, Ludlow JB, Mol A, Cevidanes L. Comparison of conventional and cone beam CT synthesized cephalograms. Dentomaxillofac Radiol. 2007;36(5):263-9.

2. Moshiri M, Scarfe WC, Hilgers ML, Scheetz JP, Silveira AM, Farman AG. Accuracy of linear measurements from imaging plate and lateral cephalometric images derived from cone-beam computed tomography. Am J Orthod Dentofacial Orthop. 2007;132(4):550-60.

3. Collins J, Shah A, McCarthy C, Sandler J. Comparison of measurements from photographed lateral cephalograms and scanned cephalograms. Am J Orthod Dentofacial Orthop. 2007;132(6):830-3.

4. Chen YJ, Chen SK, Huang HW, Yao CC, Chang HF. Reliability of landmark identification in cephalometric radiography acquired by a storage phosphor imaging system. Dentomaxillofac Radiol. 2004;33(5):301-6.

5. Farman AG, Scarfe WC. Development of imaging selection criteria and procedures should precede cephalometric assessment with cone-beam computed tomography. Am J Orthod Dentofacial Orthop. 2006;130(2):257-65.

6. Mah J, Huang J, Bumann A. The cone-beam decision in orthodontics. Proceedings of the 32nd Annual Moyers Symposium. Ann Arbor; 2006. p. 59-75.

7. Sarment DP. Dental applications for cone-beam computed tomography. Proceedings of the 32nd Annual Moyers Symposium. Ann Arbor; 2006.

8. Swennen GR, Schutyser F. Three-dimensional cephalometry: spiral multi-slice vs cone-beam computed tomography. Am J Orthod Dentofacial Orthop. 2006;130(3):410-6.

9. Kumar V, Ludlow J, Soares Cevidanes LH, Mol A. In vivo comparison of conventional and cone beam CT synthesized cephalograms. Angle Orthod. 2008;78(5):873-9.

10. Arai Y, Tammisalo E, Iwai K, Hashimoto K, Shinoda K. Development of a compact computed tomographic apparatus for dental use. Dentomaxillofac Radiol. 1999;28(4):245-8.

11. Hajeer MY, Millett DT, Ayoub AF, Siebert JP. Applications of 3D imaging in orthodontics: part I. J Orthod. 2004;31(1):62-70.

12. Hajeer MY, Millett DT, Ayoub AF, Siebert JP. Applications of 3D imaging in orthodontics: part II. J Orthod. 2004;31(2):154-62.

13. Ludlow JB, Davies-Ludlow LE, Brooks SL. Dosimetry of two extraoral direct digital imaging devices: NewTom cone beam CT and Orthophos Plus DS panoramic unit. Dentomaxillofac Radiol. 2003;32(4):229-34.

14. Motta AT. Avaliação da cirurgia de avanço mandibular por meio da superposição de modelos tridimensionais [tese]. Rio de Janeiro: Universidade Estadual do Rio de Janeiro; 2007.

15. Mozzo P, Procacci C, Tacconi A, Martini PT, Andreis IA. A new volumetric CT machine for dental imaging based on the cone-beam technique: preliminary results. Eur Radiol. 1998;8(9):1558-64.

16. Athanasiou AE, Miethke R, Van der Meij AJ. Random errors in localization of landmarks in postero-anterior cephalograms. Br J Orthod. 1999;26(4):273-84.

17. Ludlow JB, Laster WS, See M, Bailey LJ, Hershey HG. Accuracy of measurements of mandibular anatomy in cone beam computed tomography images. Oral Surg Oral Med Oral Pathol Oral Radiol Endod. 2007;103(4):534-42.

18. Chate RA. Cephalometric landmark identification within the petrous temporal region. Br J Orthod. 1987;14(1):33-41.

19. Adenwalla ST, Kronman JH, Attarzadeh F. Porion and condyle as cephalometric landmarks: an error study. Am J Orthod Dentofacial Orthop. 1988;94(5):411-5.

20. Houston WJ. The analysis of errors in orthodontic measurements. Am J Orthod. 1983;83(5):382-90.

21. Steiner CC. Cephalometrics for you and me. Am J Orthod Dentofacial Orthop. 1953;39(10):729-55.

22. Honda K, Arai Y, Kashima M, Takano Y, Sawada K, Ejima K, et al. Evaluation of the usefulness of the limited cone-beam CT (3DX) in the assessment of the thickness of the roof of the glenoid fossa of the temporomandibular joint. Dentomaxillofac Radiol. 2004;33(6):391-5.

23. Lagravere MO, Hansen L, Harzer W, Major PW. Plane orientation for standardization in 3-dimensional cephalometric analysis with computerized tomography imaging. Am J Orthod Dentofacial Orthop. 2006;129(5):601-4.

24. Papadopoulos MA, Christou PK, Athanasiou AE, Boettcher P, Zeilhofer HF, Sader R, et al. Three-dimensional craniofacial reconstruction imaging. Oral Surg Oral Med Oral Pathol Oral Radiol Endod. 2002;93(4):382-93.

25. Quintero JC, Trosien A, Hatcher D, Kapila S. Craniofacial imaging in orthodontics: historical perspective, current status, and future developments. Angle Orthod. 1999;69(6):491-506.

26. Cohen AM. Uncertainty in cephalometrics. Br J Orthod. 1984;11(1):44-8.

27. Yoon YJ, Kim KS, Hwang MS, Kim HJ, Choi EH, Kim KW. Effect of head rotation on lateral cephalometric radiographs. Angle Orthod. 2001;71(5):396-403.

28. Ludlow JB, Davies-Ludlow LE, Brooks SL, Howerton WB. Dosimetry of 3 CBCT devices for oral and maxillofacial radiology: CB Mercuray, NewTom 3G and i-CAT. Dentomaxillofac Radiol. 2006;35(4):219-26.

29. Park SH, Yu HS, Kim KD, Lee KJ, Baik HS. A proposal for a new analysis of craniofacial morphology by 3-dimensional computed tomography. Am J Orthod Dentofacial Orthop. 2006;129(5):600.e23-34.

30. Jacobson A, Jacobson RL. Radiographic cephalometry: from basics to 3-D imaging. 2nd ed. Chicago: Quintessence; 2006.

5

Evaluation of miniscrew angulation in the posterior maxilla using cone-beam computed tomographic image

Henrique M. Villela[1], Mario Vedovello Filho[1], Heloísa C. Valdrighi[1], Milton Santamaria-Jr[1], Carolina Carmo de Menezes[1], Silvia A. S. Vedovello[1]

Objective: This study aimed at evaluating whether changes in the insertion angle is a determining factor in the positioning of the miniscrews body in a region with larger interradicular space in the posterior maxilla. **Methods:** Analysis of 60 posterior maxillary quadrants were made using images obtained by means of cone-beam computed tomographic image (CBCT), with 0.076-mm voxel, which presented a real miniscrew inserted in the mesial region of the maxillary first molars, serving as reference point for the placement of the virtual miniscrews. Measurements of the distances between roots were made in three points on the body of the virtual miniscrews (A, B and C), at four different angulations, 70^c, 60°, 50° and 40° (T_1 to T_4), in relation to the long axis of the second premolar. This evaluation was made in four groups, selected in accordance with the disposition of the roots of the second premolars and first molars: Group 1 (all types of roots), Group 2 (convergent roots), Group 3 (divergent roots) and Group 4 (parallel roots). **Results:** There were no statistically significant differences in the measurements of points A, B and C, at the different angles (70°, 60°, 50° and 40°) and in the different groups ($p > 0.05$). **Conclusions:** Changes in the insertion angle is not a determinant factor in the positioning of miniscrews body in regions with larger interradicular space in posterior maxilla.

Keywords: Bone screw. Implants. Tomography. Orthodontics.

[1] Uniararas, Fundação Hermínio Ometto, Programa de Pós-graduação em Ortodontia (Araras/SP, Brazil).

» The authors report no commercial, proprietary or financial interest in the products or companies described in this article.

Silvia A. S. Vedovello
Av. Dr. Maximiliano Baruto, 500, Jardim Universitário – Araras/SP
CEP: 13.607-339 – E-mail: silviavedovello@gmail.com

INTRODUCTION

Miniscrews have brought a new perspective to orthodontic treatment due to their low cost, effectiveness and easy clinical management.[1,2,3] Although the procedure for miniscrew insertion is simple, some care must be taken with the purpose of minimizing the risks of the miniscrew body contacting the roots of teeth, such as: evaluating the bone availability in the interradicular space; use of simplified surgical guides, and the use of a safe surgical protocol.[1] The possibilities of causing damage to periodontal structure and the roots must not be underestimated. Among the problems can be included: displacement of bone into the periodontal ligament space; damage to cement; damage to dentin and pulp damage.[4-7]

One of the factors that may vary during miniscrew insertion into the maxilla is angulation, which may be more perpendicular or more angulated in relation to the vestibular bone cortical surface, or in relation to the long axis of the teeth. Some authors have recommended a more perpendicular insertion into the maxilla, since this factor would diminish the risk of the screw body contacting the roots, and generates a line of action of force closer to the center of resistance.[8] Other authors have recommended miniscrew insertion into the maxilla with an angulation of 30° to 40° in relation to the long axis of the tooth, with the purpose of minimizing the risks of the screw contacting the roots.[9-11]

Primary stability may be increased when the miniscrew is inserted at angles of 60° to 70° in relation to the bone surface, in regions with thicker cortical bone, but for this purpose a higher torque is demanded for its insertion. However, this increased angulation may cause a higher failure rate due to excessive pressure on the bone.[12] The bone density in the posterior region of the maxilla is lower than it is in the mandible, and this area also presents a thin vestibular cortical.[13-15] Studies in the mandibles of human cadavers and using finite elements method have shown that the insertion of screws at 90° in relation to the bone surface offered greater resistance and less stress on cortical bone than that of screws inserted at 60° and 30°.[16] Stability and resistance to failure do not depend on the orientation of miniscrew implantation in relation to the bone surface, however, miniscrews inserted at 90° presented greater stability in shear tests, in comparison with those inserted at 45°. This higher degree of stability occurred due to the line of action of force being positioned closer to the long axis of screws perpendicular to the bone surface.[17] Screw insertion in a more apical and angled position not only increases the risk of contact with the maxillary sinus, but also increases the risk of sliding during its insertion.[18] The miniscrew may be placed at an angle between 55° and 70° in relation to the occlusal plane, in the infrazygomatic crest region, above the maxillary first molar, with the purpose of preventing its contact with the root. However, in order for this strategy to be efficient, the miniscrew must be inserted at a distance of 14 to 16mm from the occlusal plane.[19] One of the greater risk factors of this anchorage system is inflammation of the peri-screw soft tissues, which occurs when screws are inserted into the alveolar mucosa. To prevent this from occurring, the screws must preferably be inserted into keratinized mucosa.[20,21]

During planning of screw insertion into the molar region, the location of the maxillary sinus must be observed and it perforation prevented, since it could lead to complications such as sinusitis and mucosal retention cysts.[18,22] In-depth knowledge of anatomic relations between the roots and adjacent structures, with the use of tomography, is essential to prevent root injuries; and studies to evaluate which would be the best position of the miniscrew to diminish the possibility of contact with the roots, are of fundamental importance. This is because the proximity of the miniscrew to the root is a risk factor that may lead to the loss of stability and consequent failure of this device as an orthodontic anchorage.[23,24] Studies conducted in human maxillae and mandibles, and studies in tomographies have concluded that the region between the maxillary first molar and second premolar, from the vestibular direction, represent the safest region for performing the insertion of miniscrews at the height of 6 to 8 mm from the cervical line.[9,24]

The objective of this study was to evaluate if the change in insertion angle is a determining factor in the positioning of the miniscrews body in a region with larger interradicular space in the posterior maxilla, using real miniscrews inserted in this region with clinical success, as guidance.

MATERIAL AND METHODS

This study received approval from a Ethics Committee (FHO/Uniararas, protocol # 2.081.877). The convenience sample comprised images selected from a file containing orthodontics records. These had been captured by means of cone-beam computed tomographic image (CBCT) with 0.076-mm voxel, in a Kodak 9000 3D tomograph (Kodak Dental Systems, Carestream Health, Rochester, NY, USA), which belonged to the file of one of the researchers, according to the following inclusion criteria:

» Brazilian patients of both genders.

» Who had undergone corrective orthodontic treatment.

» With real miniscrews inserted between the maxillary first molars and second premolars at an advanced stage of leveling.

» With real miniscrews inserted by the same clinician professional.

» With CBCT taken by the same tomograph.

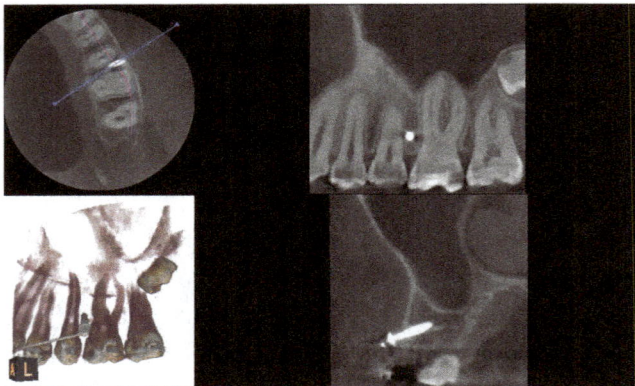

Figure 1 - CBCT visualization of three slices and 3D reconstruction.

The CBCT images of patients who did not fall within the selection criteria were excluded. The final sample consisted of 60 maxillary posterior quadrants of 35 patients, with 26 being female and 09 male, and 30 quadrants from the right and 30 from the left side.

The CBCT depicted miniscrews previously inserted in the mesial region of the maxillary first molars, which served as reference for positioning the virtual miniscrews (Fig 1). The virtual miniscrews were created, coinciding with the real miniscrews in the vestibular cortical region. This site represents the point of introduction of the miniscrew into the cortical bone and was chosen according to the orthodontic planning. Usually, this site is found in the region of keratinized mucosa, which determines the limit in height for the insertion of a miniscrew. This height may range between 6 to 8mm apical to the line of the orthodontic arch. The virtual miniscrews were created with four different angulations: 70°, 60°, 50° and 40°, in relation to the long axis of the second premolar (Fig 2).

The insertion and changes in angulation of the virtual miniscrews were performed by means of a specific software program (CS 3D imaging software, Kodak Dental Systems, Carestream Health, Rochester, NY, USA), which is a visualizer of CBCT images in DICOM (Digital Imaging and Communications in Medicine) format. The distance between the roots of the first molars and second premolars was evaluated in three specific points on the body of the virtual miniscrews, on a slice constructed parallel to the long axis of each virtual inclination. These three points were determined by measuring 2mm, 4mm and 6mm from the point of the virtual miniscrews, which presented a body length of 8mm. The measurements were determined on a slice constructed parallel to the long axis of each virtual inclination. The points were denominated as follows: A) 2mm, B) 4mm and C) 6mm from the tip of the miniscrew, respectively. These three

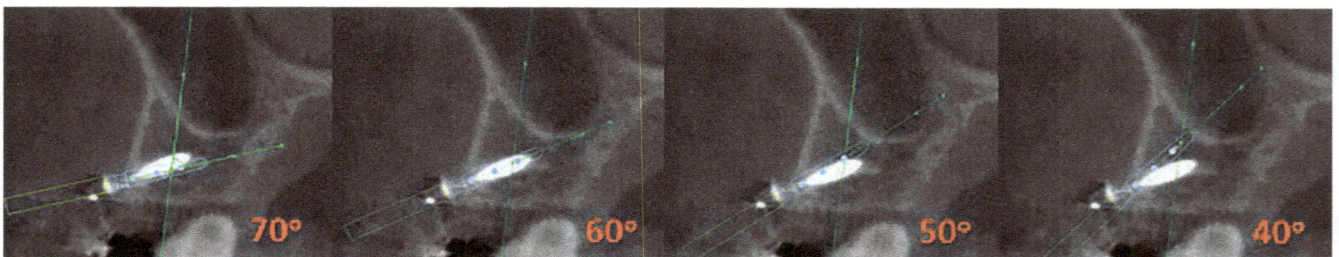

Figure 2 - Virtual miniscrews at 70°, 60°, 50° and 40° of inclination in relation to the long axis of the second premolar, in the transaxial slice.

distances were measured at the four angulations of the miniscrew, determining: $T1 = 70^0$, $T2 = 60^0$, $T3 = 50^0$ and $T4 = 40^0$ (Fig 3). Then, they were duly recorded in accordance with their location (A, B and C) and the angle (70°, 60°, 50° and 40°) (Table 1).

During CBCT evaluation the different shapes and dispositions of the roots were observed, which resulted in distinct interradicular spaces. From this observation, three groups were created, which presented interradicular spaces with different characteristics, based on the disposition of the maxillary first molar roots in relation to those of the second premolars. The groups were denominated as follows, regarding roots: convergent, divergent and parallel. The convergent roots, composed of 5 (8.33%) tomographies, presented a reduction in interradicular space in the direction towards the apices, due to convergence of the first molar roots in the direction

of the premolar roots (Fig 4). The divergent roots, composed of 21 (35%) tomographies, presented a constant and significant increase in interradicular space in the direction towards the apices (Fig 5). The parallel roots, composed of 34 (56.66%) tomographies, presented an interradicular space that remained equal in the direction towards the apex, however, with a increase in this space only in the apical third (Fig 6).

Evaluations of the spaces between the roots at the four angulations were made in the four different groups: Group 1, with all the tomographies without distinction of the types of roots; Group 2, with convergent roots; Group 3, with divergent roots; Group 4, with parallel roots.

The CBCT were numbered in alphabetical order according to the patient's first name. When there were two tomographies for a patient, one of each side, then

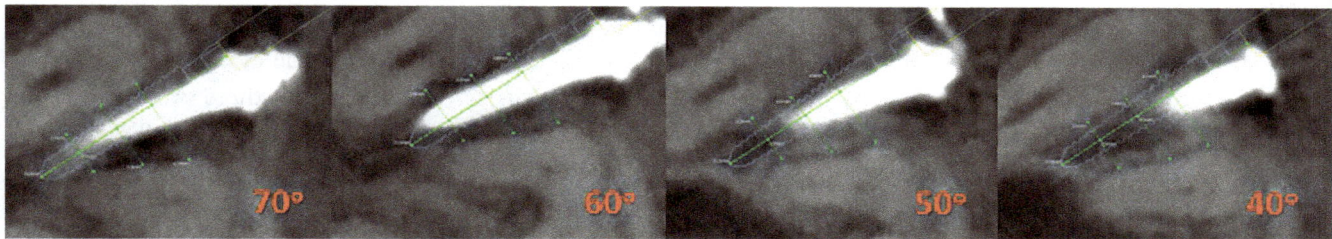

Figure 3 - Measurement of the distances between the root of the molar and premolar at points (A), (B) and (C), located at 2.0 mm, 4.0 mm and 6.0 mm, respectively, from the tip of the miniscrew at 70° (T_1), 60° (T_2), 50° (T_3) and 40° (T_4) of inclination in relation to the long axis of the second premolar, in the transaxial slice.

Table 1 - Values of measurements (A), (B) and (C) by angle in study population in all types of roots (n=60).

Points	Angles	Mean	Standard Deviation	Minimum Value	Maximum Value	P-value**
A	T_1 (70°)	3.98	0.92	2.20	6.30	
	T_2 (60°)	4.08	0.99	2.30	6.60	
	T_3 (50°)	4.22	1.10	2.10	6.60	0.25
	T_4 (40°)	4.36	1.29	2.20	8.90	
B	T_1 (70°)	3.86	0.79	2.30	5.40	
	T_2 (60°)	3.88	0.84	2.20	5.50	
	T_3 (50°)	3.94	0.89	1.80	5.90	0.47
	T_4 (40°)	4.09	1.00	1.70	6.30	
C	T_1 (70°)	4.35	0.90	2.40	6.40	
	T_2 (60°)	4.38	0.91	2.40	6.70	
	T_3 (50°)	4.45	0.97	2.40	6.90	0.39
	T_4 (40°)	4.63	1.15	2.50	7.70	

(A) 2mm, (B) 4mm and (C) 6mm from the tip of the miniscrew. ** ANOVA, $p < 0.05$.

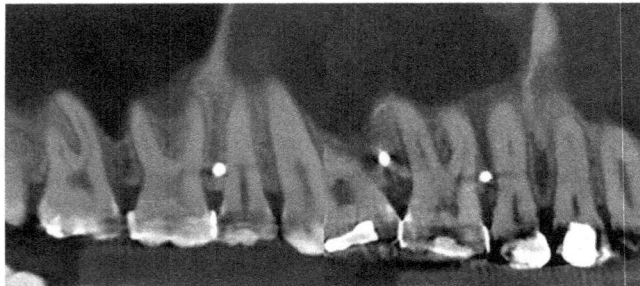

Figure 4 - Convergent roots.

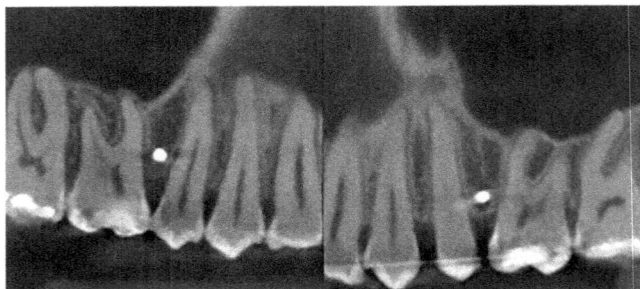

Figure 5 - Divergent roots.

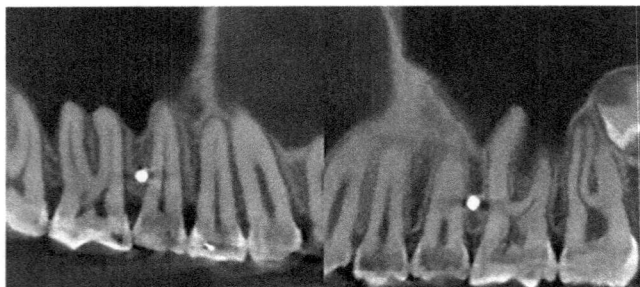

Figure 6 - Parallel roots.

the first to be numbered was the right side, and then the left side. Thus, all the tomographies had a number. For the intra-examiner test of agreement, the following tomography numbers were used: 10, 20, 30, 40, 50 and 60. All measurements were taken twice by the same operator blinded to group status, with an interval of ten days.[25] For the agreement test, the Kappa statistics were calculated and obtained 0.91, which indicates excellent agreement between exams. The value varied from 0.89 for the measurement B, 0.91 for the measurement C and 0.94 for the measurement A.

Statistical analysis

The variables were descriptively analyzed, and their measurements of central tendency and dispersion were calculated. The Kolmogorov-Smirnov test was used to analyze normality of distribution. After proof of normality of the data, the Student's-t test was used to identify differences among the groups. In the presence of three or more groups of comparisons, the option was to use the Analysis of Variance (ANOVA), followed by the Tukey test. All the analyses were performed using a level of significance of 95%.

RESULTS
Evaluation of Group 1
All the types of roots (n = 60)

The highest obtained values for the distances between roots were for measurement C, followed by A and then B, considering all types of roots and the subdivision by angles (Table 1). This first evaluation only registered the fact that in the middle portion of the miniscrew, which is found at approximately 4mm from the cortical (bone), there is the region with the smallest space between the roots. In the evaluation of Group 1 (all the roots) at different angles, there was a clear trend towards increase in the values from T_1 to T_4, although this increase was not statistically significant (Table 2).

Evaluation of Group 2 – convergent roots (n=5)

In the evaluation of Group 2 (convergent roots) at different angles, there was a trend towards reduction in the values from T_1 to T_4, although this reduction was not statistically significant. The cases of convergent roots, composed of 5 tomographies, 8.33% of the sample of 60 tomographies, on an average, presented a discrete trend towards reduction in interradicular space, when the angle was diminished; however, it was not statistically significant (Table 2).

Evaluation of Group 3 – divergent roots (n=21)

In the evaluation of Group 3 (divergent roots) at different angles, there was a trend towards increase in the values from T_1 to T_4, although this increase was not statistically significant. The cases of divergent roots, composed of 21 tomographies, 35% of the sample of 60 tomographies, on an average, presented a trend towards increase in interradicular space, particularly at Point A, when the angle was diminished. However, it was not statistically significant (Table 2).

Table 2 - Values of measurements (A), (B) and (C) by angle in a samples with convergent roots (n=05), divergent roots (n=21) and parallel roots (n=34).

Roots	Points	Angles	Mean	Standard Deviation	P-value**
Convergent	A	T_1 (70°)	2.98	0.67	0.99
		T_2 (60°)	2.92	0.69	
		T_3 (50°)	2.88	0.62	
		T_4 (40°)	2.92	0.30	
	E	T_1 (70°)	3.06	0.32	0.70
		T_2 (60°)	2.98	0.28	
		T_3 (50°)	2.76	0.58	
		T_4 (40°)	2.78	0.62	
	C	T_1 (70°)	3.80	0.72	0.99
		T_2 (60°)	3.72	0.66	
		T_3 (50°)	3.72	0.71	
		T_4 (40°)	3.78	0.77	
Divergent	A	T_1 (70°)	4.59	0.89	0.07
		T_2 (60°)	4.80	0.93	
		T_3 (50°)	5.05	0.97	
		T_4 (40°)	5.40	1.29	
	3	T_1 (70°)	4.45	0.66	0.31
		T_2 (60°)	4.52	0.70	
		T_3 (50°)	4.63	0.72	
		T_4 (40°)	4.86	0.87	
	C	T_1 (70°)	4.84	0.87	0.50
		T_2 (60°)	4.85	0.90	
		T_3 (50°)	4.98	0.94	
		T_4 (40°)	5.25	1.20	
Parallel	A	T_1 (70°)	3.75	0.74	0.79
		T_2 (60°)	3.81	0.74	
		T_3 (50°)	3.91	0.86	
		T_4 (40°)	3.92	0.86	
	B	T_1 (70°)	3.62	0.67	0.63
		T_2 (60°)	3.62	0.70	
		T_3 (50°)	3.68	0.69	
		T_4 (40°)	3.81	0.76	
	C	T_1 (70°)	4.13	0.83	0.68
		T_2 (60°)	4.19	0.83	
		T_3 (50°)	4.24	0.89	
		T_4 (40°)	4.39	1.02	

(A) 2mm, (B) 4mm and (C) 6mm from the tip of the miniscrew. ** ANOVA, $p < 0.05$.

Evaluation of Group 4 – parallel roots (n = 34)

In the evaluation of Group 4 (parallel roots) at different angles, there was a slight trend towards increase in the values from T_1 to T_4, although this increase was not statistically significant. The cases of parallel roots, composed of 34 tomographies, 56.66% of the sample of 60 tomographies, on an average, presented a slight trend towards increase in interradicular space when the angle was diminished. However, it was not statistically significant (Table 2).

The results of the evaluation of the four groups were very similar. There were cases in which an increase in space occurred when the insertion angle was reduced. However, there were also simulations in which the space did not change, and in other cases a reduction in space occurred. However, on an average, this trend towards increase or reduction was not statistically significantly. The interradicular spaces along the miniscrew did not increase similarly in all cases in which the angulation was changed from 70° to 40°. The distances between the roots varied differently according to the region of the miniscrew body.

DISCUSSION

This study evaluated miniscrews angulation in the space between the first molars and second premolars because, according to several authors, this is a region where there is greater availability of space in the maxilla from the vestibular side, which present signifcant clinical application.[9,24]

The choice of angulation is not unanimous. Some authors have recommended miniscrew insertion into the maxilla with an angulation of 30° to 40° in relation to the long axis of the tooth, with the purpose of minimizing the risks of contact of the screw with the roots.[9-11] However, other authors have recommended more perpendicular miniscrew insertion into the maxilla, because of the understanding that this factor does not increases the risk of screw contact with the root, and also provides better distribution of force on the cortical bone.[8,16,17]

The present study recorded the fact that in the middle portion of the miniscrew, which is found at approximately 4mm from the cortical (bone), there is the region with the least space between the roots. Thus, when introducing the miniscrew into the maxilla from the vestibular side, the moment of greatest risk was when the body of the miniscrew was passing through this region, which is equivalent to half of its length when using a screw with a body length of 8mm. One must pay attention to the patient's sensitivity or to an increase in resistance to the insertion when 4 to 5mm of the miniscrew body are intraosseously inserted.

When miniscrews were inserted at an angle of 50° and 40°, there was superimposition of the virtual screw body on the maxillary sinus in 24 tomographies, equivalent to 40% of the total number of evaluations. This fact must be avoided, because it may lead to complications such as sinusitis and mucosal retention cysts.[18,22] Moreover, screw insertion in a more apical and angled position not only increases the risk of contact with the maxillary sinus, but also increases the risk of sliding during its insertion.[18]

Our results differ from other findings[11] conducted in typodont teeth. To evaluate the efficiency of more angulated miniscrew insertion in contrast with the more vertical insertion, the methods of the study conducted in typodont teeth should use mannequins with different shapes and dispositions of roots and vestibular cortical (bone). When the evaluation is made in a typodont with divergent roots, it should produce different clinical results from those of simulations performed in mannequins which perhaps present convergent roots. In this study,[11] only one type of typodont was used, leading to an analysis of the efficiency in only that clinical situation, which may differ from others. Other studies in mannequins must be conducted with a minimum of three clinical situations of roots disposition (convergent roots, divergent roots and parallel roots), in order to be compared with studies carried out with tomographies.

Although the present study suggests that in a region with greater interradicular space, the angulation is not a determinant factor in the positioning of the miniscrew, clinically, this change could modify the height of the line of force action and, consequently, the orthodontic mechanics.

Reduction in the angle of placement during miniscrew insertion, with the purpose of diminishing the risks of contact of the body with the root was not shown to be efficient, considering that in 40% of the virtual miniscrews inserted at an angulation of 40° and 50°, the body was superimposed on the maxillary sinus.

Evaluation of the interradicular spaces at the three points on the miniscrew (A, B and C), performed in the four groups of types of roots (general, convergent, divergent and parallel), at four angulations (70°, 60°, 50° and 40°), was rather similar. On an average this trend towards increase or reduction in interradicular space was not statistically significantly.

CONCLUSIONS

The change in insertion angle is not a determinant factor in the positioning of miniscrews body in a region with larger interradicular space in posterior maxilla.

Author contributions

Conceived and designed the study: HMV, SASV. Data acquisition, analysis or interpretation: HMV, SASV. Writing the article: HMV, SASV. Critical revision of the article: MVF, HCV, MSJ, CCM. Final approval of the article: HMV, SASV.

REFERENCES

1. Kyung HM, Park HS, Bae SM, Sung JH, Kim IB. Development of orthodontic micro-implants for intraoral anchorage. J Clin Orthod. 2003 June;37(6):321-8; quiz 314..

2. Melsen B. Mini-Implants: Where Are We? J Clin Orthod. 2005 Sept;39(9):539-47; quiz 531-2.

3. Yang L, Li F, Cao M, Chen H, Wang X,Chen X, et al. Quantitative evaluation of maxillary inter-radicular bone with cone-beam computed tomography for biotical placement of orthodontic mini-implants. Am J Orthod Dentofacial Orthop. 2015 June;147(6):725-37.

4. Hembree M, Buschang PH, Carrillo R, Spears R, Rossouw PE. Effects of intentional damage of the roots and surrounding structures with miniscrews implants. Am J Orthod Dentofacial Orthop. 2009 Mar;135(3):280.e1-9; discussion 280-1.

5. Kadioglu O, Büyükyilmaz T, Zachrisson BU, Maino BG. Contact damage to root surfaces of premolars touching miniscrews during orthodontic treatment. Am J Orthod Dentofacial Orthop. 2008 Sept;134(3):353-60.

6. Brisceno CE, Rossouw PE, Carrillo R, Spears R, Buschang PH. Healing of the roots and surrounding structures after intentional damage with miniscrews implants. Am J Orthod Dentofacial Orthop. 2009 Mar;135(3):292-301.

7. Asscherickx K, Vannet BV, Wehrbein H, Sabzevar MM. Root repair after injury from mini-screw. Clin Oral Implants Res 2005 Oct;16(5):575-8.

8. Dobranszki A, Faber J, Scatolino IVMC, Dobranszki NPAC, Toledo AO. Analysis of factors associated with orthodontic microscrew failure. Braz Dent J. 2014;25(4):346-51.

9. Poggio PM, Incorvat C, Velo S, Cararo A. "Safe Zones": A Guide for Miniscrew Positioning in the Maxillary and Mandibular Arch. Angle Orthod. 2006 Mar;76(2):191-7.

10. Park HS, Bae SM, Kyung HM, Sung JH. Micro-implant anchorage for treatment of skeletal Class I bialveolar protrusion. J Clin Orthod. 2001 July;35(7):417-22.

11. Antoszewska J, Trześniewska P, Kawala B, Ludwig B, HS Park. Qualitative and quantitative evaluation of root injury risk potentially burdening insertion of miniscrew implants. Korean J Orthod. 2011;41(2):112-20.

12. Wilmes B, Su YY, Drescher D. Insertion Angle Impact on primary stability of orthodontic mini-implants. Angle Orthod. 2008 Nov;78(6):1065-70.

13. Choi JH, Park CH, Yi SW, Lim HJ, Hwang HS. Bone density measurement in interdental areas with simulated placement of orthodontic miniscrew implants Am J Orthod Dentofacial Orthop. 2009 Dec;136(6):766.e1-12;discussion 766-7.

14. Park HS, Lee YJ, Jeong SH, Kwon TG. Density of the alveolar and basal bones of the maxilla and the mandible. Am J Orthod Dentofacial Orthop. 2008 Jan;133(1):30-7.

15. Baumgaertel S, Hans MG. Buccal cortical bone thickness for mini-implant placement. Am J Orthod Dentofacial Orthop. 2009 Aug;136(2):230-5.

16. Woodall N, Tadepalli SC, Qian F, Grosland NM, Marshall SD, Southard TE. Effect of miniscrew angulation on anchorage resistance. Am J Orthod Dentofacial Orthop. 2011 Feb;139(2):e147-52.

17. Pickard MB, Dechow P, Rossouw PE, Buschang PH. Effects of miniscrew orientation on implant stability and resistance to failure. Am J Orthod Dentofacial Orthop. 2010 Jan;137(1):91-9.

18. Kravitz ND, Kusnoto B. Risks and complications of orthodontic miniscrews. Am J Orthod Dentofacial Orthop. 2007 Apr;131(4 Suppl):S43-51.

19. Liou EJ, Chen PH, Wang YC, Lin JC. A computed tomographic image study on the thickness of the infrazygomatic crest of the maxilla and its clinical implications for miniscrew insertion. Am J Orthod Dentofacial Orthop. 2007 Mar;131(3):352-6.

20. Antoszewska J, Papadopoulos MA, Park HS, Ludwig B. Five-year experience with orthodontic miniscrew implants: a retrospective investigation of factors influencing success rates. Am J Orthod Dentofacial Orthop. 2009 Aug;136(2):158.e1-10;discussion 158-9.

21. Park HS, Jeong SH, Kwon OW. Factors affecting the clinical success of screw implants used as orthodontic anchorage. Am J Orthod Dentofacial Orthop. 2006 July;130(1):18-25.

22. Gracco A, Tracey S, Baciliero U. Miniscrew insertion and the maxillary sinus: an endoscopic evaluation. J Clin Orthod. 2010 July;44(7):439-43.

23. Kuroda S, Yamada K, Deguchi T, Hashimoto T, Kyung HM, Takano-Yamamoto T. Root proximity is a major factor for screw failure in orthodontic anchorage. Am J Orthod Dentofacial Orthop. 2007 Apr;131(4 Suppl):S68-73.

24. Park HS, Hwangbo ES, Kwon TG. Proper mesiodistal angles for microimplant placement assessed with 3-dimensional computed tomography images. Am J Orthod Dentofacial Orthop. 2010 Feb;137(2):200-6.

25. Houston WJ, Maher RE, McElroy D, Sherriff M. Sources of error in measurements from cephalometric radiographs. Eur J Orthod. 1986 Aug;8(3):149-51.

6

Long-term evaluation of apical root resorption after orthodontic treatment using periapical radiography and cone beam computed tomography

Jairo Curado de Freitas[1], Olavo César Porto Lyra[2], Ana Helena Gonçalves de Alencar[3], Carlos Estrela[4]

Objective: To evaluate the frequency of Apical Root Resorption (ARR) after orthodontic treatment at 52-288 months using periapical radiography (PR) and cone beam computed tomography (CBCT). **Methods:** Radiographic images obtained from 58 patients, before (T_1) and after orthodontic treatment (T_2), and following 52-288 months of treatment were analyzed by three members of the Brazilian Board of Orthodontics. Apical structures were evaluated by PR images (T_2 and T_3), using Levander and Malmgren scores. The presence of ARR on CBCT images were detected only at T_3. The Kolmogorov-Smirnov test was used for statistical analyses, and the level of significance was set at 5%. Kappa statistics determined interobserver agreement. **Results:** The more frequent ARR were with scores 1 in T_2 (51.6%) and T_3 (53.1%), when evaluated by PR (p > 0.05). When compared the frequencies of ARR in T_3 among PR and CBCT images, the differences were significant for maxillary and mandibular pre-molar groups, and for mandibular molar group (p > 0.05). The teeth with highest frequency of ARR presence using CBCT images were maxillary lateral incisors (94.5%) and mandibular central incisors (87.7%), while the premolars showed the lowest frequency. The CBCT images showed that the teeth involved in orthodontic treatment with extraction present higher ARR frequency (p < 0.05). **Conclusion:** PR showed more frequency of ARR in posterior teeth groups when compared with CBCT images. ARR did not change in long-term post treatment.

Keywords: Tooth resorption. Cone beam computed tomography. Corrective orthodontics.

[1] PhD in Health Sciences, UFG.
[2] MSc in Health Sciences, UFG.
[3] Post-doc in Endodontics, Cardiff University. Professor of Endodontics, School of Dentistry, UFG.
[4] Full Professor in Endodontics, USP. Professor of Endodontics, School of Dentistry, UFG.

» The authors report no commercial, proprietary or financial interest in the products or companies described in this article.

Jairo Curado de Freitas
Praça Universitária, S/N – Setor Universitário – Goiânia/GO, Brazil
CEP: 74605-220 – E-mail: curadojf@terra.com.br

INTRODUCTION

Apical root resorption may occur after orthodontic tooth movement. Its etiology is multifactorial and may be associated with individual biological variability, genetic predisposition, effect of mechanical factors, root morphology, and tooth injuries sustained before orthodontic treatment.[1-6]

Root resorption associated with orthodontic tooth movement is classified as inflammatory because it results from inflammation of the apical periodontium and the consequent destruction of tooth structures caused by clastic activity.[7] Clinical relevance is not often mentioned when the rate of ARR is low. However, in severe ARR, structural tooth changes may result from an unfavorable combination of factors, such as anatomic, physiological and genetic variations.[8,9,10] The understanding of the pathological mechanisms of radicular resorptions due to orthodontic treatment may help to establish accurate treatment plans.

Clinically, periapical radiographs are often used for diagnosis, treatment planning and follow-up. The revolution of information technology in health investigations started with computed tomography (CT), which has been used for planning, diagnosis, treatment and prognosis of several diseases.[11,12] Cone beam computed tomography (CBCT) is a recently developed technology[13,14] with important applications in research, clinical dentistry in general, and orthodontics in particular.[15-18]

A longitudinal prospective study[19] of the progression of ARR associated with orthodontic treatment using PR showed that central incisors do not continue to lose root length during the retention phase. Furthermore, no association with gender, age, overbite, overjet, headgear use, or intrusion mechanics was found. ARR was greater in patients that had undergone extractions.

Reukers et al[20] used digitally reconstructed images of maxillary incisors and found that ARR prevalence was 63% in the group of incisors. Relevant root shortening was found in only a few cases.[10,20] In another study, orthodontically induced ARR was evaluated using panoramic radiography and CBCT, and results showed that ARR was found in 69% of the teeth when CBCT scans were used and in 44% when panoramic radiography was the imaging method.[21]

As the application of CBCT in orthodontics seems promising, it may become a useful tool for the long-term follow up of patients that may develop ARR in association with orthodontic tooth movement in different tooth groups. However, few studies have focused on that use of CBCT. This study evaluated ARR at 52 to 288 months after treatment using periapical radiography and cone beam computed tomography. The null hypothesis was that there was no difference in apical root resorption frequencies detected by periapical radiography and cone beam computed tomography.

MATERIAL AND METHODS

Patients

Fifty-eight patients, 28 male and 30 female (1,392 teeth) were selected in a database search of a private orthodontic clinic in Goiânia, GO, Brazil. Inclusion criteria were: Complete orthodontic records, radiographs, pictures, plaster models, and orthodontic treatment completed at least 52 months before. Only patients whose radiographs showed high quality were included, and no patient had any history of retreatment. Time since treatment completion was up to 52 months, and patient mean age was 12 years and 4 months (SD = 2.31).

All the patients had been treated using edgewise mechanics by the same orthodontist and were invited to return for a follow-up examination, which included a full mouth set of periapical radiographs and CBCT scanning. The study was approved by the local Ethics in Research Committee (UFG, Prot. #169/2008).

Imaging methods

Periapical radiographs were acquired using a Spectro 70X Dental X-ray unit (Dabi Atlante, Ribeirão Preto, SP, Brazil) at 70 kV, 8 mA, 0.8 mm x 0.8 mm focal spot, using Kodak Insight film (Eastman Kodak Co, Rochester, NY, USA), using bisector technique with position indicating device and exposure time in accordance with the region imaged. All films were processed automatically and developed using standard methods (Peri-Pro II, Air techniques, NY,USA).

CBCT images were acquired with a first generation i-CAT Cone Beam 3D imaging system (Imaging Sciences International, Hatfield, PA, USA). The vol-

58 patients selected			

1,392 teeth			
	T_2 PR	T_3 PR	T_3 CBCT
Extracted	78	78	78
Congenital absence	7	7	7
Excluded	39	46	2
Total	1.268	1.261	1.305

Presence of ARR - PR		
	Teeth	
Scores*	T_2	T_3
1	654	670
2	265	277
3	14	8
4	1	0
Total	934	955

Presence of ARR in T_3	PR	CBCT
Teeth	Maxilla	
Anterior	286	250
Pre-molars	136	69
Molars	85	56
	Mandible	
Anterior	266	230
Pre-molars	90	41
Molars	92	49

Evaluation	
ARR Score (PR): T_2 x T_3	
ARR Presence: PR x CBCT	

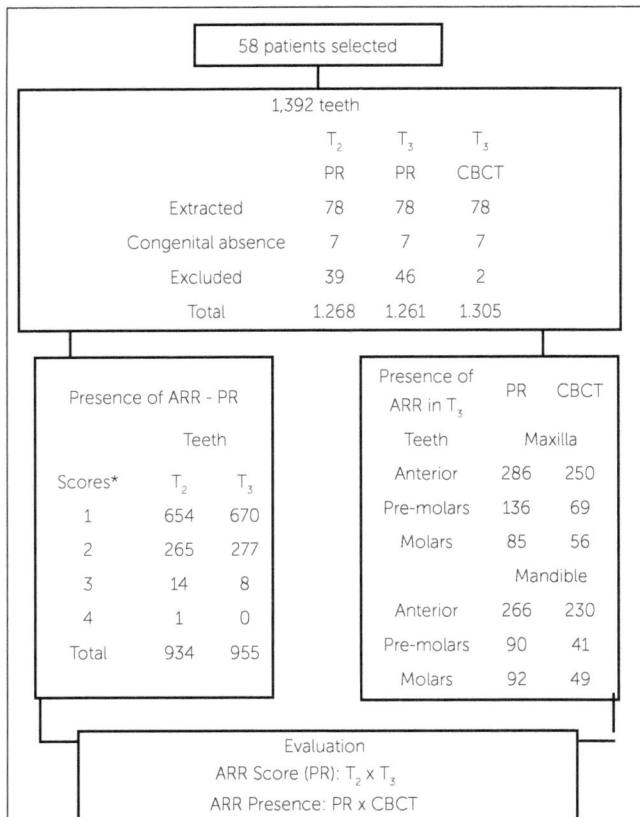

Figure 1 - Distribution of teeth according to presence or absence of ARR. (Source: modified from Levander and Malmgren[2]).

umes were reconstructed at 0.2 x 0.2 x 0.2 mm voxel size. The tube voltage was 120 kVp, and the current, 3.8 mA. Exposure time was 40 seconds. Images were examined using the scanner proprietary software (Xoran 3.1.62; Xoran Technologies, Ann Arbor, MI, USA) in a PC workstation running Microsoft Windows XP professional SP-2 (Microsoft Corp., Redmond, WA, USA), Intel® Core™ 2 Duo-6300 1.86 GHz (Intel Corporation, Santa Clara, CA, USA), NVIDIA GeForce 6200 turbo cache videocard (NVIDIA Corporation, Santa Clara, CA, USA) and an EIZO - Flexscan S2000 monitor at a resolution of 1600 x 1200 pixels (Eizo Nanao Corporation Hakusan, Ishikawa, Japan). The program tools permitted the evaluation of each tooth in three dimensions.

Evaluation methods

Periapical radiographs were analyzed at three time points: T_1 – before fixed orthodontic treatment; T_2 – after fixed orthodontic treatment; T_3 – at 52 to 288 months after treatment. Three members of the Brazilian Board of Orthodontics individually evaluated all images of PR in all teeth (except second and third molars) to detect ARR. The teeth with periapical lesions, traumatism history, and impossibility of diagnosis due to image overlapping and incomplete rhizogenes were excluded. The high number of teeth with incomplete apexes hindered the evaluation of apical structures in T_1. To evaluate interexaminer reliability, 10% of the sample was examined.

Levander and Malmgren[2] modified scoring system was used to evaluate ARR. Root apexes were classified into 5 levels of root resorption: 0= no root resorption; 1= irregular root outline; 2= apical root resorption, less than 2 mm; 3= apical root resorption, from 2 mm to one third of the original root length; 4= apical root resorption exceeding one third of original root length. The radiographs were mounted on slit sheets of cardboard and examined in a darkened room using a light box (Medalight LP-300, Universal Electronics Ind., NY, USA) at 3X magnification.

The CBCT images obtained in T_3 were evaluated by a radiology specialist with 5 years of training. CBCT was used only at T_3 because this imaging diagnostic tool was not available at the other time points.

The analysis of apical region was performed in a dynamic way into different plans (axial and cross-sectional). The thickness slices varied between 1 and 1.5 mm.

ARR presence or absence in PR and CBCT images were evaluated in all dental groups. In teeth with more than one root, the most resorbed root was selected to determine the score for that tooth.

The expected initial number of teeth was 1,392; extracted and congenitally absent teeth and teeth whose images had superposed structures (Fig 1) were excluded. The number of teeth involved or not with ARR was recorded.

The Kolmogov-Smirnov test was used to evaluate the data. The level of significance was set at 5%. Kappa statistics was used to determine interobserver agreement according to the study methods.

RESULTS

From all 58 patients, 40 had been classified, at the beginning of orthodontic treatment as Class I; 14 patients classified as Class II, division 1; 2 patients classified as Class II, division 2; 2 patients classified as Class III. Forty-nine patients used some type of intermaxillary elastics. The mean duration of treatment was 22.9 months (SD = 6.72).

The distribution of teeth in sample, showing the presence or absence of ARR, is presented in Figure 1. The radiographic images of 1,268 teeth were analyzed in T_2, 1,261 in T_3, and 1,305 CBCT images in T_3.

The frequency of ARR by PR after orthodontic treatment (T_2) and 52-288 months (T_3) is shown in Table 1. ARR more frequent score was 1, presenting 51.6% in T_2, and 53.1% in T_3. There was no significant statistical difference between T_2 and T_3, when evaluated by PR, in none of the scores.

Kappa value used to determine interobserver agreement according to modified Levander and Malmgren[2] study methods varied from 0.86 to 0.96 for PR images.

Table 2 summarizes the results of frequency (%) of teeth group most affected with ARR using PR and CBCT scans. The difference was statistically significant to pre-molar maxillary and mandibular group and to molar mandibular group, when compared the frequencies of ARR in T_2, between PR and CBCT images. The highest presence of ARR by PR was detected in these groups. So, the null hypothesis was rejected. Table 3 shows frequency (%) of teeth group most affected with ARR using CBCT scans. The maxillary lateral incisors were the teeth most affected by ARR. The second group of teeth most affected by ARR was the mandibular central incisors. The teeth group presenting less ARR was the premolars. Table 4 shows frequency (%) of ARR according to CBCT scans (T_3) and effect of extractions. The frequency of teeth with ARR was higher in the group with teeth involved in orthodontic treatments with extractions (66.7%) than in the group without extractions (45.2%). The difference was statistically significant.

Figure 2 shows periapical radiographs of the maxillary lateral incisor suggesting that apical root resorption do not change after finishing the orthodontic tooth movement in long term. Figure 3 shows presence or absence of ARR in central incisor, by PR and CBCT, while Figure 4 shows the same in upper premolar.

Table 1 - Frequency (%) of ARR after orthodontic treatment (T_2) and past 52 to 288 months follow-up according to PR.

Score	T_2 - PR	T_3 - PR	p
0	334 (26.3%)	306 (24.2%)	p > 0.05
1	654 (51.6%)	670 (53.1%)	p > 0.05
2	265 (20.9%)	277 (21.9%)	p > 0.05
3	14 (1.1%)	8 (0.6%)	p > 0.05
4	1 (0.1%)	0	p > 0.05
Total	1,268 (100%)	1,261 (100%)	p > 0.05

Table 2 - Frequency (%) of teeth group most affected with ARR using PR and CBCT scans.

Teeth	PR n (%)	CBCT n (%)	p
Maxilla			
Anterior	286 (22.7%)	250 (19.2%)	p > 0.05
Premolars	136 (10.8%)	69 (5.3%)	p < 0.05
Molars	85 (6.7%)	56 (4.3%)	p > 0.05
Mandible			
Anterior	266 (21.1%)	230 (17.6%)	p > 0.05
Premolars	90 (7.1%)	41 (3.1%)	p < 0.05
Molars	92 (7.3%)	49 (3.8%)	p < 0.05

Table 3 - Distribution of teeth most affected with ARR using CBCT scans

Teeth	Absence of ARR	Presence of ARR	Classification
Maxilla			
11/21	23 (19.8%)	93 (80.1%)	3rd
12/22	6 (5.4%)	104 (94.5%)	1st
13/23	63 (54.3)	53 (45.6%)	
14/24	45 (59.2%)	31 (40.7%)	
15/25	77 (66.9%)	38 (33.0%)	
16/26	60 (51.7%)	56 (48.2%)	5th
Mandible			
31/41	14 (12.2%)	100 (87.7%)	2nd
32/42	26 (22.4%)	90 (77.5%)	4th
33/43	76 (65.5%)	40 (34.4%)	
34/44	66 (82.5%)	14 (17.5%)	
35/45	87 (76.3%)	27 (23.6%)	
36/46	67 (57.7%)	49 (42.2%)	

Table 4 - Frequency (%) of ARR considering tooth involved in orthodontic treatment with or without extraction, analyzed by CBCT (T_3).

Enrolled teeth	Absence of ARR	Presence of ARR
Orthodontic treatment without extractions (n = 815)	446 (54.7%)	370 (45.2%)
Orthodontic treatment with extractions (n = 490)	163 (33.2%)	327 (66.7%)
p	p < 0.05	p < 0.05

p = significance of percentage differences.

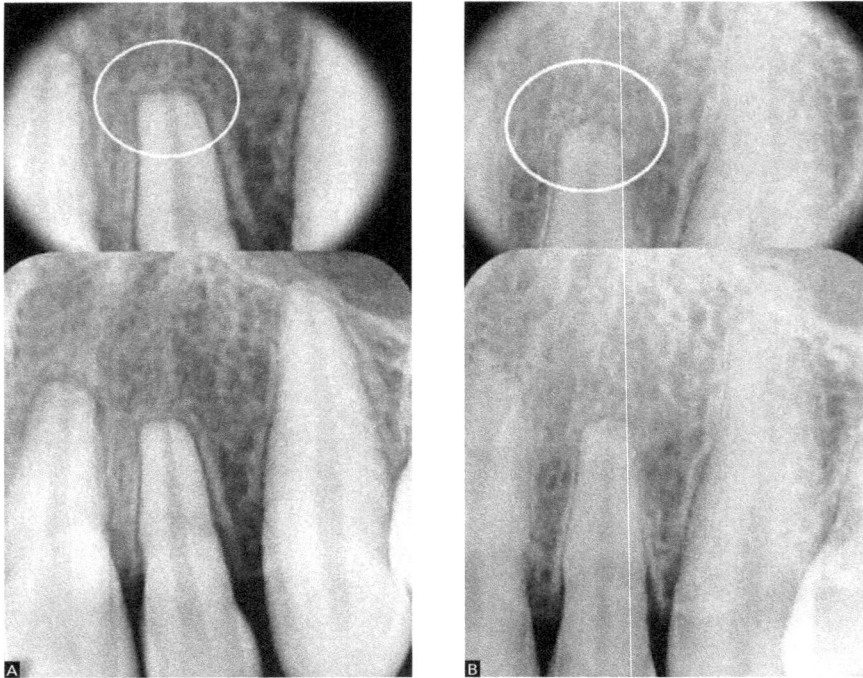

Figure 2 - Periapical radiographs of an upper left lateral incisor presenting the same ARR score after orthodontic treatment (**A**) and 288 months after treatment (**B**).

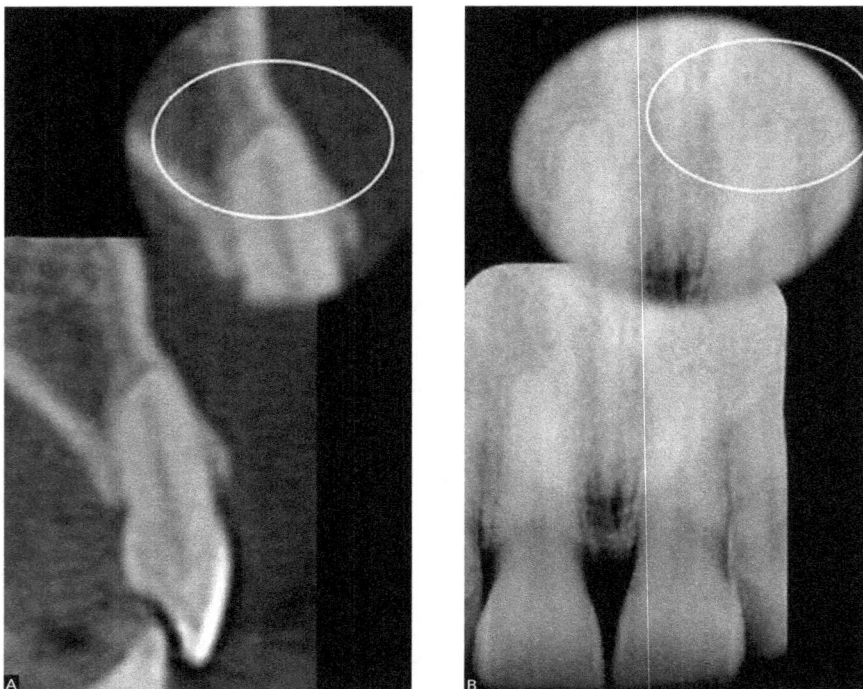

Figure 3 - CBCT scan of a maxillary left central incisor (**A**) (transverse view) shows more details of apical root resorption than periapical radiography (**B**).

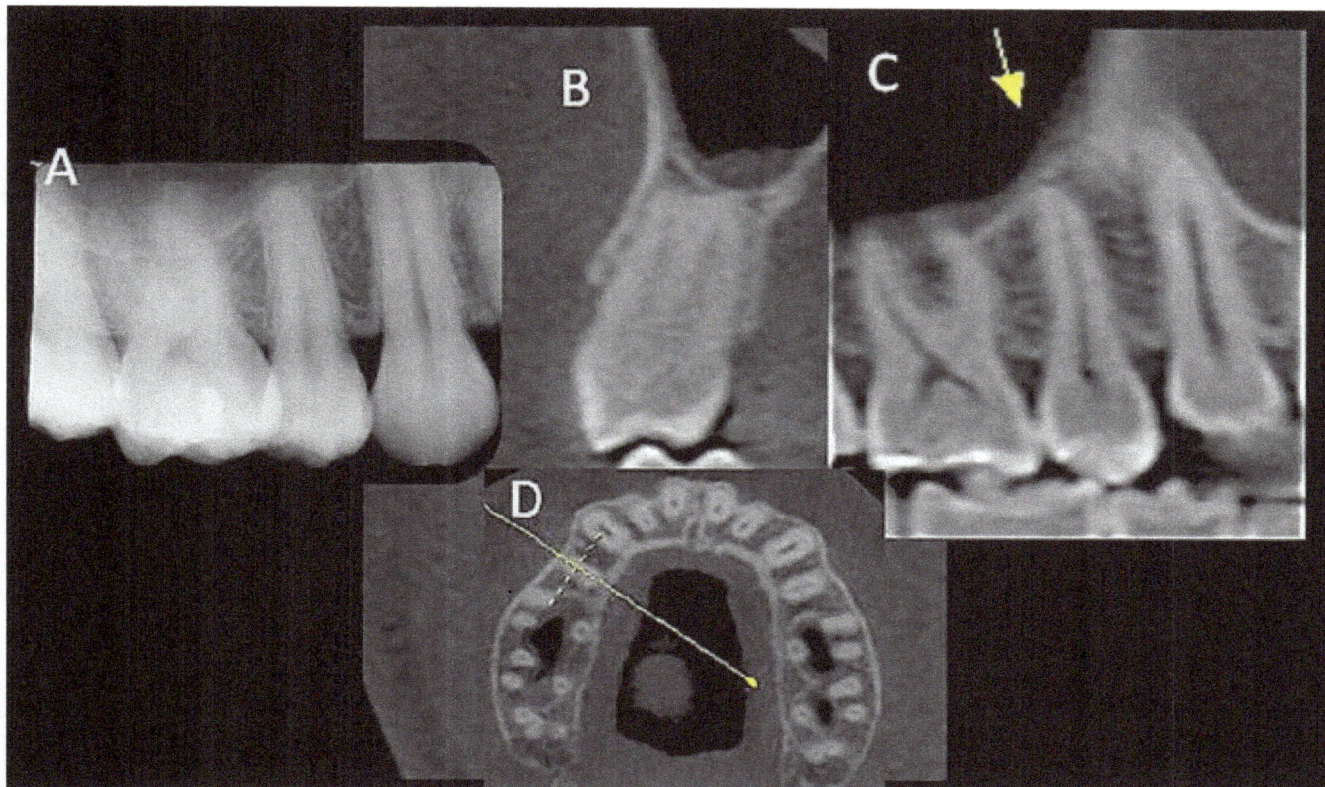

Figure 4 - Periapical radiograph of a maxillary right second premolar shows score 2 according to Levander and Malmgren system (A). The same tooth on CBCT scan presenting absence of ARR (B-D).

DISCUSSION

The advent of computed tomography brought a true revolution in medical sciences.[15-18] Particularly in dental specialties, the possibility of acquiring information from three-dimensional images of the maxillofacial region minimized the chances of underestimating lesions, such as ARR,[21,24] in dental structures.[15-18,21-25]

ARR characterize the loss of tooth structure and occurs due to several factors such as individual biological variability, genetic predisposition, mechanical factors, root morphology, and apical lesions prior to orthodontic treatment.[1-6] The extent of this resorption after orthodontic treatment influences the prognosis. Harmful consequences for the tooth may occur when severe resorption is present, even if observed in a small percentage and forward to well-planned and conducted orthodontic treatment.

Current knowledge does not allow the orthodontists to identify which patients are vulnerable to serious ARR. In a recent systematic review about ARR

associated with orthodontic treatment, Weltman et al[1] found only 11 suitable studies and the protocols were too variable to undertake a quantitative analysis. This revision reflects the timing of the published research about ARR. No study allowed consistent evidence about the longevity of teeth with severe resorption.[28]

The frequency of ARR, after completion of orthodontic treatment (T_2) and after 52 to 288 months (T_3), was determined by PR images (Table 1). The most frequent ARR score were 1, which did not show significant difference between T_2 (51.6%) and T_3 (53.1%). This study is in agreement with previous findings.[9,10] Copland and Green[9] (using lateral cephalometric radiograms) examined 45 individuals to investigate whether ARR in maxillary central incisors associated with orthodontic treatment continues after the end of the active treatment. Mean time between treatment end and final cephalometric radiogram was 2 years 4 months (28 months). When active treatment stopped, further ARR practically stopped, too.

Remington et al[10] conducted a retrospective study (using periapical radiography) to evaluate ARR in 100 patients at a mean 14.1 years (169 months) after orthodontic treatment. They found no apparent changes after appliance removal, except remodeling of rough and sharp edges (Fig 2).

Despite method differences between several studies[9,10] and our investigation, some important aspects should be analyzed: The mean duration of treatment was 22.9 months; the variation of follow-up time was 52 to 288 months, mean time between treatment end and the final cephalometric radiogram was 1.1 months, range was 0 to 7 months, the evaluation was made according to teeth groups; the scoring system of ARR detected by PR was the one described by Levander and Malmgren,[2] while the presence or absence of ARR was detected by CBCT images.

The results of CBCT and PR images at T_3, (52-288 months after treatment) revealed differences between the two imaging methods (Table 2). When comparing the frequencies of ARR in T_3, the difference was significant for the group of upper and lower premolars, and for the group of mandibular molars. In these dental groups a greater presence of ARR by PR images was detected. The results suggest that PR, due to limitations, tends to overestimate the ARR into posterior teeth groups (Figs 3 and 4). These findings might be assigned to the fact that analyses were made according to teeth groups. In different teeth group, the apical morphological variations, surrounding bone density (thick or thin bone cortex), x-ray angulations, radiographic contrast and overlapping of anatomic structures may affect radiographic interpretations.[26]

Advanced technologies that may potentially aid in establishing diagnoses, such as CBCT, bring up challenges that might only be overcomed when its properties and limitations are fully understood. Developing new software may greatly improve the acquisition and reconstruction of CBCT scans. In this study, a map-reading approach was used to examine all planes of the root apex, as suggested in a recent study[27] which showed that it promotes the perfect management of CBCT images and might reveal abnormalities not detected in conventional PR. For both imaging methods, extra care was taken to ensure an optimal interpretation environment.

Dudic et al[21] compared ARR in 275 teeth of 22 orthodontic patients using panoramic radiography and CBCT and the scoring system develop by Levander and Malmgren.[2] They found significant differences between the two methods and for all degrees of ARR. Panoramic radiography underestimated ARR after orthodontic treatment. CBCT imaging should be used to help to monitor patients at risk for developing severe root resorption during orthodontic movement. Our results were similar, but we evaluated ARR after a long-term follow-up of orthodontic treatment using PR and CBCT images.

Maxillary lateral incisors (94.5%) and mandibular central incisors (87.7%) were the most affected teeth (Table 3). ARR analysis, using CBCT. forward to the most affected teeth has not been compared with other literature data by a lack of studies. Newman[5] investigated possible etiological factors of external root resorption and found that maxillary incisors, maxillary premolars, and mandibular second premolars had the greatest incidence of apical resorption. This sequence differed from that found in other studies about root resorption.[29,30] In the present study, premolar were the least affected teeth by ARR when evaluated through CBCT image. Hemley[29] through PR showed that the teeth more susceptible to ARR were central incisors (9.1%). The lower central incisors were more likely to be affected than upper ones. Sharpe et al[30] found a higher frequency of ARR using PR in the central upper central incisors (52.7%) followed by lower ones (45.7%).

In this study, it was found that the most affected teeth are the anterior teeth, as demonstrated in other studies.[5,9,10,28] It might be suggested that a radiographic control of this dental group during and after orthodontic treatment is benefic for detecting of ARR.[9]

Tooth extraction was shown to be a risk factor for ARR during orthodontic tooth movement (Table 4). The frequency of teeth with ARR was higher in the tooth involved in orthodontic treatment with extractions (66.7%) than the group without extractions (45.2%) analyzed by CBCT (p < 0.05). One explanation for these results may be the fact that, in orthodontic treatment with extractions, extensive movements are needed. Our results are in agreement with those reported by Marques et al,[28] who found that the main factors directly involved in severe resorption were extraction of premolars, triangle-shaped roots and root resorption before treatment. Those authors also found a high prevalence of severe root resorptions in Brazilian patients treated with the edgewise method; differently from our findings.

CBCT is not commonly available in most dental offices. The analysis of the cost-effectiveness of 3D imaging in clinical routine should include the caution with radiation dose, variability of radiation between scanners and the lack of a standard recommended dose in some countries.

Silva et al[22] compared the radiation doses of conventional panoramic and cephalometric imaging with the doses of 2 different CBCT units and a multi-slice computed tomography (CT) unit in orthodontic practice. They concluded that conventional imaging still emits the lowest dose of radiation, and when three-dimensional imaging is required in orthodontic practice, CBCT scans should be preferred over CT imaging.

It is presumed that a new technology with potential to assist in diagnosis, such as CBCT, set new challenges until there is a complete understanding of their properties and limitations. New machines with low radiation doses and new software to reduce metal artifacts in CBCT image reconstruction should be developed. Further longitudinal studies should determine the behavior of severe ARR due to orthodontic movement.

CONCLUSION

PR showed more frequency of ARR in posterior teeth groups when compared with CBCT images. ARR did not change in long-term post treatment.

Acknowledgments

This study was supported in part by grants from the National Council for Scientific and Technological Development (CNPq grants 302875/2008-5 and CNPq grants 474642/2009 to C.E.).

REFERENCES

1. Weltman B, Vig KW, Fields HW, Shanker S, Kaizar EE. Root resorption associated with orthodontic tooth movement: a systematic review. Am J Orthod Dentofacial Orthop. 2010;137(4):462-76.
2. Levander E, Malmgren O. Evaluation of the risk of root resorption during orthodontic treatment: a study of upper incisors. Eur J Orthod. 1988;10(1):30-8.
3. Al-Qawasmi RA, Hartsfield JK Jr, Everett ET, Flury L, Liu L, Foroud TM, et al. Genetic predisposition to external apical root resorption. Am J Orthod Dentofacial Orthop. 2003;123(3):242-52.
4. Harris EF, Kineret SE, Tolley EA. A heritable component for external apical root resorption in patients treated orthodontically. Am J Orthod Dentofacial Orthop. 1997;111(3):301-9.
5. Newman WG. Possible etiologic factors in external root resorption. Am J Orthod. 1975;67(5):522-39.
6. McLaughlin KD. Quantitative determination of root resorption during orthodontic treatment [abstract]. Am J Orthod. 1964;50(2):143.
7. Consolaro A, Consolaro MF. The orthodontic root resorption is inflammatory, the phenomenon are genetically regulated although not hereditarily transmitted. Rev Dental Press Ortod Ortop Facial. 2009;14(4):25-32.
8. Levander E, Malmgren O, Eliasson S. Evaluation of root resorption in relation to two orthodontic treatment regimes. A clinical experimental study. Eur J Orthod. 1994;16(3):223-8.
9. Copeland S, Green L J. Root resorption in maxillary central incisors following active orthodontic treatment. Am J Orthod. 1986;89(1):51-5.
10. Remington DN, Joondeph DR, Artun J, Riedel RA, Chapko MK. Long-term evaluation of root resorption occurring during orthodontic treatment. Am J Orthod Dentofacial Orthop. 1989;96(1):43-6.
11. Ambrose J. Computerized transverse axial scanning (tomography): Part 2. Clinical application. Br J Radiol. 1973;46:1023-47.
12. Hounsfield GN. Computerized transverse axial scanning (tomography): Part 2. Clinical application. Br J Radiol. 1973;46:1016-22.
13. Arai Y, Tammisalo E, Hashimoto K, Shinoda K. Development of a compact computed apparatus for dental use. Dentomaxillofac Radio. 1999(28):245-8.
14. Mozzo P, Procacci C. Tacconi A. Martini PT, Andreis IA. A new volumetric CT machine for dental imaging based on the cone-beam technique: preliminary results. Eur Radiol. 1998;8:1558-64.
15. Scarfe WC, Farman AG, Sukovic P. Clinical applications of cone-beam computed tomography in dental practice. J Can Dent Assoc. 2006;72(1):75-80.
16. Farman AG. Applying DICOM to dentistry. J Digit Imaging. 2005;18(1):23-7.
17. Farman AG, Scarfe WC. Development of imaging selection criteria and procedures should precede cephalometric assessment with cone-beam computed tomography. Am J Orthod Dentofacial Orthop. 2006;130(2):257-65.
18. De Vos W, Casselman J, Swennen GRJ. Cone-beam computerized tomography (CBCT) imaging of the oral and maxillofacial region: a systematic review of the literature. Int J Oral Maxillofac Surg. 2009;38(6):609-25.
19. Spence TM. A prospective study of apical root resorption during orthodontic treatment and into retention. Am J Orthod Dentofac Orthop 2001;119(4):A1.
20. Reukers E, Sanderink G, Kuijpers-Jagtman AM, van't Hof M. Assessment of apical root resorption using digital reconstruction. Dentomaxillofac Radiol. 1989;27(1):25-9.
21. Dudic A, Giannopoulou C, Leuzinger M, Kiliaridis S. Detection of apical root resorption after orthodontic treatment by using panoramic radiography and cone-beam computed tomography of super-high resolution. Am J Orthod Dentofacial Orthop. 2009;135(4):434-7.
22. Silva MA, Wolf U, Heinicke F, Bumann A, Visser H, Hirsch E. Cone-beam computed tomography for routine orthodontic treatment planning: a radiation dose evaluation. Am J Orthod Dentofacial Orthop. 2008;133(5):640.e1-5.
23. Estrela C, Bueno MR, Leles CR, Azevedo B, Azevedo JR. Accuracy of cone beam computed tomography and panoramic and periapical radiography for detection of apical periodontitis. J Endod. 2008;34(3):273-9.
24. Estrela C, Bueno MR, Alencar AH, Mattar R, Neto JV, Azevedo BC, Estrela CRA. Method to evaluate inflammatory root resorption by using cone beam computed tomography. J Endod. 2009;35(11):1491-7.
25. Kau CH, Bozic M, English J, Lee R, Bussa H, Ellis RK. Cone-beam computed tomography of the maxillofacial region – an update. Int J Med Robot. 2009;5(4):366-80.
26. Huumonen S, Orstavik D. Radiological aspects of apical periodontitis. Endod Topics. 2002;1(1):3-25.

27. Bueno MR, Estrela C, Figueiredo JAP, Azevedo BC. Map-reading strategy to diagnose root perforations near metallic intracanal posts by using cone beam computed tomography. J Endod. 2011;37(1):85-90.

28. Marques LS, Ramos-Jorge ML, Rey AC, Amond MC, Ruellas ACO. Severe root resorption in orthodontic patients treated with the edgewise method: prevalence and predictive factors. Am J Orthod Dentofacial Orthop. 2010;137(3):384-8.

29. Hemley S. The incidence of root resorption of vital permanent teeth. J Dent Res. 1941;20(2):133.

30. Sharpe W, Reed B, Subtelny JD, Poison A. Orthodontic relapse, apical root resorption, and crestal alveolar bone levels. Am J Orthod Dentofacial Orthop. 1987;91(3):252-8.

7

Changes in alveolar bone support induced by the Herbst appliance: A tomographic evaluation

João Paulo Schwartz[1], Taisa Boamorte Raveli[1], Humberto Osvaldo Schwartz-Filho[2], Dirceu Barnabé Raveli[3]

Objective: This study evaluated alveolar bone loss around mandibular incisors, induced by the Herbst appliance. **Methods:** The sample consisted of 23 patients (11 men, 12 women; mean age of 15.76 ± 1.75 years), Class II, Division 1 malocclusion, treated with the Herbst appliance. CBCT scans were obtained before treatment (T_0) and after Herbst treatment (T_1). Vertical alveolar bone level and alveolar bone thickness of mandibular incisors were assessed. Buccal (B), lingual (L) and total (T) bone thicknesses were assessed at crestal (1), midroot (2) and apical (3) levels of mandibular incisors. Student's t-test and Wilcoxon t-test were used to compare dependent samples in parametric and nonparametric cases, respectively. Pearson's and Spearman's rank correlation analyses were performed to determine the relationship of changes in alveolar bone thickness. Results were considered at a significance level of 5%. **Results:** Mandibular incisors showed no statistical significance for vertical alveolar bone level. Alveolar bone thickness of mandibular incisors significantly reduced after treatment at B1, B2, B3, T1 and significantly increased at L2. The magnitude of the statistically significant changes was less than 0.2 mm. The changes in alveolar bone thickness showed no statistical significance with incisor inclination degree. **Conclusions:** CBCT scans showed an association between the Herbst appliance and alveolar bone loss on the buccal surface of mandibular incisors; however, without clinical significance.

Keywords: Periodontium. Activator appliances. Cone-beam computed tomography.

[1] PhD resident, Universidade Estadual Paulista (UNESP), Department of Orthodontics, Araraquara, São Paulo, Brazil.

[2] Adjunct Professor, Universidade Federal do Paraná (UFPR), Department of Stomatology, Curitiba, Paraná, Brazil.

[3] Professor, Universidade Estadual Paulista (UNESP), Department of Orthodontics, Araraquara, São Paulo, Brazil.

» The authors report no commercial, proprietary or financial interest in the products or companies described in this article.

João Paulo Schwartz
Rua Rio Grande do Sul, n. 368, apt 203
Curitiba – Paraná – 80620-080 – Brazil
E-mail: joaoschwartz@hotmail.com.br

INTRODUCTION

Angle Class II relationship is the malocclusion most commonly found in the orthodontic practice;[1] approximately one third of all patients present Class II, Division 1 malocclusion,[2] and mandibular deficiency is the primary etiological factor.[2]

Clinical practice and researches have shown that the Herbst appliance is effective in correcting Class II malocclusion.[3,4] The Herbst appliance is a fixed functional appliance that induces dentoalveolar changes and buccal movement of mandibular incisors.[5-11]

Compensatory orthodontic treatment of Class II malocclusion requires mandibular incisors to be proclined. Due to this fact, alveolar bone around incisors should be considered. The presence of harmful habits can alter the periodontal status and, in association with proclined mandibular incisors, could result in gingival recession.[12,13]

Evaluation of orthodontic treatment effects produced by the Herbst appliance has been performed by periapical, panoramic and cephalometric radiographs. Buccal and lingual alveolar bone plates are not correctly visualized in two-dimensional radiographs due to overlapping images. Cone-beam computed tomograph (CBCT) scans allow evaluation of periodontal tissue support tridimensionally. Researchers have been recently studying alveolar bone changes induced by orthodontic tooth movement with different voxel sizes.[14-17]

Knowledge of changes in periodontal tissue support induced by tooth movement is important, and there are no studies in the literature relating alveolar bone changes induced by the Herbst appliance by means of CBCT scans.

This research aimed at evaluating alveolar bone changes around mandibular incisors, induced by orthodontic treatment with the Herbst appliance.

MATERIAL AND METHODS

This retrospective study was reviewed and approved by the Ethics Committee of Universidade Estadual Paulista (FOAr-UNESP), School of Dentistry, Araraquara, São Paulo, Brazil. Patients were selected in local public schools. A total of 30 patients who presented skeletal Class II, Division 1 malocclusion were invited to participate in the study, following the inclusion criteria. Five patients refused to participate and two left the study before its conclusion. A total of 23 patients (11 men, 12 women; mean age of 15.76 ± 1.75 years) were sequentially treated by an orthodontist at the Department of Universidade Estadual Paulista (FOAr-UNESP), School of Dentistry, Araraquara, São Paulo, Brazil.

Skeletal Class II, Division 1 malocclusion was diagnosed by facial and occlusal analyses. Inclusion criteria were: convex profile; straight nasolabial angle; short mentocervical line; molar and canines in bilateral Class II relationship, equal or higher than the half of a cusp; overjet equal or greater than 5 mm; absence of posterior crossbite; absence of dental crowding; and complete permanent dentition, except third molars.[18] Exclusion criteria were: syndromic patient, extreme vertical growth pattern and prior orthodontic treatment.[18]

Patients used banded Herbst appliance until eight months of treatment were completed (mean 8.50 ± 0.70 months), with single mandibular advancement until incisors were in an edge–to–edge relationship.[8,18] The telescopic mechanism used was the Flip-Lock Herbst™ (TP Orthodontics, Inc.) model constituted by connectors, tubes and pistons.

A transpalatal fixed bar was used for upper anchorage, secured to first molars. The bar was made of 1.2-mm steel wire, 2 mm distant from the palate and with an extension of 1.2-mm steel wire to the second molar.[18] In the lower arch, a Nance lingual arch modified for the Herbst appliance was attached to first molars. It was made of 1.2-mm steel wire and located 3 mm distant from incisors lingual face. Anchorage appliances were constructed by the same technician.[18]

To evaluate alveolar bone loss around mandibular incisors, induced by the Herbst appliance, CBCT scans were obtained before treatment (T_0) and after treatment (T_1). Patients were scanned in an upright position with maximum intercuspation. To this end, i-CAT™ Classic (Imaging Sciences International, Hatfield, PA, USA) was used, with a 17 x 13.3 cm field of view, 120 kVp tube voltage, 18.45 mA tube current and 0.4 mm isometric voxel. CBCT scans were examined by means of Dolphin™ Imaging software (Dolphin Imaging and Management Solutions, Chatsworth, Calif., USA) by means of multiplanar reconstruction (axial, sagittal and coronal) and two-dimensional reconstruction of lateral cephalogram.

Tables 1 and 2 show reference points and measurements used to evaluate alveolar bone height and thickness (Fig 1). The coronal and sagittal cursor was adjusted in the tooth long axis (incisal edge center to root apex), according to the tooth of interest [19] (Fig 2). Buccal and

Table 1 - Reference points and definitions used to evaluate alveolar bone height and thickness.

Points	Definitions
1	Incisal edge
2	Root apex
3	Lingual CEJ
4	Buccal CEJ
5	Lingual alveolar crest
6	Buccal alveolar crest
7	Lingual symphysis crestal level
8	Lingual root crestal level
9	Buccal root crestal level
10	Buccal symphysis crestal level
11	Lingual symphysis midroot
12	Lingual root midroot level
13	Buccal root midroot level
14	Buccal symphysis midroot level
15	Lingual symphysis apical level
16	Lingual root apical level
17	Buccal root apical level
18	Buccal symphysis apical level

Table 2 - Definitions of measurements used to evaluate alveolar bone height and thickness.

Measurements	Definitions
Vertical bone lingual (VBL')	Distance between points 3 and 5
Vertical bone buccal (VBL)	Distance between points 4 and 6
Lingual bone crestal level (L1)	Distance between points 7 and 8
Buccal bone crestal level (B1)	Distance between points 9 and 10
Total bone crestal level (T1)	Distance between points 7 and 10
Lingual bone midroot level (L2)	Distance between points 11 and 12
Buccal bone midroot level (B2)	Distance between points 13 and 14
Total bone midroot level (T2)	Distance between points 11 and 14
Lingual bone apical level (L3)	Distance between points 15 and 16
Buccal bone apical level (B3)	Distance between points 17 and 18
Total bone apical level (T3)	Distance between points 15 and 18
Long Axis	Distance between points 1 and 2

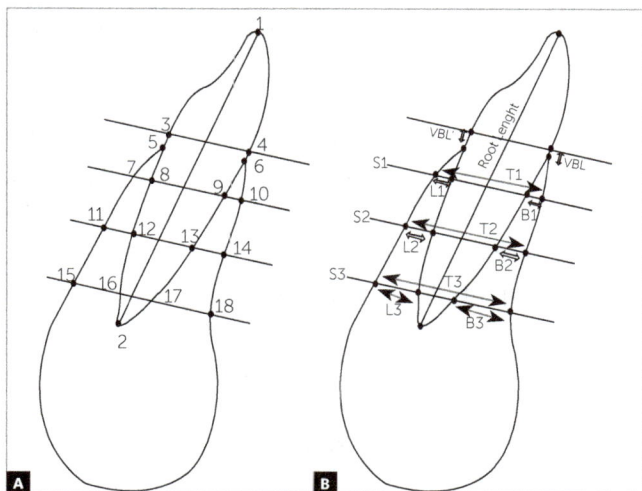

Figure 1 - Reference points (A) and measurements (B) used to evaluate alveolar bone height and thickness.

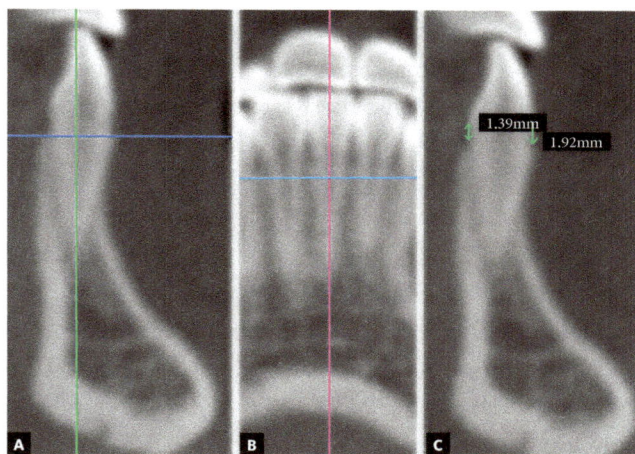

Figure 2 - Measurements used to evaluate alveolar bone height. Sagittal multiplanar reconstruction, coronal cursor adjusted in tooth long axis (A). Coronal multiplanar reconstruction, sagittal cursor adjusted in tooth long axis (B). Buccal and lingual alveolar bone height (C).

lingual alveolar bone heights were evaluated in sagittal multiplanar reconstruction. Measurement was taken from the most superior point of crestal alveolar bone to the cemento-enamel junction (CEJ), being a parallel line to the tooth long axis[14] (Fig 2).

Buccal (V), lingual (L) and total (T) bone thicknesses were assessed in each tooth by axial multiplanar reconstruction in three levels.[17] Axial slices were 3 mm distant from each other, and so was the reference point CEJ, being the three slices established at sagittal multiplanar reconstruction parallel to CEJ (Fig 1). The most buccal and lingual points were established at the alveolar bone plate and tooth root to measure buccal bone thickness (buccal bone point to buccal tooth root point), lingual bone thickness (lingual bone point to lingual tooth root point) and total bone thickness (buccal bone point to lingual bone point) in the three axial levels (Fig 3).

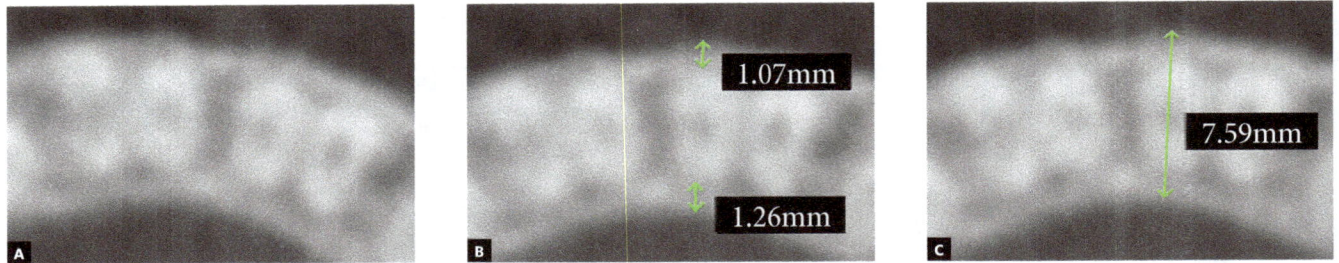

Figure 3 - Measurements used to evaluate alveolar bone thicknesses. Axial multiplanar reconstruction (**A**). Buccal and lingual bone thickness (**B**). Total bone thickness.

Measurements were reevaluated randomly after two weeks by the same blinded examiner. The error of the method was evaluated by Intraclass Correlation Coefficient (ICC). Shapiro-Wilk test was used to assess normal distribution, and Student's t-test as well as Wilcoxon t-test were used to compare dependent samples in parametric and nonparametric cases, respectively. Pearson's and Spearman's rank correlation analyses were performed to determine the relationship of changes in alveolar bone thickness. Results were considered at a significance level of 5%. Statistical analysis was performed by means of SPSS™ (SPSS Inc, Chicago, III) and GraphPad Prism™ (GraphPad Prism Inc, San Diego, USA).

RESULTS

Systematic intraexaminer error indicated excellent reliability (ICC = 0.91). Table 3 shows the means and standard deviations for cephalometric measurements at T_0 and T_1 for all subjects. Significant differences were found in SNB, ANB, WITS and IMPA measurements, showing the changes induced by the Herbst appliance. Table 4 shows means and standard deviations of changes in alveolar bone around mandibular incisors at T_0 and T_1. There were no statistical differences for buccal and lingual vertical alveolar bone level of mandibular incisors during treatment.

There was statistical significant difference for buccal and total alveolar bone thickness at the crestal level, showing a reduction of mean values from T_0 to T_1. Alveolar bone thickness at the midroot level showed statistical significant difference for lingual and buccal surfaces, with an increase and reduction of means during treatment, respectively. Mean alveolar bone thickness at the apical level decreased, showing a significant difference from T_0 to T_1 (Table 4). Alveolar bone thickness increased at the midroot level and reduced at the crestal level, midroot and apical levels for lingual and buccal sides, respectively.

The magnitude of statistically significant changes for alveolar bone thickness was less than 0.2 mm (Table 4). There was no statistically significant correlation between incisor inclination degree and extension of changes in alveolar bone thickness around mandibular incisors (Table 5).

Table 3 - Mean, standard deviation (SD) and level of significance (p) of cephalometrics measures.

Measurements	T_0 (Mean ± SD)	T_1 (Mean ± SD)	p value
SNA (degrees)	81.69 ± 4.11	81.62 ± 3.81	0.836
SNB (degrees)	77.66 ± 3.88	78.49 ± 3.66	0.027*
ANB (degrees)	4.34 ± 2.16	3.47 ± 2.17	0.000**
WITS (mm)	4.49 ± 2.76	3.47 ± 2.72	0.010*
IMPA (degrees)	98.39 ± 7.00	103.00 ± 7.90	0.000**
$\overline{1}.1$ (degrees)	116.60 ± 9.99	116.90 ± 9.07	0.805

*p <0.05; **p <0.001.

Table 4 - Mean, standard deviation (SD) and level of significance (P) of alveolar bone height and thickness in the lower incisors.

Measurements	T_0 (Mean ± SD)	T_1 (Mean ± SD)	T_1-T_0 (Mean ± SD)	p value
Buccal height (VBL) (mm)	1.41 ± 0.43	1.54 ± 0.53	0.13 ± 0.07	0.090
Lingual height (VBL') (mm)	1.43 ± 0.50	1.52 ± 0.50	0.09 ± 0.00	0.132
Lingual crestal (L1) (mm)	0.76 ± 0.40	0.70 ± 0.42	-0.06 ± 0.01	0.300
Buccal crestal (B1) (mm)	0.60 ± 0.26	0.44 ± 0.25	-0.16 ± 0.00	0.000***
Total crestal (T1) (mm)	7.03 ± 0.73	6.90 ± 0.74	-0.13 ± 0.00	0.010*
Lingual midroot (L2) (mm)	1.16 ± 0.52	1.36 ± 0.65	0.20 ± 0.09	0.000***
Buccal midroot (B2) (mm)	0.78 ± 0.42	0.60 ± 0.40	-0.18 ± 0.01	0.000***
Total midroot (T2) (mm)	7.06 ± 0.92	7.08 ± 0.96	0.02 ± 0.02	0.862
Lingual apical (L3) (mm)	1.85 ± 0.87	1.98 ± 0.86	0.13 ± 0.00	0.078
Buccal apical (B3) (mm)	1.98 ± 0.93	1.84 ± 0.87	-0.14 ± 0.04	0.035*
Total apical (T3) (mm)	7.66 ± 1.35	7.69 ± 1.35	0.03 ± 0.00	0.705

*$p < 0.05$; ***$p < 0.001$.

Table 5 - Pearson's and Spearman's rank correlation analysis between mandibular incisors inclination and alveolar bone changes.

Variable	Pearson's correlation		Spearman's correlation	
	Coefficient	p value	Coefficient	p value
Buccal height (VBL) (mm)	0.209	0.337	0.208	0.339
Lingual height (VBL') (mm)	0.401	0.057	0.272	0.208
Lingual crestal (L1) (mm)	0.143	0.514	0.051	0.815
Buccal crestal (B1) (mm)	-0.314	0.143	-0.248	0.253
Total crestal (T1) (mm)	-0.085	0.698	-0.098	0.653
Lingual midroot (L2) (mm)	0.409	0.052	0.385	0.069
Buccal midroot (B2) (mm)	-0.157	0.474	0.036	0.868
Total midroot (T2) (mm)	0.141	0.519	0.226	0.297
Lingual apical (L3) (mm)	-0.005	0.980	-0.227	0.296
Buccal apical (B3) (mm)	0.168	0.441	0.189	0.385
Total apical (T3) (mm)	0.313	0.145	0.360	0.360

DISCUSSION

This CBCT study evaluated alveolar bone loss around mandibular incisors, induced by the Herbst appliance. Patients with a mean age of 15.76 years comprised the group to simulate the postpubertal period, a stage during which Class II treatment with the Herbst appliance shows more dentoalveolar than skeletal response.[4] Cephalometric measurements SNB, ANB, WITS and IMPA showed significant statistical differences (Table 3), confirming appliance effectiveness and changes induced by the mechanic of mandibular advancement during correction of skeletal Class II malocclusion. These results are similar to related articles in the literature.[5-11]

Alveolar bone support is essential to teeth stability and periodontal health. Optimal stability of mandibular incisors is considered when the tooth is positioned in the medullary portion of the alveolar bone and it is found in good balance with labial and lingual musculature.[20] The mandibular symphysis is an anatomical structure that limits the buccal and lingual movement of incisors, shows thin alveolar bone plate and is susceptible to periodontal disease.[21] Previous studies have shown that excessive inclination of incisors buccally or lingually must be avoided, thereby preventing alveolar bone loss and consequent loss of tooth bone support.[22,23,24] This shows the importance of our study because there is no literature evaluating the effect of forward movement of mandibular incisors induced by the Herbst appliance in alveolar bone tridimensionally.

Lingual alveolar bone thickness presented statistically significant difference and increased at the midroot level (Table 3). Buccal bone thickness presented statistically significant difference and reduced at the crestal, midroot and apical levels (Table 3). Even with the use of anchorage with a lingual arch modified for the Herbst appliance, distant from incisors lingual surface, and a transpalatal fixed bar at the upper arch, mandibular incisors proclined significantly. There was a statistically significant decrease in total bone thickness at the crestal level (Table 3). Changes in total bone thickness are related to changes in inclination and intrusion extension of mandibular incisors.[17,25] As previously mentioned, there is no literature that reports assessing alveolar bone thickness induced by the Herbst appliance by means of CBCT scans; therefore, there are no parameters for comparison of our results.

Alveolar bone thickness with statistically significant changes was less than 0.2 mm, and this result is similar to that achieved by Lee et al[14] who evaluated alveolar bone loss around mandibular incisors with similar protocols of tomographic image acquisition. A limitation of this study could be that the magnitude of statistically significant changes is smaller than the voxel size. However, Yodthong, et al[17] evaluated alveolar bone thickness during maxillary incisors retraction with 0.125-mm voxel resolution, and found mean alveolar bone changes similar to our study. Moreover, the mean alveolar bone thickness and vertical level are larger than the voxel size, similarly to Kook et al[13] and Lee et al.[14] One of the discussions regarding tomographic image acquisition for evaluation of alveolar bone is voxel size. Tomographic image accuracy to measure bone thickness around mandibular anterior teeth under different resolutions showed no significant statistical difference between voxel protocols.[26] Despite statistically significant alveolar bone changes induced by the Herbst appliance, the minimal thickness reduction at the buccal surface of mandibular incisors has no clinical significance in patients in good periodontal health and without harmful habits.

Orthodontic proclination of mandibular incisors by the Herbst appliance does not result in gingival recession.[27] There is no association between buccal movement of mandibular incisors and the occurrence of gingival recession.[12] The periodontal status must be evaluated regarding health, the amount of keratinized gingiva, mucogingival problems and harmful habits, such as smoking.[28] The association between these periodontal conditions pre- or postorthodontic treatment, with proclination of mandibular incisors, could result in gingival recession.

There was no statistical difference between the inclination degree of mandibular incisors and changes in alveolar bone (Table 5). Alveolar bone change is related to biomechanical phenomena and is influenced by many factors, including periodontal environment, gingival type and oral habit of patient.[29] Thus, it might be possible that the extent of alveolar bone change is not mathematically or directly correlated with the degree of incisor inclination.

Regarding tomographic image acquisition, the accuracy of CBCT scans under different voxel resolutions (0.125 and 0.4 mm) for linear measurement of alveolar bone thickness around mandibular incisors was evaluated and there was no significant statistical difference between these voxel protocols.[26] However, when alveolar bone thickness is larger than the voxel size (0.4 mm), measurements are susceptible to be overestimated, and when it is close or smaller than the voxel size, it tends to be underestimated.[30] Alveolar bone changes smaller than the voxel size could be a limitation of our study.

In spite of the clinical relevance of the present results, we cannot underestimate that this is a retrospective study with methodological limitations. Therefore, further prospective studies must be performed with a larger sample size, including a control group, tomographic image acquisition, protocols (smaller voxel size, smaller field of view, higher spatial resolution and smaller noise from scatter) and long-term evaluations of alveolar bone remodeling after the end of treatment.

CONCLUSION

Tridimensional evaluation by means of CBCT scans revealed an association between the Herbst appliance and alveolar bone loss at the buccal surface of mandibular incisors; however, thickness of bone changes was minimal and clinically irrelevant.

REFERENCES

1. Ast DB, Carlos JP, Cons NC. The prevalence and characteristics of malocclusion among Senior High School Students in Upstate New York. Am J Orthod. 1965 Jun;51(6):437-45.

2. McNamara JA Jr. Components of Class II malocclusion in children 8-10 years of age. Angle Orthod. 1981 July;51(3):177-202.

3. Pancherz H. Dentofacial orthopedics or orthognathic surgery: is it a matter of age? Am J Orthod Dentofacial Orthop. 2000 May;117(5):571-4.

4. Ruf S, Pancherz H. When is the ideal period for Herbst therapy-early or late? Semin Orthod. 2003 Mar;9(1):47-56.

5. Barnett GA, Higgins DW, Major PW, Flores-Mir C. Immediate skeletal and dentoalveolar effects of the crown-or banded type Herbst appliance on Class II division 1 malocclusion. Angle Orthod. 2008 Mar;78(2):361-9.

6. El-Fateh T, Ruf S. Herbst treatment with mandibular cast splints: revisited. Herbst treatment with mandibular cast splints--revisited. Angle Orthod. 2011 Sept;81(5):820-7.

7. Obijou C, Pancherz H. Herbst appliance treatment of Class II, division 2 malocclusions. Am J Orthod Dentofacial Orthop. 1997 Sept;112(3):287-91.

8. Pancherz H. The mechanism of Class II correction in Herbst appliance treatment. A cephalometric investigation. Am J Orthod. 1982 Aug;82(2):104-13.

9. Pancherz H. Treatment of class II malocclusions by jumping the bite with the Herbst appliance. A cephalometric investigation. Am J Orthod. 1979 Oct;76(4):423-42.

10. von Bremen J, Pancherz H, Ruf S. Reduced mandibular cast splints an alternative in Herbst therapy? A prospective multicentre study. Eur J Orthod. 2007 Dec;29(6):609-13.

11. Weschler D, Pancherz H. Efficiency of three mandibular anchorage forms in Herbst treatment: a cephalometric investigation. Angle Orthod. 2005 Jan;75(1):23-7.

12. Kalha A. Gingival recession and labial movement of lower incisors. Evid Based Dent. 2013 Mar;14(1):21-2.

13. Kook YA, Kim G, Kim Y. Comparison of alveolar bone loss around incisors in normal occlusion samples and surgical skeletal class III patients. Angle Orthod. 2012 July;82(4):645-52.

14. Lee KM, Kim YI, Park SB, Son WS. Alveolar bone loss around lower incisors during surgical orthodontic treatment in mandibular prognathism. Angle Orthod. 2012 July;82(4):637-44.

15. Lund H, Gröndahl K, Gröndahl HG. Cone beam computed tomography for assessment of root length and marginal bone level during orthodontic treatment. Angle Orthod. 2010 May;80(3):466-73.

16. Lund H, Gröndahl K, Gröndahl HG. Cone beam computed tomography evaluations of marginal alveolar bone before and after orthodontic treatment combined with premolar extractions. Eur J Oral Sci. 2012 Jun;120(3):201-11.

17. Yodthong N, Charoemratrote C, Leethanakul C. Factors related to alveolar bone thickness during upper incisor retraction. Angle Orthod. 2013 May;83(3):394-401.

18. Schwartz JP, Raveli TB, Almeida KCM, Schwartz-Filho HO, Raveli DB. Cone Beam Tomography study of apical root resorption induced by Hebst Appliance. J Appl Oral Sci. 2015 Oct;23(5):479-85.

19. Timock AM, Cook V, McDonald T, Leo MC, Crowe J, Benninger BL, et al. Accuracy and reliability of buccal bone height and thickness measurements from cone-beam computed tomography imaging. Am J Orthod Dentofacial Orthop. 2011 Nov;140(5):734-44.

20. Sarikaya S, Haydar B, Ciğer S, Ariyürek M. Changes in alveolar bone thickness due to retraction of anterior teeth. Am J Orthod Dentofacial Orthop. 2002 July;122(1):15-26.

21. Yamada C, Kitai N, Kakimoto N, Murakami S, Furukawa S, Takada K. Spatial relationships between the mandibular central incisor and associated alveolar bone in adults with mandibular prognathism. Angle Orthod. 2007 Sept;77(5):766-72.

22. Ten Hoeve A, Mulie RM. The effect of antero-postero incisor repositioning on the palatal cortex as studied with laminagraphy. J Clin Orthod. 1976 Nov;10(11):804-22.

23. Vardimon AD, Oren E, Ben-Bassat Y. Cortical bone remodeling/tooth movement ratio during maxillary incisor retraction with tip versus torque movements. Am J Orthod Dentofacial Orthop. 1998 Nov;114(5):520-9.

24. Wainwright WM. Faciolingual tooth movement: its influence on the root and cortical plate. Am J Orthod. 1973 Sept;64(3):278-302.

25. Bimstein E, Crevoisier RA, King DL. Changes in the morphology of the buccal alveolar bone of protruded mandibular permanent incisors secondary to orthodontic alignment. Am J Orthod Dentofacial Orthop. 1990 May;97(5):427-30.

26. Patcas R, Müller L, Ullrich O, Peltomäki T. Accuracy of cone-beam computed tomography at different resolutions assessed on the bony covering of the mandibular anterior teeth. Am J Orthod Dentofacial Orthop. 2012 Jan;141(1):41-50.

27. Ruf S, Hansen K, Pancherz H. Does orthodontic proclination of lower incisors in children and adolescents cause gingival recession? Am J Orthod Dentofacial Orthop. 1998 July;114(1):100-6.

28. Aziz T, Flores-Mir C. A systematic review of the association between appliance-induced labial movement of mandibular incisors and gingival recession. Aust Orthod J. 2011 May;27(1):33-9.

29. Helm S, Petersen PE. Causal relation between malocclusion and periodontal health. Acta Odontol Scand. 1989 Aug;47(4):223-8.

30. Sun Z, Smith T, Kortam S, Kim DG, Tee BC, Fields H. Effect of bone thickness on alveolar bone-height measurements from cone-beam computed tomography images. Am J Orthod Dentofacial Orthop. 2011 Feb;139(2):117-27.

8

Dentoalveolar mandibular changes with self-ligating *versus* conventional bracket systems: A CBCT and dental cast study

Marcio Rodrigues de Almeida[1], Cristina Futagami[2], Ana Cláudia de Castro Ferreira Conti[3], Paula Vanessa Pedron Oltramari-Navarro[1], Ricardo de Lima Navarro[4]

Objective: The aim of the present study was to compare dentoalveolar changes in mandibular arch, regarding transversal measures and buccal bone thickness, in patients undergoing the initial phase of orthodontic treatment with self-ligating or conventional bracket systems. **Methods:** A sample of 25 patients requiring orthodontic treatment was assessed based on the bracket type. Group 1 comprised 13 patients bonded with 0.022-in self-ligating brackets (SLB). Group 2 included 12 patients bonded with 0.022-in conventional brackets (CLB). Cone-beam computed tomography (CBCT) scans and a 3D program (Dolphin) assessed changes in transversal width of buccal bone (TWBB) and buccal bone thickness (BBT) before (T_1) and 7 months after treatment onset (T_2). Measurements on dental casts were performed using a digital caliper. Differences between and within groups were analyzed by Student's t-test; Pearson correlation coefficient was also calculated. **Results:** Significant mandibular expansion was observed for both groups; however, no significant differences were found between groups. There was significant decrease in mandibular buccal bone thickness and transversal width of buccal bone in both groups. There was no significant correlation between buccal bone thickness and dental arch expansion. **Conclusions:** There were no significant differences between self-ligating brackets and conventional brackets systems regarding mandibular arch expansion and changes in buccal bone thickness or transversal width of buccal bone.

Keywords: Orthodontic appliances. Corrective orthodontics. Orthodontic brackets.

[1] Full professor of Orthodontics, Universidade Norte do Paraná (UNOPAR), Londrina, Paraná, Brazil.

[2] MSc in Orthodontics, Universidade Norte do Paraná (UNOPAR), Londrina, Paraná, Brazil.

[3] Professor of Orthodontics, Universidade do Sagrado Coração (USC), Bauru, São Paulo, Brazil.

[4] PhD in Orthodontics, Universidade de São Paulo (USP), São Paulo, São Paulo, Brazil.

Marcio Rodrigues de Almeida
Avenida Paris, 675 Jardim Piza, Londrina -PR - Brazil
CEP: 86041-120 - E-mail: marcioralmeida@uol.com.br

» The authors report no commercial, proprietary or financial interest in the products or companies described in this article.

INTRODUCTION

The ongoing search for innovation in Orthodontics has boosted the emergence or re-emergence of appliances so as to offer patients more comfort, shorter treatment time, improved post-treatment stability, and fewer side effects. Self-ligating brackets (SLB) came back into scene in the seventies, arising strong expectancy, and became popular in the nineties. Much empirical and anecdotal evidence as well as advantages were attributed to these appliances: increased patient comfort, better oral hygiene, increased patient cooperation, less chair time, shorter treatment time, greater patient acceptance, expansion, and less dental extractions.[1-6]

Correcting dental crowding without extractions or interproximal reductions requires an increase in arch perimeter in order to allow excellent teeth alignment. In the absence of distal movements, the dimensional changes of the arch involve transversal and buccal dental expansion.[7] It is a well-known fact that both self-ligating and conventional ligating brackets (CLB) when used for non-extraction treatment of dental crowding produce dentoalveolar expansion. The amount of transversal increase depends on the mechanics applied in each case.[7-11]

Before the introduction of computerized tomography, it was not possible to visualize the buccal bone due to superposition that occurred in 2D radiographs.[12,13] To achieve successful orthodontic treatment, the limits of orthodontic movement must be respected, in order to prevent iatrogenic effects to the sustaining and protection periodontium, such as gingival recessions, dehiscence and bone fenestrations. Studies prior to cone-beam computed tomography (CBCT) scans assessed only radiographs and dental casts, both of which used to be regarded as gold standards. Improvements in CBCT scans revealed it to be a reliable method, which offers an excellent visualization of the actual structures.[14,15] Timock et al[16] investigated the accuracy and reproducibility of measurements of alveolar bone height and thickness by means of CBCT imaging. They found good precision and accuracy for both measurements.[16]

The transversal response of the mandibular dental arch treated with CLB has been widely studied in the literature, especially the dentoalveolar response on dental casts.[7,10,17,18] However, little is known regarding CBCT scans used to assess the mandibular alveolar bone of the posterior region, where buccal bone can be detected and quantified.[19] This study aims at testing the null hypothesis that there is no difference, regarding changes in transversal width and buccal bone thickness in the mandibular arch, between patients undergoing the initial phase of orthodontic treatment (7 months) with SLB and CLB systems.

MATERIAL AND METHODS

This research protocol was approved by Universidade Norte do Paraná (UNOPAR, Londrina/PR, Brazil) Institutional Review Board. Patients and guardians were fully informed about the study and its implications, and signed a consent form.

For this prospective study, power analysis showed that a sample size of 12 patients in each group would give 80% probability to detect a real difference of 1.4 mm in intermolar distance and 0.2 mm in bone thickness, with a 95% ($p < 0.05$) significance level.[20] The sample for the present prospective randomized study was treated at Universidade Norte do Paraná (UNOPAR, Londrina, PR, Brazil) from 2009 to 2012. All patients had complete orthodontic records taken at the beginning (T_1) of treatment and 7 months after treatment onset (T_2), including study models and CBCT scans. In selecting the sample, the following inclusion criteria were applied: patients with Angle Class I malocclusion, moderate-to-severe lower dental crowding (3.0 to 7.0 mm), absence of diastema, absence of posterior crossbite, complete permanent teeth (except for third molars). Patients were randomly divided into two groups: SLB and CLB. Out of the selected individuals, none were excluded after treatment onset. Premolars extraction and tooth wear were not included in the proposed treatment.

Group 1 (G1) comprised 13 patients treated with 0.022 x 0.027-in slot SLB (EasyClip Aditek, Cravinhos/SP, Brazil), with initial mean age of 18.58 years (SD = 5.43). Group 2 (G2) comprised 12 patients treated with 0.022 x 0.028-in slot CLB (3M Unitek, Monrovia, Calif., USA), with initial mean age of 21.61 years (SD = 6.69). The archwires for Group 2 were tied to the brackets by means of a metallic ligature. Patients were orthodontically treated during initial leveling and alignment for six months, following the same sequence of round archwires: 0.013, 0.014 and 0.016-in nickel-titanium archwires, according to the manufacturers's (Aditek) prescription (Damon system). Each archwire remained in place for two months.

Cone-beam computed tomography scans were obtained from all patients at two time intervals prior to orthodontic treatment onset and 7 months after it. All CBCT scans were carried out by a single experienced radiologist using the same scanner (i-Cat Imaging Sciences International, Hatfield, Pennsylvania, USA) set up as follows: 22 x 16 cm fov, 40 sec, 120 kVp, 36 mA. This scanner has high-resolution sensors and affords 0.4-mm voxel images.[21]

CBCT scans were analyzed by one single operator who assessed mandibular bone changes by means of Dolphin 3D software (Version 11.5®, Dolphin Imaging & Management Solutions, Chatsworth, Calif., USA) with a level of sensitivity set at 25%.

Coronal slices were selected for the bone measurements (Fig 1) and 1-mm thick cross-sections were made through the first molar (M1), second premolar (P2) and first premolar (P1), in the right and left mandibular arches. As for coronal slices, the mid portion of teeth (molars and premolars) was chosen. The point selected for buccal bone measurement was the most external prominence of the buccal bone (EBB) in the root most apical portion (apex). At this same height, a point was projected from the parallel projection of the cusp point. The distance between the two points was determined as BBT, buccal bone thickness (Figs 2 and 3). Thus, changes in BBT were calculated by subtracting T_1 from T_2 values. For transversal width of the buccal bone, the EBB point was used on the right and left sides. The distance between right and left EBB was the transversal width of buccal bone (TWBB) (Fig 1). Similarly, TWBB changes were calculated by subtracting T_1 from T_2 values. In order to confirm whether transversal width and bone thickness measurements were taken on the same coronal slices, the mid region of each posterior teeth was used as reference to ensure consistency of slices.

Intermolar distances, intersecond premolar distances, and interfirst premolar distances were measured in dental casts (Fig 4) by means of a previously calibrated digital caliper (Mitutoyo Caliper, Japan). In order to measure the transversal distances, buccal cusp tips were selected for first and second mandibular premolars, while mesiobuccal cusp tips were selected for first molars.

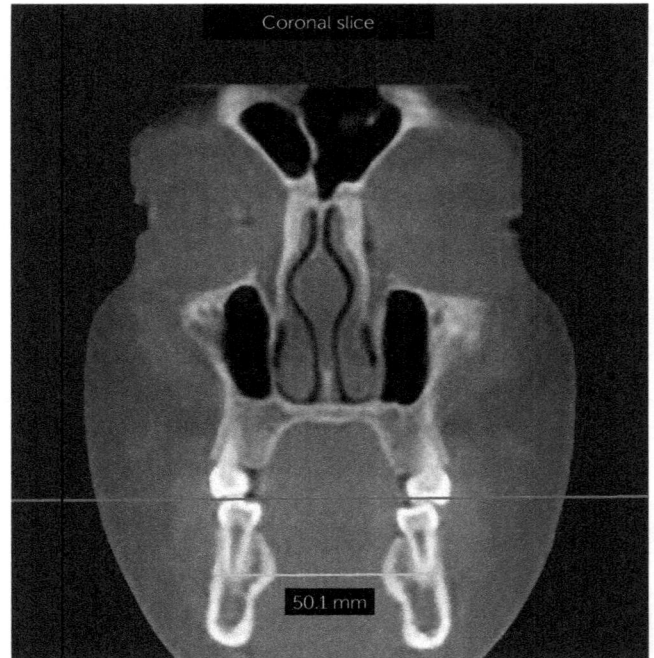

Figure 1 - Coronal slice and transversal width of buccal bone (TWBB).

Statistical analysis

To assess intra and interexaminer reliability, ten CBCT scans were randomly selected and remeasured four weeks apart by two operators. Intraexaminer error was assessed by means of paired t-test and Dahlberg's formula. Interexaminer reliability was assessed by intraclass correlation coefficient (ICC). Data were tested for normal distribution by means of Kolmogorov-Smirnov test. As data were normally distributed, parametric tests were applied. Results were described by parameters of mean and standard deviation of T_1 and T_2 measurements for both groups. Independent t-tests were used to compare the initial demographic data of both groups. Paired and unpaired t-tests were used to compare intra and intergroup changes. Finally, Pearson correlation coefficient was calculated to further explore the association between dental expansion and expansion of TWBB. In all statistical tests, the significance level was set at 5%.[22] All statistical analyses were performed with SPSS software for Windows version 17.0 (SPSS Inc, Chicago Ill.).

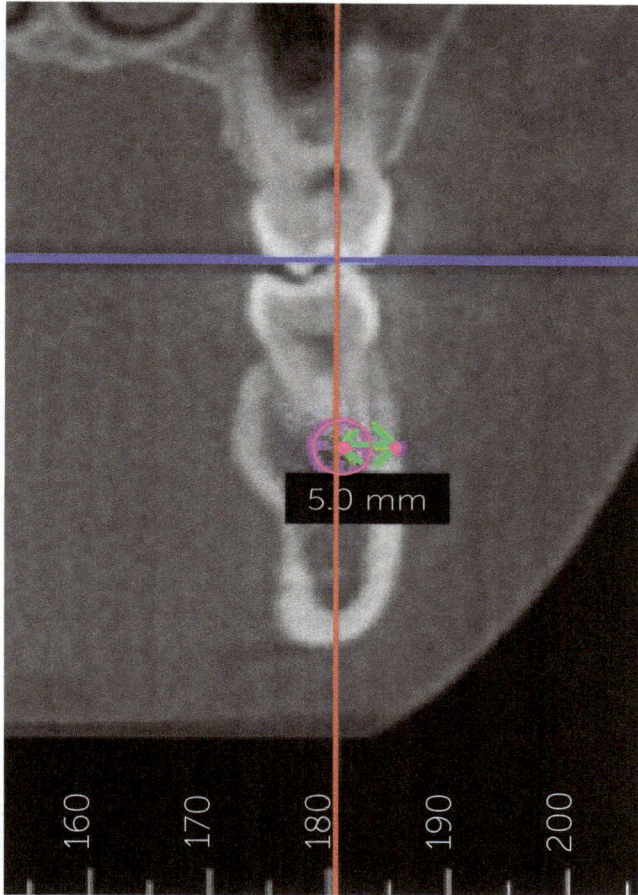

Figure 2 - Buccal bone thickness (BBT) measurements.

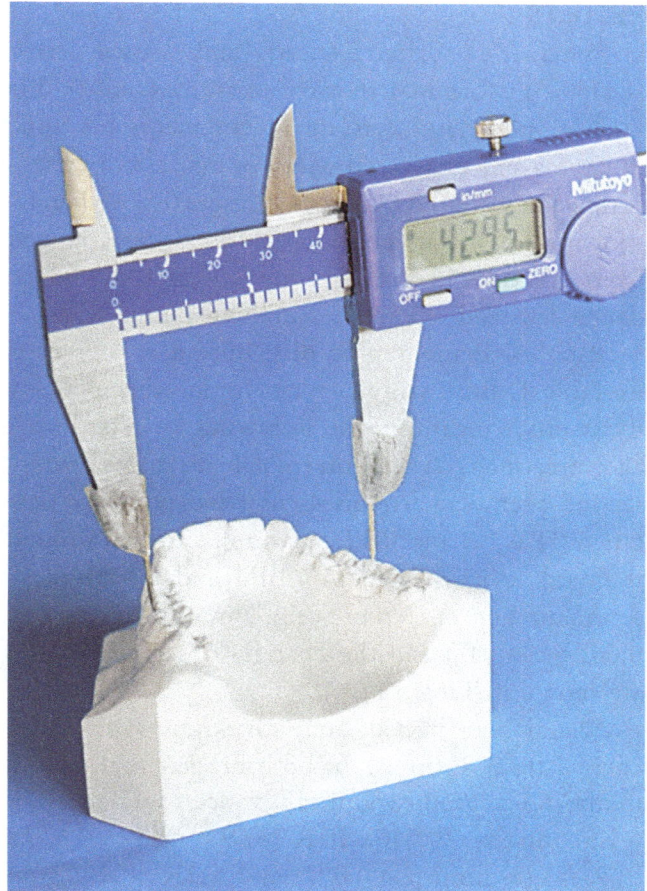

Figure 4 - Intermolar width measured on a dental cast by means of a digital caliper.

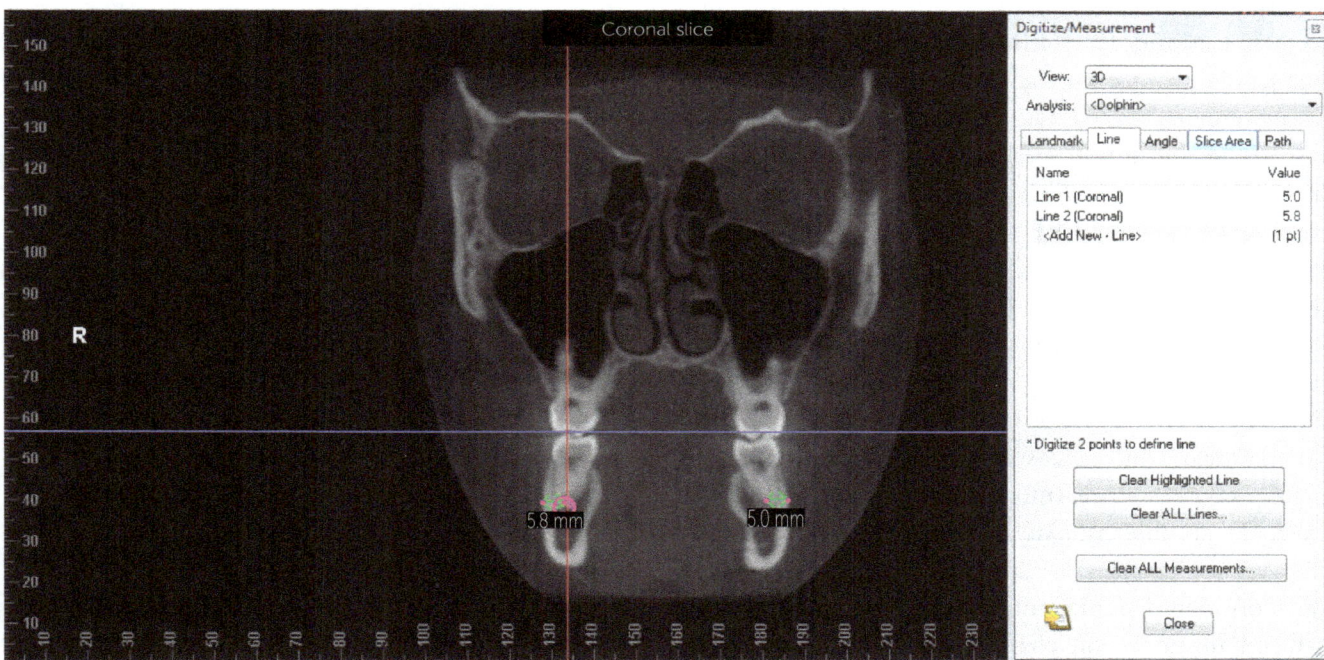

Figure 3 - Example of measurements for buccal bone thickness (BBT) of mandibular first molars.

RESULTS

Systematic (paired t-test) and casual error (Dahlberg's formula) showed no intraexaminer difference. Intraclass correlation coefficients for bone thickness and transversal width of buccal bone measurements were 0.89 and 0.98, respectively, thereby showing acceptable reliability. Random error ranged from 0.30 to 0.56 mm and from 0.53 to 1.08 mm for dental casts and CBCT measurements, respectively.

Patients' demographic distribution is presented in Table 1. Both samples were comparable at treatment onset regarding the following aspects: initial age, treatment time, intermolar distances, intersecond premolar distances, interfirst premolar distances, TWBB and BBT measurements. Means and standard deviation values for BBT and TWBB measurements at pretreatment (T_1), 7 months after treatment onset (T_2) and the changes observed (T_2-T_1) are shown in Tables 2 to 4.

Mandibular buccal bone thickness (BBT) decreased from T_1 to T_2 for both bracket types. BBT in the CLB group significantly decreased for P1L (-1.51 mm; p = 0.016), P1R (-0.9 mm; p = 0.039), P2R (-1.09 mm; p = 0.007) and M1R (-0.79 mm; p = 0.008). BBT in the SLB group significantly decreased for P1R (-0.88 mm, p = 0.019), P2L (-0.64 mm; p = 0.002), P2R (-1.09 mm, p < 0.001) and M1R (-0.54 mm; p = 0.025). However, changes in TWBB measurements showed a slight decrease and were not considered statistically significant in either one of the groups: for the CLB group, the following measurements decreased: P1 (-0.21 mm; p = 0.613), P2 (-0.66 mm; p = 0.222) and M1 (-0.31 mm; p = 0.611); as for the SLB group, the following measurements decreased: P1 (-0.56 mm; p = 0.076) and P2 (-0.01 mm; p = 0.980), with an increase in M1 (0.10 mm; p = 0.750).

Comparison between BBT and TWBB measurements from T_1 to T_2 revealed no significant differences between groups (Table 4). Additionally, no significant differences were found when comparing dental casts at treatment onset (T_1) and 7 months later (T_2) (Table 5). An average increase of dental transversal distances occurred from T_1 to T_2, which was considered significant. Bracket type had no significant influence on changes in mandibular dental arch. Differences between SLB and CLB for interfirst

Table 1 - Patients' demographic distribution.

	SLB (G1) (n = 13)	CLB (G2) (n = 12)	P
Initial mean age (years)	18.58 ± 5.43	21.61 ± 6.69	0.221
Treatment time (days)	210.15 ± 41.44	218.17 ± 46.60	0.654
CBCT scans			
P1L BBT (mm)	2.34 ± 2.59	2.31 ± 1.32	0.972
P1R BBT (mm)	2.65 ± 2.23	2.44 ± 1.21	0.788
P2L BBT (mm)	4.64 ± 2.38	4.02 ± 3.56	0.613
P2R BBT (mm)	4.82 ± 2.71	4.92 ± 2.11	0.927
M1L BBT (mm)	6.24 ± 2.29	6.49 ± 2.10	0.783
M1R BBT (mm)	6.70 ± 2.78	6.87 ± 1.48	0.856
P1 TWBB (mm)	40.37 ± 2.43	38.94 ± 2.58	0.175
P2 TWBB (mm)	49.35 ± 4.44	49.17 ± 4.07	0.928
M1 TWBB (mm)	59.04 ± 4.86	59.16 ± 4.45	0.956
Dental cast measurements (mm)			
4-4 width (mm)	33.95 ± 1.87	33.37 ± 2.36	0.749
5-5 width (mm)	38.42 ± 2.18	38.57 ± 2.69	0.888
6-6 width (mm)	44.85 ± 1.68	44.37 ± 2.76	0.612

M1 = first molar, P2 = second premolar and P1 = first premolar.

Table 2 - Mean and standard deviation at the beginning of treatment (T_1) and 7 months after treatment onset (T_2), regarding changes in buccal bone thickness and transversal width of buccal bone (CBCT measurements) for the CLB group.

Measurements	T_1	T_2	Diff.	P value
P1L BBT (mm)	2.31 ± 1.32	0.80 ± 1.86	-1.51	0.016*
P1R BBT (mm)	2.44 ± 1.21	1.54 ± 1.46	-0.90	0.039*
P1 TWBB (mm)	38.94 ± 2.58	38.73 ± 2.88	-0.21	0.613
P2L BBT (mm)	4.02 ± 3.56	3.14 ± 2.31	-0.88	0.165
P2R BBT (mm)	4.92 ± 2.11	3.83 ± 2.01	-1.09	0.007*
P2 TWBB (mm)	49.17 ± 4.07	48.52 ± 3.72	-0.66	0.222
M1L BBT (mm)	6.49 ± 2.10	6.18 ± 1.55	-0.31	0.292
M1R BBT (mm)	6.87 ± 1.48	6.08 ± 1.76	-0.79	0.008*
M1 TWBB (mm)	59.16 ± 4.45	58.90 ± 4.34	-0.26	0.611

* P < 0.05. M1 = first molar, P2 = second premolar and P1 = first premolar.

Table 3 - Mean and standard deviation at the beginning of treatment (T_1) and 7 months after treatment onset (T_2), regarding changes in buccal bone thickness and transversal width of buccal bone (CBCT measurements) SLB group.

Measurements	T_1	T_2	Diff.	P value
P1L BBT (mm)	2.34 ± 2.59	1.69 ± 1.64	-0.66	0.177
P1R BBT (mm)	2.65 ± 2.23	1.77 ± 2.01	-0.88	0.019*
P1 TWBB (mm)	40.37 ± 2.43	39.82 ± 2.67	-0.55	0.076
P2L BBT (mm)	4.64 ± 2.38	4.00 ± 2.42	-0.64	0.002*
P2R BBT (mm)	4.82 ± 2.71	3.73 ± 2.40	-1.09	<0.001**
P2 TWBB (mm)	49.35 ± 4.44	49.34 ± 4.13	-0.01	0.980
M1R BBT (mm)	6.24 ± 2.29	5.93 ± 2.43	-0.32	0.158
M1R BBT (mm)	6.70 ± 2.78	6.16 ± 2.63	-0.54	0.025*
M1 TWBB (mm)	59.04 ± 4.86	58.94 ± 4.79	-0.10	0.750

* P < 0.05. ** P < 0.01. M1 = first molar, P2 = second premolar and P1 = first premolar.

Table 4 - Means and standard deviation at the beginning of treatment (T_1) and 7 months after treatment onset (T_2) measured by CBCT and comparing CLB and SLB groups.

Measurements	SLB (G1) (n = 13)	CLB (G2) (n = 12)	Diff.	P value
P1L BBT (mm)	-0.66 ± 1.65	-1.51 ± 1.84	0.85	0.234
P1R BBT (mm)	-0.88 ± 1.17	-0.90 ± 1.34	0.02	0.964
P1 TWBB (mm)	-0.56 ± 1.04	-0.21 ± 1.38	-0.35	0.475
P2L BBT (mm)	-0.64 ± 0.57	-0.88 ± 2.06	0.25	0.681
P2R BBT (mm)	-1.09 ± 0.83	-1.09 ± 1.16	0.00	0.995
P2 TWBB (mm)	-0.01 ± 1.10	-0.66 ± 1.76	0.65	0.275
M1L BBT (mm)	-0.32 ± 0.75	-0.31 ± 0.97	0.01	0.992
M1R BBT (mm)	-0.54 ± 0.77	-0.79 ± 0.85	0.25	0.452
M1 TWBB (mm)	-0.10 ± 1.15	-0.26 ± 1.72	0.16	0.537

M1 = first molar, P2 = second premolar and P1 = first premolar.

Table 5 - Means and standard deviation at the beginning of treatment (T_1) and 7 months after treatment onset (T_2) measured in dental casts and comparing CLB and SLB groups.

Measurements	SLB (G1) (n = 13)	CLB (G2) (n = 12)	Diff.	p value
4-4 width	1.27 ± 1.95	1.87 ± 2.30	-0.60	0.489
5-5 width	2.10 ± 1.00	1.75 ± 1.33	0.35	0.465
6-6 width	0.92 ± 0.88	0.46 ± 0.77	0.46	0.180

Table 6 - Pearson correlation coefficient between transversal width of buccal bone (TWBB) and dental expansion within the two bracket system groups.

Measurements	r	P
P1 TWBB	0.15	0.467
P2 TWBB	0.28	0.176
M1 TWBB	0.09	0.676

M1 = first molar, P2 = second premolar and P1 = first premolar.

premolar width, intersecond premolar width and intermolar width were -0.6 mm (p = 0.489), 0.35 mm (p = 0.465) and 0.46 mm (p = 0.180), respectively.

Furthermore, no statistically significant association was found between transversal width of buccal bone (TWBB) and dental expansion (Table 6).

DISCUSSION

In this sample, patients were treated by different dentists, but in order to obtain more reliable results, measurements were made by only one previously calibrated examiner. The error of the method used to assess intra and interexaminer reliability proved to be small. No significant differences were found between measurements made by two operators at two different time points. Interexaminer analysis showed that errors ranged from 0.30 to 1.08 mm. This may have occurred due to high resolution images offering excellent view without overlapping structures.

A disadvantage of the CBCT method is its greater radiation dose in comparison to conventional radiographs (periapical and panoramic). However, CBCT is an invaluable tool in orthodontic research. Good to excellent reliability of CBCT scans used for detection of bone defects was demonstrated by Misch et al.[23] Furthermore, when compared to bidimensional radiographs, CBCT showed great reliability and offered advantages when detecting and quantifying bone fissures and fenestrations, as well as periodontal defects in the buccal bone.[24]

Mandibular arch bone expansion studies with CBCT scans comparing SLB and CLB are rare in the literature. And few studies have assessed the maxillary arch response to SLB and CLB systems.[19] Nonetheless, some studies compared arch expansion on dental casts and on digitized models, which may offer great accuracy.[7,10,11] Claims have been made that SLB can result in broader arch forms in comparison to CLB.[4] Thus, this study aimed at testing the null hypothesis that there are no significant differences in the amount of expansion of the mandibular arch (dental and alveolar bone changes) during the first 7 months of alignment and leveling when either SLB or CLB systems are used, as demonstrated by analysis on CBCT and dental casts.

According to Birnie,[25] Damon divulged his theory that by using SLB with low friction and light forces more stable biological results could be produced. Damon,[4] based on empirical and anedotical evidence, attributed advantages to self-ligating brackets, among which is the passive expansion of the arches. The Damon SLB system claims that post-treatment computed tomography images show transverse arch development and normal alveolar bone on buccal surface. Low friction and low force are purported to be good to physiologically rebuild the alveolar bone.[26]

The three-dimensional capability of CBCT makes it possible to noninvasively assess alveolar bone changes for mandibular posterior teeth. We found that BBT and TWBB measurements decreased from T_1 to T_2 for both groups. A significant difference occurred for the majority of measurements regarding BBT from T_1 to T_2 for both groups. There was significant difference for the following measurements, from T_1 to T_2, regarding BBT changes: CLB group — P1L (-1.51 mm, p = 0.016), P1R (-0.90 mm, p = 0.039), P2R (-1.09 mm, p = 0.007), M1R (-0.79 mm, p = 0.008); SLB group — P1R (-0.88 mm, p = 0.019), P2L (-0.64 mm, p = 0.002), P2R (-1.09 mm, p < 0.001), M1R (-0.54 mm, p = 0.025). However, no significant differences were found between groups. Furthermore, no significant differences from T_1 to T_2 were observed between and within groups for TWBB.

The results of the present study confirm findings in the literature showing similar behaviors for both brackets, particularly with regard to dental expansion assessed by means of dental casts. Mandibular arch alignment resulted in transverse expansion irrespective of the appliance system used. Interfirst premolar distances, measured on dental casts with a digital caliper in both groups, increased (SLB, 1.27 mm; CLB, 1.87 mm). This result is similar to those found by Fleming et al,[7] with an increase of 0.85 mm and 1.17 mm for SLB and CLB, respectively. However, the change was not significantly different between the two bracket systems. Further corroborating these findings, Vajaria el al[11] also found expansion in interfirst premolar distances. As for intersecond premolar distances, there was an increase of 2.10 mm for SLB and 1.75 mm for CLB; however, this increase was similar for both groups. Once again, the results yielded by the present study are similar to those obtained by Fleming et al[7] (SLB= 1.43 mm, and CLB= 1.72 mm). Nevertheless, contrary to our findings, Vajaria et al[11] found a larger increase for the self-ligating group (4.35 mm in comparison to 2.6 mm for the conventional group). Regarding intermolar distances, there was an increase ranging from 1.4 to 2.4 mm for SLB, and from 0.43 to 1.85 mm for CLB.[7,9,10,11,17,27,28] On the other hand, a

decrease in intermolar distance was observed in only one study in which cases were treated by means of premolar extractions.[28] We found nonsignificant increases of mandibular first intermolar width for both SLB and CLB groups, and there was no significant difference between the two bracket groups. The present study showed molar expansion of 0.92 mm and 0.46 mm for SLB and CLB, respectively. This result is in accordance with the study by Vajaria et al.[11] Nonetheless, Pandis et al[10,17] and Fleming et al[7] found that SLB expanded more than CLB in the molars region, and this difference was considered statistically significant.

When the Pearson correlation coefficient was assessed, we found that the alveolar buccal bone did not follow dental expansion. Therefore, the statements wherein self-ligating brackets produce physiological and passive movements of the arches were not confirmed in this study, at least 7 months after orthodontic treatment onset. Regarding buccal bone changes, it seems that self-ligating appliances do not offer any advantages over the conventional bracket system. Thus, the null hypothesis of the present study was accepted; in other words, no significant differences were found between self-ligating and conventional brackets systems regarding mandibular buccal bone plate expansion or dentoalveolar expansion.

CONCLUSIONS

» There is no difference between patients treated with self-ligating brackets or conventional brackets, regarding mandibular dentoalveolar expansion.

» There is no difference between patients treated with self-ligating brackets or conventional brackets, regarding buccal bone plate changes (mandibular buccal bone thickness and transversal width of buccal bone).

» There were no significant correlations between buccal bone plate changes and dentoalveolar expansion within groups.

REFERENCES

1. Stolzenberg J. The efficiency of the Russell attachment. Am J Orthod Oral Surg. 1946;32:572-82.

2. Berger J. Self-ligation in the year 2000. J Clin Orthod. 2000;34:74-81.

3. Harradine N. The history and development of self-ligating brackets. Semin Orthod. 2008;14(1):5-18.

4. Damon DH. The Damon low-friction bracket: a biologically compatible straight-wire system. J Clin Orthod. 1998;32(11):670-80.

5. Fleming PS, DiBiase AT, Lee RT. Self-ligating appliances: evolution or revolution? J Clin Orthod. 2008;42:641-51.

6. Rinchuse DJ, Miles PG. Self-ligating brackets: present and future. Am J Orthod Dentofacial Orthop. 2007;132(2):216-22.

7. Fleming PS, DiBiase AT, Sarri G, Lee RT. Comparison of mandibular arch changes during alignment and leveling with 2 preadjusted edgewise appliances. Am J Orthod Dentofacial Orthop. 2009;136(3):340-7.

8. Fleming PS, Johal A. Self-ligating brackets in orthodontics. A systematic review. Angle Orthod. 2010;80(3):575-84.

9. Chen SS, Greenlee GM, Kim JE, Smith CL, Huang GJ. Systematic review of self-ligating brackets. Am J Orthod Dentofacial Orthop. 2010;137(6):726.e1-726.e18; discussion -7.

10. Pandis N, Polychronopoulou A, Eliades T. Self-ligating vs conventional brackets in the treatment of mandibular crowding: a prospective clinical trial of treatment duration and dental effects. Am J Orthod Dentofacial Orthop. 2007;132(2):208-15.

11. Vajaria R, Begole E, Kusnoto B, Galang MT, Obrez A. Evaluation of incisor position and dental transverse dimensional changes using the Damon system. Angle Orthod. 2011;81(4):647-52.

12. Tai K, Park JH, Mishima K, Shin JW. 3-dimensional cone-beam computed tomography analysis of transverse changes with Schwarz appliances on both jaws. Angle Orthod. 2011;81(4):670-7.

13. Yagci A, Veli I, Uysal T, Ucar FI, Ozer T, Enhos S. Dehiscence and fenestration in skeletal Class I, II, and III malocclusions assessed with cone-beam computed tomography. Angle Orthod. 2012;82(1) 67-74.

14. Mah JK, Huang JC, Choo H. Practical applications of cone-beam computed tomography in orthodontics. J Am Dent Assoc. 2010;141 Suppl 3:7S-13S.

15. Sun Z, Smith T, Kortam S, Kim DG, Tee BC, Fields H. Effect of bone thickness on alveolar bone-height measurements from cone-beam computed tomography images. Am J Orthod Dentofacial Orthop. 2011;139(2):e117-27.

16. Timock AM, Cook V, McDonald T, Leo MC, Crowe J, Benninger BL, et al. Accuracy and reliability of buccal bone height and thickness measurements from cone-beam computed tomography imaging. Am J Orthod Dentofacial Orthop. 2011;140(5):734-44.

17. Pandis N, Polychronopoulou A, Makou M, Eliades T. Mandibular dental arch changes associated with treatment of crowding using self-ligating and conventional brackets. Eur J Orthod. 2010;32(3):248-53.

18. Tecco S, Tete S, Perillo L, Chimenti C, Festa F. Maxillary arch width changes during orthodontic treatment with fixed self-ligating and traditional straight-wire appliances. World J Orthod. 2009;10(4):290-4.

19. Cattaneo P, Treccani M, Carlsson K, Thorgeirsson T, Myrda A, Cevidanes L, et al. Transversal maxillary dento-alveolar changes in patients treated with active and passive self-ligating brackets: a randomized clinical trial using CBCT-scans and digital models. Orthod Craniofac Res. 2011;14(4):222-33.

20. Pandis N, Polychronopoulou A, Eliades T. Sample size estimation: an overview with applications to orthodontic clinical trial designs. Am J Orthod Dentofacial Orthop. 2011;140(4):e141-6.

21. Leite V, Conti AC, Navarro R, Almeida MR, Oltramari-Navarro P, Almeida R. Comparison of root resorption between self-ligating and conventional preadjusted brackets using cone beam computed tomography. Angle Orthod. 2012;82(6):1078-82.

22. Houston WJ. The analysis of errors in orthodontic measurements. Am J Orthod. 1983;83(5):382-90.

23. Misch KA, Yi ES, Sarment DP. Accuracy of cone beam computed tomography for periodontal defect measurements. J Periodontol. 2006;77(7):1261-6.

24. Mol A, Balasundaram A. In vitro cone beam computed tomography imaging of periodontal bone. Dentomaxillofac Radiol. 2008;37(6):319-24.

25. Birnie D. The Damon passive self-ligating appliance system. Semin Orthod. 2008;16:19-35.

26. Yu YL, Qian YF. The clinical implication of self-ligating brackets. Shanghai Kou Qiang Yi Xue. 2007;16:431-5.

27. Fleming PS, DiBiase AT, Lee RT. Randomized clinical trial of orthodontic treatment efficiency with self-ligating and conventional fixed orthodontic appliances. Am J Orthod Dentofacial Orthop. 2010;137(6):738-42.

28. Scott P, DiBiase AT, Sherriff M, Cobourne MT. Alignment efficiency of Damon3 self-ligating and conventional orthodontic bracket systems: a randomized clinical trial. Am J Orthod Dentofacial Orthop. 2008;134(4):470.e1-8.

9

Cone beam tomographic study of facial structures characteristics at rest and wide smile, and their correlation with the facial types

Luciana Flaquer Martins[1], Julio Wilson Vigorito[2]

Objective: To determine the characteristics of facial soft tissues at rest and wide smile, and their possible relation to the facial type. **Methods:** We analyzed a sample of forty-eight young female adults, aged between 10, 19 and 40 years old, with a mean age of 30.9 years, who had balanced profile and passive lip seal. Cone beam computed tomographies were performed at rest and wide smile postures on the entire sample which was divided into three groups according to individual facial types. Soft tissue features analysis of the lips, nose, zygoma and chin were done in sagittal, axial and frontal axis tomographic views. **Results:** No differences were observed in any of the facial type variables for the static analysis of facial structures at both rest and wide smile postures. Dynamic analysis showed that brachifacial types are more sensitive to movement, presenting greater sagittal lip contraction. However, the lip movement produced by this type of face results in a narrow smile, with smaller tooth exposure area when compared with other facial types. **Conclusion:** Findings pointed out that the position of the upper lip should be ahead of the lower lip, and the latter, ahead of the pogonion. It was also found that the facial type does not impact the positioning of these structures. Additionally, the use of cone beam computed tomography may be a valuable method to study craniofacial features.

Keywords: Diagnosis. Cone beam computed tomography. Smile.

[1] Visiting professor, Ciodonto College.
[2] Full professor of Orthodontics, University of São Paulo (USP).

» The authors report no commercial, proprietary or financial interest in the products or companies described in this article.

Luciana Flaquer Martins
Rua das Caneleiras, 1074. B. Jardim, Santo André/SP —Brazil — CEP: 09.090-050
E-mail: luflaquer@uol.com.br

Cone beam tomographic study of facial structures characteristics at rest and wide smile, and their correlation...

69

INTRODUCTION

One of the first facial esthetic concepts in Orthodontics was conceived by Angle,[1] who related perfect tooth intercuspation to the existing harmony between dental skeletal and facial structures. Case[2] has stated that even in face of lack of tooth contact and adequate masticatory function cases, patients could occasionally present reasonable facial esthetics. He also observed that all "beautiful" faces exhibited the following features: passive labial seal, good relation between the zygoma and the upper lips, lower lips slightly retracted in relation to the upper lips, and protruded chin.

Diagnosis and orthodontic planning were developed based on cephalometric studies, using lines, planes and angles aiming at quantifying the features of the craniofacial complex in addition to determining normality parameters and goals to be achieved at the end of the orthodontic treatment.[3-6]

From the 70's onwards, esthetic parameters assessments have been described as essential to treatment planning, associating Orthodontics to Orthognatic Surgery. Nevertheless, using cephalometric radiographs only is considered insufficient, since soft tissue characteristics would be better visualized by pictures.[7-12]

The incorporation of cone beam computed tomography (CBCT) techniques to Dentistry allowed comparison between soft and hard tissue structures, without overlaps or magnifications, providing data that correspond to the patient's real measurements.[14,15]

The possibility of a better appreciation of craniofacial structures improved not only the accuracy in landmarks demarcation, but also the precision of conventional cephalometric analysis[16,17,18,19,20,21] and it is likely that new assessment techniques might come up and change the current craniofacial analysis paradigms.[16,17,19]

Our purpose in this paper was to assess the soft tissue features of the face, nose, lips, zygoma and chin, both at rest and during wide smile positions, and their possible relation to the facial type. In order to accomplish that, we used cone beam computed tomographies, once they provide us with a better visualization and a more comprehensive approach for orthodontic diagnosis when compared with traditional methods.[18-21]

MATERIAL AND METHODS

The project for this article was approved by the University of Sao Paulo College of Dentistry Institutional Review Board, under report number 17/2008. This research assessed 48 female subjects aged between 19.10 and 40 years old, with a mean age of 30.9 years old, caucasian, who had passive lip seal . None of the patients had previously taken part on research activities, facial surgeries (plastic or orthognatic) and had never undergone any facial esthetic intervention.

Facial Index was used to determine each patient's facial type. Patients' faces were photographed with facial soft tissues at rest and with guided NHP,[22] according to Vigorito e Martins.[26]

Each patient's image was inserted into the Radiocef Studio 2 computer software (Radio Memory Ltda, Belo Horizonte — Brazil), by means of which the facial type was obtained according to the anthropometric Facial Index.

Calculations were done using the following formula:

$$\text{N'-Me'x } 100 \: / \: \text{ZiR'-ZiL'}$$

Once Facial Index had been determined, patients were classified as brachifacial, mesofacial or dolicofacial according to the following parameters:[23,26]

- Brachifacial: between 80.0 and 84.9%.
- Mesofacial: between 85.0 and 89.9%.
- Dolicofacial: between 90.0 and 95.0% or higher.

Following the aforementioned proportions, sample was subdivided into three groups with sixteen subjects each (Brachifacial, Mesofacial and Dolicofacial).

After the facial type had been determined, cone beam computed tomographies were taken by an i-Cat (Imaging Sciences International Hatfield, PA — USA) digital tomography scanner, at two stages: 1- With facial soft tissues at rest; 2- Wide smile.

All measurements were obtained through the i-CAT Vision (Imaging Sciences International Hatfield, PA — USA) computer software at the MPR visualization screen, (multi-plane reconstruction).

For the purpose of this study, true horizontal determination was chosen by means of a single intracranial landmark (Sela), tracing a perpendicular line departing from it, this being the true vertical.[24] This technique, together with guided natural head position, is suggested to avoid that possible variations between intracranial planes and lines diverge from the true horizontal line.[23,24]

For frontal assessment visualization, the 3DVR 5.0 (Imaging Sciences International Hatfield, PA — USA) 3D computer software was used.

Variables used in tomographic soft tissue cephalometric assessment

Axial section (Fig. 1):

1) Zygomatic thickness (Zygoma point; zygomatic soft tissue point, left and right sides); 2) Nose width (left and right alar); 3) Base of the nose width (left to right nasal base)

Sagittal section (Fig. 2):

1) Snv-Ul (upper lip position in relation to the vertical subnasal line); 2) Snv-Ll (lower lip position in relation to the vertical subnasal line); 3) Snv-Pog' (pogonion position in relation to the vertical subnasal line); 4) H-nose (distance from the tip of the nose to line H); 5) Nose height (distance from pro-nasal to the true horizontal line); 6) Collumela height (distance from collumela to true horizontal); 7) Upper lip height (distance from the stomion to subnasal point); 8) Lower lip height (distance from stomion to mental lip point); 9) Upper lip thickness (distance between vertical prosthion to the tip of the upper lip); 10) Lower lip thickness (distance from vertical infradentale to the tip of lower lip); 11) Distance between labial apexes (distance between upper and lower lip width lines); 12) E-Ll (distance from line E and the lower lip).

Frontal view (Figs 4 and 5):

1) Upper lip vermilion height (distance between the most central upper lip point to the stomion, marked over the midline); 2) Lower lip vermilion height (distance between the stomion and the inferior portion of the lower lip, marked over the midline); 3) Distance between right and left labial comissures; 4) Labial height (distance between the upmost part of the upper lip and the lowest part of the lower lip, marked over the midline); 5) Labial index (proportional distance between comissures and labial height, at rest); 6) Smile index (proportional distance between the comissures and labial height, at wide smile); 7) Teeth exposure area.

STATISTICAL METHOD

Facial structures movements were calculated for each patient by subtracting the value at rest from the

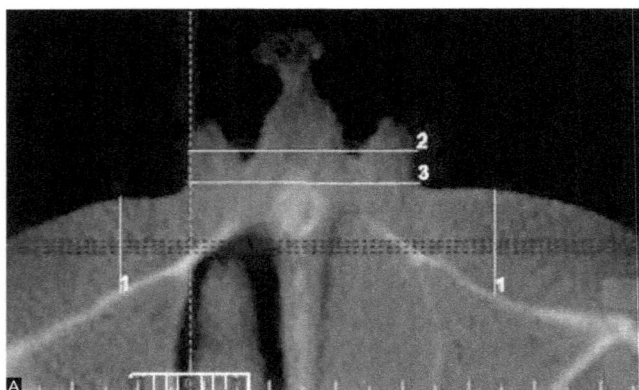

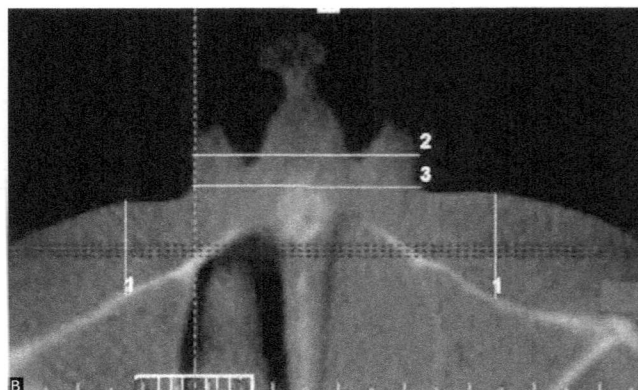

Figure 1 - Variables studied in axial section at rest (**A**) and wide smile (**B**).

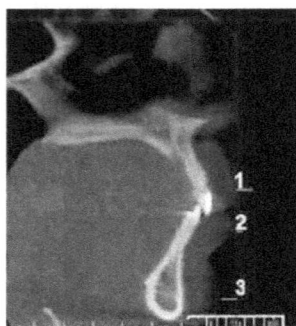

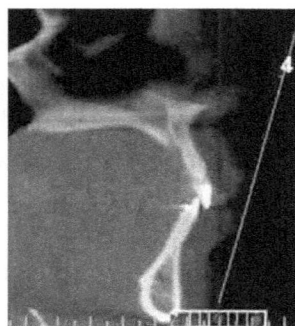

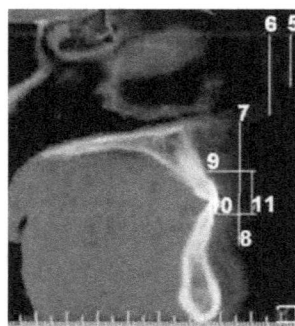

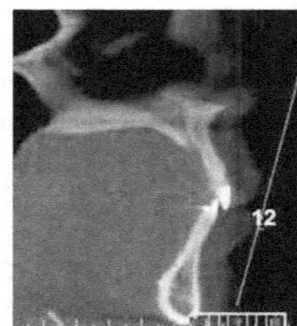

Figure 2 - Variables studied in sagittal section at rest.

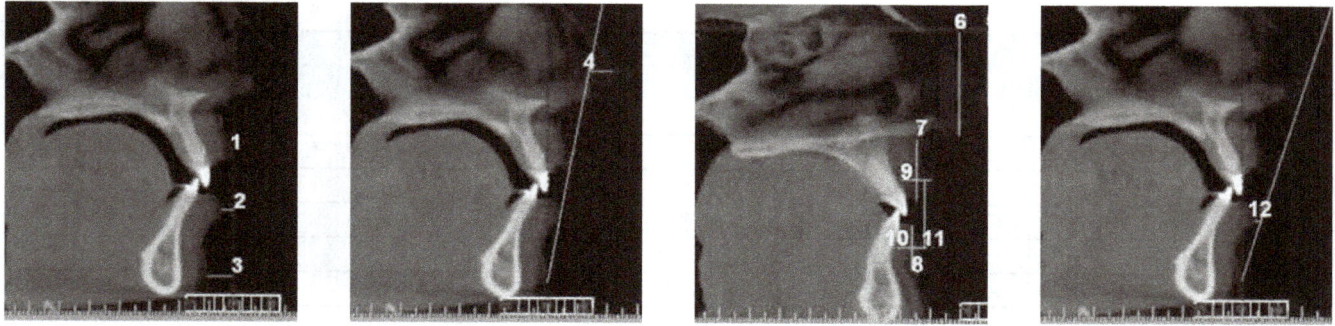

Figure 3 - Variables studied in sagittal section during wide smile.

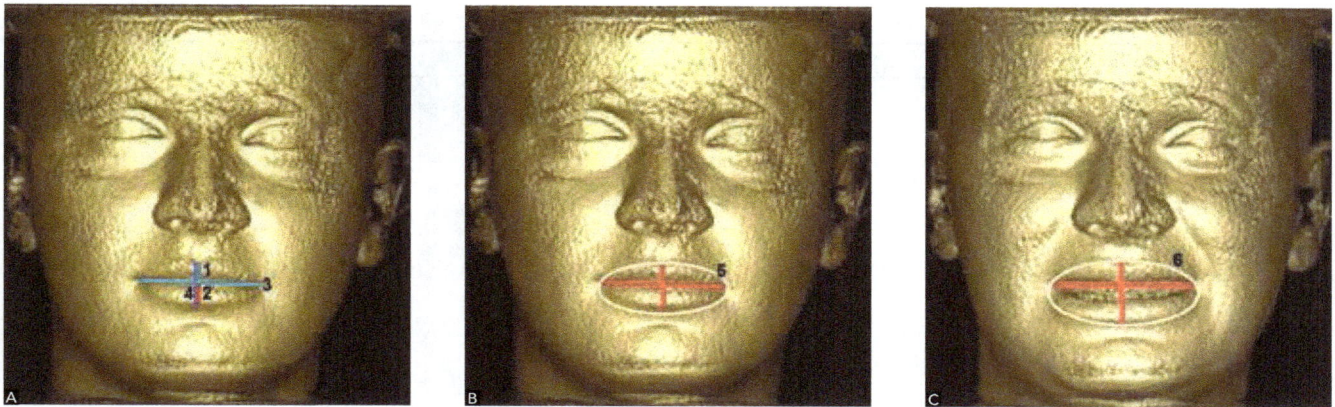

Figure 4 - Variables studied in tridimensional view of the face at rest (A and B) and during wide smile (C).

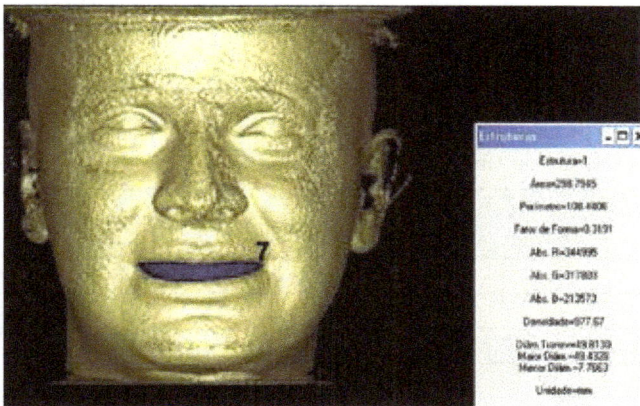

Figure 5 - Tooth exposure area, calculated by tridimensional view of the face during wide smile.

wide smile value. Each facial movement measurement was compared between facial types by means of analysis of variance (one-way ANOVA),[25] followed by Bonferroni[25] multiple comparisons when the ANOVA presented statistically significant differences while checking which facial types presented distinct facial movement.

In order to assess the relationship between smile index and teeth exposure area, Pearson's correlations were calculated separately for each face type, for the whole sample.

RESULTS

Results are shown in Tables 1 to 8.

Table 1 - ANOVA analysis of variance of the difference between facial types at rest and wide smile, in axial tomographic section.

Variable	Facial type						P
	Brachifacial		Mesofacial		Dolicofacial		
	Mean ± SD	n	Mean ± SD	n	Mean ± SD	n	
Left zygomatic thickness	5.11 ± 2.48	16	3.93 ± 2.28	16	3.11 ± 1.64	16	0.04
Right zygomatic thickness	5.25 ± 2.34	16	3.83 ± 2.22	16	3.17 ± 1.84	16	0.027
Nose width	4.42 ± 3.54	16	3.74 ± 2.83	16	3.12 ± 2.59	16	0.479
Nasal base width	5.24 ± 2.68	16	4.3 ± 1.93	16	4.13 ± 2.12	16	0.336

Table 2 - Bonferroni analysis of measurements presenting statistically significant differences between rest and wide smile, in axial tomographic section.

Variable	Comparison		Mean difference	Standard Error	P	CI (95%)	
						Lower	Upper
Left zygomatic thickness	Brachifacial	Mesofacial	1.18	0.76	0.388	-0.72	3.08
	Brachifacial	Dolicofacial	2	0.76	0.036	0.1	3.9
	Mesofacial	Dolicofacial	0.82	0.76	0.87	-1.08	2.72
Right zygomatic thickness	Brachifacial	Mesofacial	1.42	0.76	0.203	-0.47	3.3
	Brachifacial	Dolicofacial	2.08	0.76	0.026	0.2	3.97
	Mesofacial	Dolicofacial	0.66	0.76	1	-1.22	2.55

Table 3 - ANOVA analysis of variance of the difference between facial types at rest and wide smile, in sagittal tomographic section.

Variable	Facial type						P
	Brachifacial		Mesofacial		Dolicofacial		
	Mean ± SD	n	Mean ± SD	n	Mean ± SD	n	
Nose Height	-0.24 ± 3.57	16	-0.1 ± 3.53	16	0.67 ± 4.25	16	0.767
Collumela Height	-0.23 ± 3.13	16	-0.01 ± 4.17	16	0.18 ± 4.54	16	0.959
Upper Lip Height	-4.78 ± 2.23	16	-4.51 ± 1.97	16	-4.84 ± 1.71	16	0.879
Lower Lip Height	-0.85 ± 1.64	16	-1.26 ± 1.99	16	-1.97 ± 1.98	16	0.245
Upper Lip Thickness	-4.66 ± 1.37	16	-3.39 ± 1.58	16	-3.56 ± 1.21	16	0.027
Lower Lip Thickness	-5.2 ± 1.74	16	-5.11 ± 1.58	16	-4.62 ± 1.66	16	0.57
Distance between Labial Apexes	6.59 ± 2.4	16	8.33 ± 2.81	16	7.51 ± 1.96	16	0.137
Upper Lip Position	-3.2 ± 1.42	16	-1.32 ± 1.76	16	-2.23 ± 1.54	16	0.007
Lower Lip Position	-3.86 ± 2.23	16	-3.13 ± 2.03	16	-4.11 ± 2.24	16	0.417
Pogonion	-0.74 ± 2.99	16	1.29 ± 3.28	16	-1.01 ± 3.02	16	0.083
Line E-Li	-2.89 ± 4.46	16	-4.28 ± 2.13	16	-2.94 ± 1.83	16	0.35
H-Nose	5.96 ± 1.93	16	5.87 ± 2.8	16	4.13 ± 5.86	16	0.335

Table 4 - Bonferroni analysis of measurements presenting statistically significant differences between rest and wide smile, in sagittal section.

Variable	Comparison		Mean difference	Standard Error	p	CI (95%)	
						Lower	Upper
Upper Lip Thickness	Brachifacial	Mesofacial	-1.27	0.49	0.04	-2.49	-0.04
	Brachifacial	Dolicofacial	-1.11	0.49	0.089	-2.33	0.12
	Mesofacial	Dolicofacial	0.16	0.49	1	-1.06	1.39
Upper Lip Position	Brachifacial	Mesofacial	-1.87	0.56	0.005	-3.26	-0.48
	Brachifacial	Dolicofacial	-0.96	0.56	0.274	-2.35	0.43
	Mesofacial	Dolicofacial	0.91	0.56	0.335	-0.48	2.3

Table 5 - ANOVA analysis of variance of the difference between facial types at rest and wide smile, in frontal view.

Variable	Facial type						p
	Brachifacial		Mesofacial		Dolicofacial		
	Mean ± SD	n	Mean ± SD	n	Mean ± SD	n	
Distance between comissures	12.37 ± 5.75	16	9.6 ± 4.04	16	9.6 ± 4.85	16	0.197
Labial Height	5.75 ± 3.32	16	7.09 ± 3.3	16	7.77 ± 2.88	16	0.198
Upper lip Vermilion Height	-1.29 ± 1.21	16	-1.25 ± 0.99	16	0.09 ± 0.93	16	0.001
Lower lip Vermilion Height	-0.81 ± 1.04	16	-0.93 ± 0.75	16	-0.37 ± 0.43	16	0.113
Labial/Smile Index	-0.02 ± 0.42	16	-0.25 ± 0.25	16	-0.27 ± 0.26	16	0.059

Table 6 - Bonferroni analysis of upper lip vermilion height presenting statistically significant differences between facial types at rest and wide smile, in frontal view.

Variable	Comparison		Mean difference	Standard Error	p	CI (95%)	
						Lower	Upper
Upper lip vermilion Height	Brachifacial	Mesofacial	-0.04	0.37	1	-0.96	0.89
	Brachifacial	Dolicofacial	-1.38	0.37	0.002	-2.3	-0.45
	Mesofacial	Dolicofacial	-1.34	0.37	0.002	-2.26	-0.42

Table 7 - ANOVA analysis of variance of teeth exposure area between different facial types, in frontal view.

Variable	Facial type						
	Brachifacial		Mesofacial		Dolicofacial		p
	Mean ± SD	n	Mean ± SD	n	Mean ± SD	n	
Teeth exposure area	288.7 ± 158.4	16	435.04 ± 101.38	16	431.9 ± 102.14	16	0.002

Table 8 - Bonferroni analysis of teeth exposure area that presented statistically significant difference between facial types at rest and wide smile, in frontal view.

Variable	Comparison		Average Difference	Standard Error	p	IC (95%)	
						Lower	Upper
Teeth exposure area	Brachifacial	Mesofacial	-146.37	43.69	0.005	-255.01	-37.73
	Brachifacial	Dolicofacial	-143.21	43.69	0.006	-251.85	-34.57
	Mesofacial	Dolicofacial	3.16	43.69	1	-105.48	111.8

DISCUSSION

Considering the fact that the methodology applied to assess facial soft tissues is considerably different from the methodologies described in the literature, the discussion of this paper is restricted to a description of the findings, supplying data so that further researches may be developed and compared to the present one.

For the study of axial section tomographic images, for both rest and wide smile positions, measurements presented no statistically significant difference between the three facial types.

In the dynamic assessment of these structures, determined by the axial section, it was verified that neither the nose width nor the nose base width suffered any changes in different facial types. On the other hand, soft tissues thickness around the zygomatic structures was influenced by wide smile position when comparing different facial types, suggesting that brachifacial subjects present greater muscle movement, translated by increased thickness around the zygoma if compared with dolicofacial subjects (Tables 1 and 2).

When comparing all variables assessed by the sagittal section, both at rest and wide smile, no statistically significant differences were found between facial types.

However, it was found that at both rest and wide smile, upper lip, lower lip and pogonion positions remained invariable: the lower lip with discrete retrusion if compared with the upper lip, and the pogonion slightly retruded if compared with the lower lip, as reported by the literature.[2,4,5,8,24]

Except for the tip of the nose, the nasal collumela and the pogonion, dynamic assessment revealed that height and width of both upper and lower lips as well as the esthetic positioning of these structures, presented significant difference between the two phases (Table 3). Except for upper lip thickness and positioning, which tend to thin out as the smile expands in brachifacial subjects, other measurements did not particularize any facial type.

In frontal view, at rest and wide smile, lips and their features were analyzed and no statistical difference was found between measurements and the facial types.

Dynamic assessment of different variables in frontal view revealed a peculiar behavior with regard to the facial types, as follows:

» Brachifacial, the distance between lip comissures and lip height presented significant alteration. Lower lip vermilion height decreased due to vertical muscle contraction (Table 4).

» Mesofacial, all variables studied revealed significant alteration (Table 4).

» Dolicofacial, wide smile measurements were higher than at rest, but the difference between smile and labial indexes pointed out that rest measurements exceeded the wide smile ones. (Table 4).

The dynamic behavior between labial and smile indexes presented a statistical significant difference for mesofacial and dolicofacial types, with labial index exceeding the smile index. These results demonstrate that although muscle movements take place during wide smile, they do not equally involve vertical and horizontal lip distancing, with a larger distance for horizontal distancing if compared with the vertical one.

Bonferroni analysis of upper lip vermilion height (Table 5) revealed that the upper lip vermilion height was greater for brachifacial patients than for dolicofacial ones, and when comparing dolicofacial with mesofacial subjects, this parameter was higher for mesofacial individuals

On comparing the tooth exposure area variable between facial types, as an attempt to distinguish their features, it was observed that there was a statistical significant difference (Table 6) that, when submitted to Bonferroni analysis (Table 7), demonstrated that brachifacial subjects presented lower values if compared with mesio and dolicofacial ones, with no significant difference between the two latter patterns.

Observation of tooth exposure behavior in comparison with the smile index showed no relation between those two variables (Table 8). That confirms the fact that the range of lip movement does not impact total tooth exposure.

CONCLUSION

The results obtained from this research led to the conclusion that in balanced faces, the facial type does not distinguish lip, nose, pogonion or zygoma positioning in soft tissues, neither at rest nor at wide smile position.

That reinforces the importance of orthodontic planning that in addition to being based on bone structures relation, facial growth and dental intercuspation, should also be able to assess soft tissue accommodation towards dental and skeletal tissues as well as facial esthetics, always seeking for the balance between these structures as a final goal of the treatment.

The use of cone beam computed tomography may be a great adjuvant in diagnostic studies that attribute equal weight to both hard and soft tissues analysis, since it allows the assessment of lateral, sagittal and coronal views as well as frontal and profile appreciations of the facial soft tissues.

REFERENCES

1. Angle EH. Treatment of malocclusion of the teeth. 7a ed. Philadelphia: SS White; 1907.
2. Case CS. Orthodontic principles of diagnosis and general rules of treatment of all malocclusions. Chicago: CS Case; 1921.
3. Tweed CH. The Frankfort-mandibular plane angle in orthodontic diagnosis, classification, treatment planning, and prognosis. Am J Orthod Oral Surg. 1946;32(4):175-230.
4. Downs WB. Analysis of the dentofacial profile. Angle Orthod. 1956;26(4):191-212.
5. Holdaway RA. Changes in relationships of points A and B during orthodontic treatment. Am J Orthod. 1956;42(3):176-93.
6. Ricketts RM. Planning treatment on the basis of the facial pattern and an estimate of its growth. Angle Orthod. 1957;27(1):14-37.
7. Legan HL, Burstone CJ. Soft tissue cephalometric analysis for orthognathic surgery. J Oral Surg. 1980;38(10):744-51.
8. Lündstrom A, Forsberg CM, Peck S, McWilliam J. A proportional analysis of the soft tissue facial profile in young adults with normal occlusion. Angle Orthod. 1992;62(2):127-33; discussion 144-4.
9. Cox NJ, van der Linden FPGM. Facial harmony. Am J Orthod Dentofacial Orthop. 1971;60(2):175-83.
10. Wylie GA, Fish LC, Epker BN. Cephalometrics: a comparison of five analyses currently used in the diagnosis of dentofacial deformities. Int Adult Orthodon Orthognath Surg. 1987;2(1):15-36.
11. Jacobson A. Planning for orthognathic surgery-art or science? Int J Adult Orthod Orthognath Surg. 1990;5(4):217-24.
12. Matteson SR, Deahl ST, Alder ME, Nummikoski PV. Advanced imaging methods. Crit Rev Oral Biol Med. 1996;7(4):346-95.
13. Farman AG, Scarfe WC, Hilgers MJ, Bida O, Moshiri M, Sukovic P. Dentomaxillofacial cone beam CT for orthodontic assessment. Int Congress Series. 2005;1281:1187-90.
14. Sukovic P. Cone beam computed tomography in craniofacial imaging. Orthod Craniofac Res. 2003;6(1):31-6.
15. Schulze D, Heiland M, Schmelzle R, Rother UJ. Diagnostic possibilities of cone beam computed tomography in facial skeleton. Int Cong Series. 2004;1268:1179-83.
16. Halazonetis DJ. From 2-dimensional cephalograms to 3-dimensional computed tomography scans. Am J Orthod Dentofacial Orthop. 2005;127(5):627-37.
17. Farman AG, Scarfe WC, Hilgers MJ, Bida O, Moshiri M, Sukovic P. Dentomaxillofacial cone beam CT for orthodontic assessment. Int Congress Series. 2005;1281:1187-90.
18. Rino-Neto J, Accorsi MAO, Ribeiro A, Paiva JB, Cavalcanti MGP. Imagens craniofaciais em ortodontia: O estágio atual da documentação ortodôntica tridimensional. Ortodontia SPO. 2006;39(2):144-54.
19. Garib DG, Raymundo Jr R, Raymundo MV, Raymundo DV, Ferreira SN. Tomografia computadorizada de feixe cônico (Cone beam): entendendo este novo método de diagnóstico por imagem com promissora aplicabilidade na Ortodontia. Rev Dental Press Ortod Ortop Facial. 2007;12(2):139-56.
20. Kumar V, Ludlow JB, Cevidanes LH. Comparison of conventional and cone beam CT synthesized cephalograms. Dentomaxillofac Radiol. 2007;36(5):263-9.
21. Ludlow JB, Gubler M, Cevidanes L, Mol A. Precision of cephalometric landmark identification: Cone-beam computed tomography vs conventional cephalometric views. Am J Orthod Dentofacial Orthop. 2009;136(3):312.e1-10; discussion 312-3.
22. Paiva JB, Rino-Neto J, Lopes KB. Análise do lábio superior após o tratamento ortodôntico. Ortodontia. 2004;37(2):8-13.
23. Daruge E, Zalaff CF. A biometria aplicada na identificação. RGO. 1985;33(2):153-5.
24. Lopes KB. Avaliações tegumentares, esqueléticas e dentárias do perfil facial [dissertação]. São Paulo (SP): Universidade de São Paulo; 2004.
25. Neter J, Kutner MH, Nachtsheim CJ, Wasserman W. Applied linear statistical models. Ilinois: Richard D Irwing; 1996.
26. Vigorito JW, Martins LF. Análise fotométrica aplicada na determinação do tipo facial. Dental Press J Orthod. 2012;17(5):71-5.

10

Nasal septum changes in adolescent patients treated with rapid maxillary expansion

Tehnia Aziz[1], Francis Carter Wheatley[2], Kal Ansari[3], Manuel Lagravere[4], Michael Major[5], Carlos Flores-Mir[6]

Objective: To analyze cone-beam computed tomography (CBCT) scans to measure changes in nasal septal deviation (NSD) after rapid maxillary expansion (RME) treatment in adolescent patients. **Methods:** This retrospective study involved 33 patients presenting with moderate to severe nasal septum deviation as an incidental finding. Out of these 33 patients, 26 were treated for transverse maxillary constriction with RME and seven, who did not undergo RME treatment, were included in the study as control group. CBCT scans were taken before appliance insertion and after appliance removal. These images were analyzed to measure changes in nasal septum deviation (NSD). Analysis of variance for repeated measures (ANOVA) was used. **Results:** No significant changes were identified in NSD regardless of the application or not of RME treatment and irrespective of the baseline deviation degree. **Conclusion:** This study did not provide strong evidence to suggest that RME treatment has any effect on NSD in adolescent patients; however, the results should be interpreted with caution, due to the small sample size and large variation amongst individual patient characteristics.

Keywords: Nasal septum. CBCT. Rapid maxillary expansion. Rapid palatal expansion.

[1] Private practice, Edmonton, Alberta, Canada.

[2] Graduate student in Computer Sciences, Boston University, Boston, Massachusetts, USA.

[3] Assistant professor, University of Alberta, Department of Surgery, Edmonton, Alberta, Canada.

[4] Assistant professor, University of Alberta, Department of Dentistry, Edmonton, Alberta, Canada.

[5] Clinical assistant professor, University of Alberta, Department of Dentistry, Edmonton, Alberta, Canada.

[6] Professor, University of Alberta, Department of Dentistry, Edmonton, Alberta, Canada.

» The authors report no commercial, proprietary or financial interest in the products or companies described in this article.

Carlos Flores-Mir
Division of Orthodontics, University of Alberta,
5-528 Edmonton Clinic Health Academy
11405 87 Ave, T6G 1C9 Edmonton, Canada
E-mail: cfl @ualberta.ca

INTRODUCTION

The reciprocal effects of nasal breathing on craniofacial development have been intensively investigated in the literature. According to Moss' functional theory, nasal respiration enables normal growth and development of the craniofacial structures.[1] Moss hypothesized that undisturbed nasal airflow is a continuous stimulus for lowering the palate and for lateral maxillary growth, thereby indicating a close relationship between nasal breathing and dentofacial morphology.

Nasal septal deviation (NSD) is defined as deviation of either the bony or cartilaginous septum or both from the facial midline. In humans, it has been hypothesized that significant nasal obstruction caused by NSD can affect nasal airflow and increase nasal airway resistance.[2] Resultant impaired nasal breathing can lead to preferential mouth breathing which, if chronic, may cause craniofacial alterations. These potential changes consist of a long face syndrome characterized by narrow maxilla, steep mandibular plane, retrognathic mandible, increased lower facial height, lip incompetence, constricted alar bases and typically malocclusion consisting of a posterior crossbite.[2]

Rapid maxillary expansion (RME) is routinely used in Orthodontics to treat transverse maxillary constriction, posterior dental crossbite and crowding.[3] Considering that maxillary bones form the periphery of the nasal cavity, it has been proposed that opening the mid palatal suture through RME could also result in lateral displacement of the nasal walls, thereby increasing nasal cavity dimensions.[4]

The earliest report of RME having an effect on nasal septal changes came in 1975 when it was discovered that RME treatment in a patient cohort also appeared to improve NSD.[5] More recently, a 94% reduction in septal deviation was reported in children aged 5-9 years old, presenting with transverse maxillary constriction treated with RME.[6] NSD correction was noted in the lower and middle half of the nasal cavity when compared to a nonexpansion control group.

Although several studies have investigated the effect of RME on nasal cavity size and airway,[5,7-11] there is a paucity of research on the changes caused by RME in the nasal septum. To our knowledge, only three studies have conducted a two-dimensional cephalometric analysis[5,6,12] to assess nasal septal changes produced during RME. All of them used coronal views from posterior anterior radiographs. Two studies reported favorable improvement of septal deviation after RME[5,6] treatment in growing patients, while one[12] study reported no change in nongrowing patients aged 15-19 years old. However, these studies had some major limitations. There was lack of standardization in study design and the nasal septum was measured at one single radiographic image instead of its entirety by assessing different points along the septum. It was also unclear whether both pre- and postexpansion radiographs measured the septal change at a set landmark. Although improvement in nasal septum was reported after expansion, it was not clear whether the change was the same at each anatomical location along the nasal septum.

Considering the importance of nasal breathing for the development of craniofacial structures, it would be beneficial to ascertain whether RME can reliably improve NSD and hence its detrimental effects on nasal breathing. Therefore, the objective of this study is to analyze three-dimensional changes of the nasal septum resulting from maxillary expansion in an adolescent patient sample. The use of three-dimensional imaging should overcome some of the limitations observed in previously conducted research.

MATERIAL AND METHODS

This retrospective study fulfilled all ethical requirements and was approved by the Health Research Ethics Board at the University of Alberta.

Patient samples were obtained from a previously conducted randomized clinical trial[14] at the Department of Dentistry at University of Alberta during an 18-month period. A total of 33 patients with varying degrees of NSD at T_1 (prior to rapid maxillary expansion [RME] treatment) were selected from an available pool of CBCT scans of 120 patients through a brief visual inspection of the entire nasal septum of each patient. Patients with nasal septum deviation were identified from transverse and coronal views of cone-beam computed tomographic (CBCT) records taken prior to treatment with RME (or without RME for control patients).

Based on a previous publication,[13] septal deviation was considered moderate to severe (clinically meaningful deviation) if the deflection of the nasal septum from the mid-sagittal plane was greater than 9 degrees, and mild (not clinically meaningful deviation) if deviation was less than or equal to 8 degrees in any isolated CBCT scan.

The final sample consisted of:
» 14 patients treated with RME with moderate to severe NSD at T_1 (more than 9 degrees);
» 12 patients treated with RME with mild NSD at T_1 (less than 9 degrees);
» 7 untreated patients with RME with moderate to severe NSD at T_1 (control group).

The BAME (bone anchored maxillary expansion) sample had a mean age of 14.2 ± 1.3 years, the TAME (tooth anchored maxillary expansion) sample had a mean age of 14.1 ± 1.4 years and finally the control sample had a mean age of 12.9 ± 1.2 years. Individual matching was not possible due to unequal sample sizes.

RME was carried out until posterior dental cross-bite overcorrection by 20% was achieved (maxillary lingual cusps overlapping with lingual inclines of mandibular buccal cusps). After active expansion treatment, the screw was fixated with a composite resin into the turn-key mechanism of the appliance. The appliance was retained for a total of six months from the time of insertion. CBCT scans taken at T_1 (at baseline, before expansion) and T_2 (after appliance removal) were analyzed for this study. (For more detailed information on the methods of the previously conducted randomized trial please refer to reference[14]).

All CBCT scans were taken with either a NewTom (18 patients) or an i-CAT (15 patients). Images were converted into DICOM format software with a voxel size of 0.25 mm. All images at T_1 and T_2 for each patient were then uploaded to OsiriX DICOM Viewer (v. 5.8, 32 bit, Pixmeo, Geneva, Switzerland).

Based on a previous publication,[15] the following steps were followed:
1. Landmarks were identified in the 3-D viewer/2-D orthogonal MPR mode in OsiriX for each patient in sagittal view (Table 1, Fig 1).
2. Based on the landmarks identified on sagittal view, three axial (A1, A2, A3) and four coronal DICOM landmarks (C1, C2, C3, C4) for each patient at each time point were isolated (Fig 1).
3. These landmarks were: the most anterior point of nasal bone (A1, C1), perpendicular plate and vomer junction (A2, C4), anterior nasal spine (C2), crista galli (C3), halfway point between anterior nasal spine and perpendicular plate/vomer junction (A3).

The landmarks were chosen due to their ease of identification based on anatomical locations and because

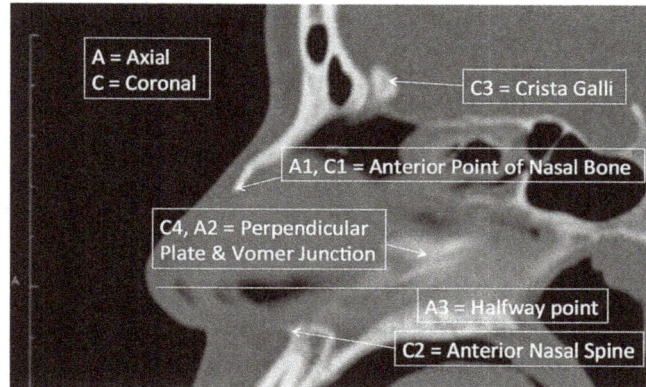

Figure 1 - Description and location of landmarks in sagittal view for axial and coronal image generation.

Table 1 - Descriptions of landmarks in sagittal view for image generation.

Axial (A) and coronal (C) landmarks	Anatomical location
A1	Most anterior point of nasal bone (axial view).
A2	Point that depicts the junction of perpendicular plate of ethmoid bone and vomer (axial view).
A3	Midway point between A2 (C4) and C2. Anatomically found between the anterior nasal spine and vomer/perpendicular plate of ethmoid junction in vertical direction (axial view).
C1	Anterior point of nasal bone (coronal view)
C2	Most anterior point of anterior nasal spine (coronal view).
C3	Mid point of crista galli (coronal view).
C4	Junction of perpendicular plate of ethmoid bone and vomer (coronal view).

Although A2 and C4 are the same landmarks in sagittal view, on A2 slice, nasal septum is measured in anterior to posterior. On C4 slice, it is measured from to inferior to superior view.

they could reasonably cover the boundaries of normal septal anatomy in anterior-posterior and inferior to superior directions. Landmark A3 was the only landmark not identified by an anatomical structure.[15] A total of 14 images for every patient was analyzed considering T_1 and T_2. These images were then transferred to MATLAB (MathWorks R2013b, Natick, Massachusetts) for NSD analysis. One researcher registered the time point (T_1 or T_2 DICOM image) in the MATLAB software, but was blinded to the degree of septal deviation or whether it was a treatment or a control patient. This software enabled the septum to be systematically traced and analyzed.

During analysis in MATLAB, the axial images (images A1, A2, A3) were traced from anterior to posterior direction. For example, for axial image A1, the nasal septum was systematically traced by placing points approximately 1-2 mm apart along its anterior posterior course. Similarly, in coronal images (C1, C2, C3, C4), the nasal septum was traced in entirety from superior to inferior direction by placing points 1-2 mm apart.

The data from NSD measurements from MATLAB software were automatically transferred to a comma separated value (csv) spreadsheet. Once data analysis was complete, data were further copied to an Excel spreadsheet for ease of statistical analysis with SPSS program.

For the present study, NSD was quantified based on the "degree of tortuosity" or the ratio of length of the curve to the length of an imaginary line in the mid sagittal plane (Fig 2 – red arrow points to ratio). In other words, the degree of tortuosity is an absolute measurement of the degree of septal deviation from the midline at each identified landmark in both coronal and/or axial views.

STATISTICAL TESTS
Reliability and measurement error

Intrarater reliability and measurement error were conducted for identification of landmarks in sagittal view in OsiriX and then as NSD tracing in MATLAB (from the selected DICOMs based on landmark identification/image isolation in OsiriX). All measurements were repeated three times with at least five days apart.

Landmark identification was done in OsiriX with X, Y and Z coordinates noted for anterior point of the nasal bone (landmarks A1/C1), vomer and perpendicular plate junction (landmarks A2/C4), anterior nasal spine (C2), crista galli (landmark C3), and halfway point between anterior nasal spine and vomer/perpendicular plate junction (A3). Nasal septum tracing and NSD measurement ratio in MATLAB for each image (A1, A2, A3, C1, C2, C3 and C4) were also recorded.

Intraclass correlation with consistency under two-way mixed model was tabulated in SPSS for both landmark identification and nasal septum measurements.

Main study statistical tests

Statistical analysis was carried out with the aid of SPSS (version 21) using alpha = 0.05. Analysis of

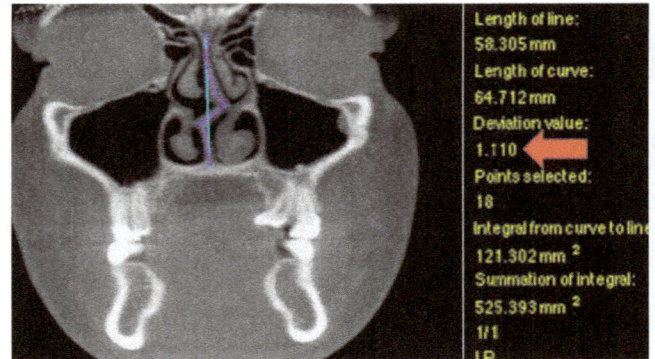

Figure 2 - MATLAB analysis for degree of tortuosity.

variance for repeated measures (ANOVA) was performed with two within-subject factors and one between-subject factor. Baseline septal deviation of "mild" and "moderate to severe" was considered between subjects factor. Time (T_1 and T_3; two levels) and landmark (A1, A2, A3, C1, C2, C3 and C4, 7 levels) were the two within-subject factors.

RESULTS

The intraclass correlation coefficients and corresponding confidence interval (95%) for both OsiriX landmark identification and MATLAB NSD measurements are listed in Tables 2 and 3. Location of most landmarks indicated good agreement[16] between parameters by high ICC values (> 0.8). Minimum, maximum and mean measurement error for both OsiriX landmark identification and MATLAB NSD ratios are listed in Tables 4 and 5. Mean measurement error in OsiriX was in the range of 0.5-2.2 mm with A3 having the largest error in all coordinates (1.96 to 2.2 mm). Difference between landmark coordinates in OsiriX measured at three different time points for reliability was not greater than 4 mm. MATLAB NSD ratios at all landmarks were less than 0.02.

There was no significant difference in NSD according to time [$F_{(1.24)} = 0.2$, $p = 0.659$]. There was also lack of evidence for differences in NSD at images A1, A2, A3, C1, C2, C3, C4 with time (time*landmark location) [$F_{(2.93, 70.24)} = 0.205$, $p = 0.889$].

Table 2 - Intrarater reliability for OsiriX landmark/image identification.

Landmark/image	X coordinate	Y coordinate	Z-coordinate
A1/C1	0.980 (0.943 – 0.995)	0.974 (0.925 – 0.993)	0.994 (0.983 – 0.998)
A2/C4	0.963 (0.897 – 0.990)	0.974 (0.926 – 0.993)	0.986 (0.959 – 0.996)
A3	0.941 (0.839 – 0.984)	0.929 (0.810 – 0.980)	0.988 (0.965 – 0.997)
C2	0.980 (0.943 – 0.995)	0.978 (0.937 – 0.994)	0.990 (0.971 – 0.997)
C3	0.998 (0.993 – 0.999)	0.973 (0.924 – 0.993)	0.986 (0.959 – 0.996)

Table 3 - Intrarater reliability for MATLAB NSD measurements.

Image	ICC	Confidence interval
A1	0.948	(0.871 – 0.983)
A2	0.993	(0.982 – 0.998)
A3	0.872	(0.702 – 0.957)
C1	0.947	(0.867 – 0.983)
C2	0.914	(0.791 – 0.972)
C3	0.904	(0.771 – 0.969)
C4	0.941	(0.854 – 0.981)

Table 4 - Measurement error in millimeters for OsiriX landmark/image identification.

Landmark/image	X coordinate	Y coordinate	Z coordinate
A1/C1	1.11 (0 – 2.24)	1.23 (0.38 – 2.77)	1.23 (0.41 – 2.67)
A2/C4	1.32 (0.3 – 3.64)	1.44 (0.37 – 2.73)	1.78 (0.09 – 3.43)
A3	1.96 (0.67 – 3.71)	2.2 (1.25 – 3.27)	2.03 (0.48 – 3.49)
C2	1.58 (0.56 – 3.25)	1.52 (0.23 – 3.14)	1.61 (0.13 – 3.65)
C3	0.52 (0.28 – 0.84)	1.89 (0.59 – 3.51)	1.64 (0.41 – 3.61)

Table 5 - Measurement error for MATLAB NSD ratio..

Image	Mean ratio
A1	0.0016
A2	0.0042
A3	0.0069
C1	0.0025
C2	0.0023
C3	0.0166
C4	0.0090

Partial eta square was 0.008 for time★spatial image accounting for only 0.8% of variance explained by the effect of RME on NSD. Baseline septal deviation of mild or moderate to severe had no effect change at spatial landmarks with time (baseline deviation★spatial image★time) [F (2.93, 70.24) = 1.85, p = 0.147, accounting for only 7% of variance in NSD].

DISCUSSION

The purpose of this retrospective study was to investigate the effect of RME treatment on patients presenting with nasal septal deviation. RME alone was conducted in these patients for the treatment of transverse maxillary deficiency, whereby NSD was discovered as an incidental finding on their CBCT scans prior to treatment.

There is no "gold standard" test to diagnose septal deviation[17] and different protocols for measuring septal deviation have been identified in the literature. The degree of tortuosity measurement was used in this study to compare the length of the curve of the deviated septum to the length of an ideal straight septum. This measurement solely measured the nasal septum in isolation and did not classify or include other confounding nasal pathology that could be the reason for septal deviation, such as turbinate hypertrophy or mucosal swelling. Therefore, this measurement method was well suited to the objective of our study.

Landmark identification in OsiriX and NSD ratios in MATLAB were indicative of good reliability. It was ascertained that identifying the location of landmark A3 with certainty was challenging. It was the only landmark that was not associated with a hard tissue anatomical structure, and rough approximation in space was made on all DICOMS without a ruler to accurately measure the half way point between anterior nasal spine and the vomer, and perpendicular plate junction. Although reliability at A3 for both OsiriX and MATLAB was suggestive of good reliability, a mean measurement error close to 4 mm was reported in x, y and z coordinates.

Owing to the retrospective nature of the study and the available CBCT records of patients that have undergone RME, sample size was less than ideal. Nevertheless, our findings were similar to a recently conducted study[12] in two dimensions, whereby no change in nasal septal deviation was identified pre- and postmaxillary expansion. On the other hand, this study was different than the previous one,[12] since the analysis of septal deviation was based on three-dimensional measurements on CBCT as opposed to two-dimensional on a posterior-anterior cephalogram. To date, this study appears to be the only one comparing the effects of RME on NSD using three-dimensional analysis of CBCT scans.

The main finding of this investigation was that rapid maxillary expansion had no effect on patients that had nasal septal deviation at baseline, as measured at images in axial and coronal views. Furthermore, mild or severe baseline deviation had no statistically significant effect on NSD change, as measured at set landmarks. The time difference between T_1 and T_2 in the treatment group was similar to that of the control

group; neither one of the groups had statistically significant changes in NSD over a 6-month period. It could be challenging to identify the true effect of RME treatment on NSD due to relatively small sample size and individual patient variation. In fact, four patients out of a sample of 26 (15%) depicted subjective visual improvement, as determined by one author in NSD from RME at mostly the coronal location of C3 (one at A3) (Figs 6 to 9). All four presented with baseline deviation of moderate to severe, but it is unclear as to why others with severe deviation and similar characteristics did not have a similar change. This is parallel to the conclusions of Harvolds primate study[18] whereby, even though the experiment protocol and sample characteristics were standardized, the animals responded and adapted to nasal obstruction quite differently. In fact, based on the statistical model, only 7% of variance in NSD could be attributed to RME treatment.

It has been proposed[19] that early intervention with RME (i.e., before palatal suture starts closing) in prepubescence would result in greater skeletal than dental change. Given that all patients in this study were adolescents, it is possible that lack of statistically significant change in NSD was the result of subjects having more advanced craniofacial development. In addition, increased bone density (calcification) of surrounding craniofacial structures in adolescence can offer greater resistance to skeletal change from RME. In contrast, in patients with mixed and deciduous dentition, studies[20,21] have reported the effect of RME to be attributed to between one half to two-thirds skeletal change. In fact, the studies[5,6] that reported favorable effects of RME on NSD consisted of patients recruited prior to their adolescent growth spurt.

Although there is a lack of studies examining the effect of RME on NSD, there are several studies[5,7-10] investigating the influence of RME treatment on nasal airway. However, there still lies a great deal of ambiguity in the literature with respect to nasal airway changes from RME due to conflicting findings. This ambiguity could be attributed due to different expansion protocols, different measurement methods to assess nasal airway change, patients with varying degrees of skeletal maturation, individual patient variation with or without concurrent pathologies, such as infections and allergies causing mucosal edema.

LIMITATIONS

This study did not provide strong evidence to suggest that RME treatment has any effect on NSD in adolescent patients, but the results should be interpreted with caution, due to the small sample size and large variation amongst individual patient characteristics. In this sense, this could be considered a pilot study testing this novel methodology.

Although potential differences between bone- or tooth-anchoraged expansion appliances over NSD could not be considered because of the limited number of subjects per group, the reality is that the expansion anchorage site may be of little real impact, as stated in the previous RCT[14] using the larger sample of 120 subjects in which dentoalveolar and skeletal changes were pretty similar regardless of expansion anchorage.

CONCLUSIONS

This study did not provide strong evidence to suggest that RME treatment has any effect on NSD in adolescent patients; however, the results should be interpreted with caution, due to the small sample size and large variation amongst individual patient characteristics.

Authors contribution

Conceived and designed the study: TA, KA, ML, MM, CFM. Drafted the study: TA, CFM. Data acquisition, analysis or interpretation: TA, FCW, KA, MM, CFM. Wrote the article: TA, ML, MM, CFM. Critical revision of the article: TA, FCW, KA, ML, MM, CFM. Final approval of the article: TA, FCW, KA, ML, MM, CFM.

REFERENCES

1. Moss-Salentijn L. Melvin L. Moss and the functional matrix. J Dent Res. 1997 Dec;76(12):1814-7.
2. Vig KW. Nasal obstruction and facial growth: the strength of evidence for clinical assumptions. Am J Orthod Dentofacia. Orthop. 1998 Jun;113(6):603-11.
3. Proffit WR, Fields Jr HW, Sarver DM. Contemporary orthodontics. 5th ed. St. Louis: Elsevier Mosby; 2013.
4. Warren DW, Hershey HG, Turvey TA, Hinton VA, Hairfield WM. The nasal airway following maxillary expansion. Am J Orthod Dentofacial Orthop. 1987 Feb;91(2):111-6.
5. Gray LP. Results of 310 cases of rapid maxillary expansion selected for medical reasons. J Laryngol Otol. 1975 Jun;89(6):601-14.
6. Farronato G, Giannini L, Galbiati G, Maspero C. RME: influences on the nasal septum. Minerva Stomato.. 2012 Apr;61(4):125-34.
7. Enoki C, Valera FC, Lessa FC, Elias AM, Matsumoto MA, Anselmo-Lima WT. Effect of rapid maxillary expansion on the dimension of the nasal cavity and on nasal air resistance. Int J Pediatr Otorhinolaryngol. 2006 Jul;70(7):1225-30.
8. Kiliç N, Oktay H. Effects of rapid maxillary expansion on nasal breathing and some naso-respiratory and breathing problems in growing children: a literature review. Int J Pediatr Otorhinolaryngol. 2008 Nov;72(11):1595-601.
9. Baratieri C, Alves M Jr, Souza MM, Araújo MTS, Maia LC. Does rapid maxillary expansion have long-term effects on airway dimensions and breathing? Am J Orthod Dentofacial Orthop. 2011 Aug;140(2):146-56.
10. Bicakci AA, Agar U, Sökücü O, Babacan H, Doruk C. Nasal airway changes due to rapid maxillary expansion timing. Angle Orthod. 2005 Jan;75(1):1-6.
11. Baccetti T, Franchi L, Cameron CG, McNamara JA Jr. Treatment timing for rapid maxillary expansion. Angle Orthod. 2001 Oct;71(5):343-50.
12. Altug-Atac AT, Atac MS, Kurt G, Karasud HA. Changes in nasal structures following orthopaedic and surgically assisted rapid maxillary expansion. Int J Oral Maxillofac Surg. 2010 Feb;39(2):129-35.
13. Setlur J, Goyal P. Relationship between septal body size and septal deviation. Am J Rhinol Allergy. 2011 Nov-Dec;25(6):397-400.
14. Lagravère MO, Carey J, Heo G, Toogood RW, Major PW. Transverse, vertical, and anteroposterior changes from bone-anchored maxillary expansion vs traditional rapid maxillary expansion: a randomized clinical trial. Am J Orthod Dentofacial Orthop. 2010 Mar;137(3):304.e1-12; ciscussion 304-5.

15. Lin JK, Wheatley FC, Handwerker J, Harris NJ, Wong BJ. Analyzing nasal septal deviations to develop a new classification system: a computed tomography study using MATLAB and OsiriX. JAMA Facial Plast Surg. 2014 May-Jun;16(3):183-7.
16. Portney L, Watkins M. Foundations of clinical research: applications to practice. Upper Saddle River: Prentice Hall; 2008.
17. Aziz T, Biron VL, Ansari K, Flores-Mir C. Measurement tools for the diagnosis of nasal septal deviation: a systematic review. J Otolaryngol Head Neck Surg. 2014 Apr 24;43:11.
18. Harvold EP, Tomer BS, Vargervik K, Chierici G. Primate experiments on oral respiration. Am J Orthod. 1981 Apr;79(4):359-72.
19. Lagravere MO, Major PW, Flores-Mir C. Long-term skeletal changes with rapid maxillary expansion: a systematic review. Angle Orthod. 2005 Nov;75(6):1046-52.
20. Haas AJ. Palatal expansion: just the beginning of dentofacial orthopedics. Am J Orthod. 1970 Mar;57(3):219-55.
21. Monini S, Malagola C, Villa MP, Tripodi C, Tarentini S, Malagnino I, et al. Rapid maxillary expansion for the treatment of nasal obstruction in children younger than 12 years. Arch Otolaryngol Head Neck Surg. 2009 Jan;135(1):22-7.

11

Assessing the predictability of ANB, 1-NB, P-NB and 1-NA measurements on Steiner cephalometric analysis

Ana Cláudia Laureano Navarro[1], Luiz Sérgio Carreiro[2], Claudenir Rossato[3],
Ricardo Takahashi[2], Carlos Eduardo de Oliveira Lima[2]

Objective: To evaluate, in the initial and final stages of corrective orthodontic treatment, the predictability of the ANB, 1-NB, PNB and 1-NA during case individualization, which considers the characteristics of the patient, professional experience and the mechanics to be used. **Methods:** Ninety patients were selected at the State University of Londrina (UEL, Brazil), presenting Angle Class I and II malocclusions, treated with and without extraction of four premolars and divided into three groups: Horizontal, balanced and vertical. The cephalometric variables were evaluated in the initial, prognosis and final stages of treatment in order to observe the behavior of the estimates, or how they were higher or lower than the values obtained. **Results:** It was noticed the influence of the facial pattern on the behavior of the measures examined, the values proposed for the ANB were statistically different from values obtained at the end of the treatment; in the vertical group the final value was the one that most approached the proposed value; regarding 1-NB the values proposed with the Steiner analysis for the balanced and vertical groups were not achieved. For P-NB, there was no difference between genders. For 1-NA it was observed that the values obtained at the end of treatment differ from estimates in the three groups. **Conclusions:** The limitations of the estimates of the measures do not invalidate its clinical or teaching use, if aware of its deficiencies, the analysis can be used with restrictions.

Keywords: Growth and development. Radiography. Tooth movement.

[1] Specialist in Orthodontics, Londrina State University.
[2] Associate Professor, Londrina State University
[3] Assistant Professor, Londrina State University

Ana Cláudia Laureano Navarro
Rua Jorge Velho, 784 Vila Ipiranga - Londrina-PR, Brazil
CEP 86010-600 – E-mail: lsc@sercomtel.com.br

INTRODUCTION

With the development of the cephalostat and the consequent standardization of the radiographs, in 1931, it became possible to carry out several cephalometric analyses based on average angular and linear values, obtained from individuals with normal occlusion and a satisfactory facial profile.[4,12] These values allow for comparisons with those from the patient, verifying the skeletal and dental pattern and the structures that show discrepancies from the norms, thus making diagnosis and the development of individualized treatment plans possible.[27]

In the mid 40's, Tweed included the movement of the lower incisors in the planning of clinical cases, with the purpose of obtaining an ideal occlusion after an orthodontic treatment. He described that these teeth should present a 90° angle to the mandibular plane, with a tolerable variation of around +5°.

In 1948, Downs[6] determined nine angular and one linear measurement, which described the skeletal and dental patterns of Caucasian North Americans, with an excellent clinical occlusion, thus carrying out the first systematic cephalometric analysis. For the author, despite the considerable variation in type and facial pattern, in order for individuals to present a good functional and esthetic balance, they should possess certain common characteristics of the profile.

Realizing that most orthodontists did not call upon cephalometry as a clinical diagnosis resource, since they saw it as a purely scientific instrument used for research purposes, Steiner,[25-28] in the following decade, proposed an analysis based, empirically, on the dentoalveolar compensatory mechanism, which helped professionals to determine the nature of the bad occlusion, making the development of treatment plans more objective. Using the analyses of Downs, Margolis, Riedel, Thompson, and Wylie, combined with some of his own cephalometric values, he established his own analysis for young leucoderms of Anglo-Saxon origin from the United States.

When arguing the value of Steiner's analysis, one must bear in mind the references and the choices available at that time. Jaw functional orthopedics was incipient and not very propagated amongst American orthodontists, therefore, it did not emphasize orthopedic problems such as the lower facial height, the relative length of the jaw and mandible, the facial convexity angle or the measurements of the posterior cranial base.[25-28]

Steiner's analysis was well accepted by many researchers who, mindful of the occurrence of variations related to the different ethnic and racial groups,[27,28] set out to verify if the values proposed by Steiner could be applied to different population groups. Several studies, mainly in relation to the dental patterns proposed by Steiner (1-NA = 4 mm and 1-NB = 4 mm), have demonstrated different values from the proposed norm.[1,9,16,21,23,29] Some authors, concerned with better analyzing and planning their cases, established the ideal cephalometric norms and the acceptable compromises of this analysis to different racial and ethnic groups.[29]

To develop a treatment plan, along with anamnesis and clinical analysis, some diagnostic elements are fundamental, as study models, intraoral x-rays, extraoral X-rays (panoramic and cephalometric) and intraoral and extraoral photographs. Each diagnostic element presents different ways of evaluation. For that purpose, we have used Steiner's analysis to estimate the qualitative and quantitative growth, with a view to establish treatment goals, thus becoming an important tool for the elaboration of treatment plans. Despite being an important tool for the clinician, it presents a certain degree of subjectivity, when it comes to estimating each patient's growth.

The result of an orthodontic treatment can sometimes be distorted by the stubbornness of some researchers who insist on the fact that the statistical averages should match the final objective of the treatment. This has determined the elaboration of this study with the purpose of analyzing, in the final phase of corrective orthodontic treatment, the predictability of the measurements ANB, 1-NB, P-NB, and 1-NA, estimated on the individualization of Steiner's analysis, considering horizontal, balanced and vertical growth patterns.

MATERIAL AND METHODS
Material
Sample collection

We randomly evaluated 300 patient files obtained from the Londrina State University Orthodontics Specialization Course databank and analyzed two lateral cephalometric radiographs from each file, totaling 600 x-rays from patients with Class I and Class II Angle malocclusions, who had their treatment ended. From the initial total of 300 files we selected 90, from which 36 were male and 54 female, to compose the final sample.

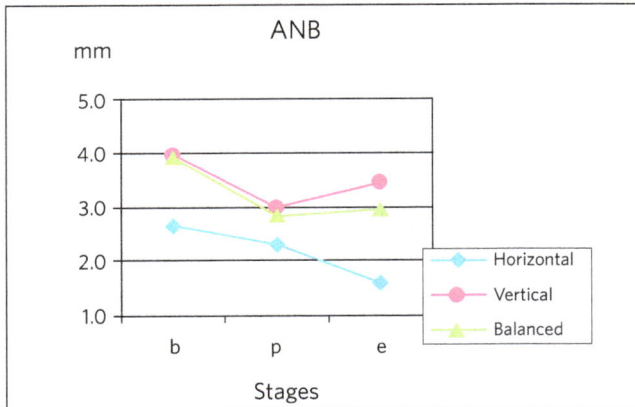

Figure 1 - Average behavior for ANB at the beginning (b) and at the end (e) of treatment, mediated by the proposed value (p).

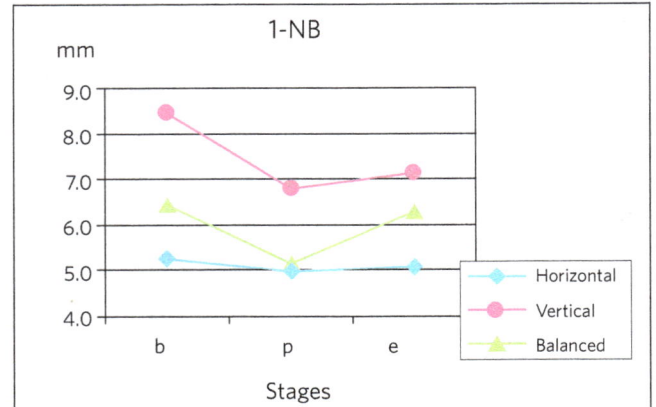

Figure 2 - Average behavior for 1-NB at the beginning (b) the end (e) treatment, mediated by the proposed value (p).

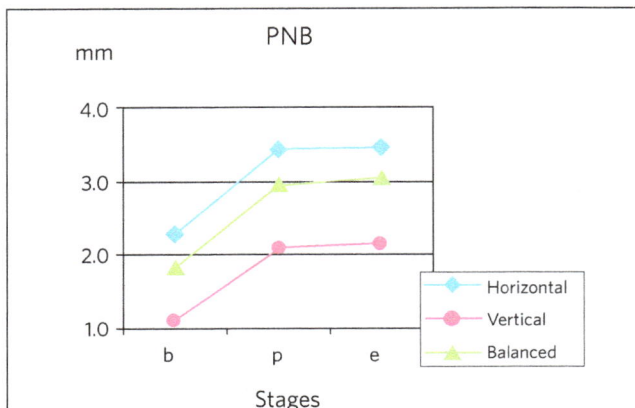

Figure 3 - Average behavior of PNB at the beginning (b), at the end (e) of treatment, mediated by the proposal (p).

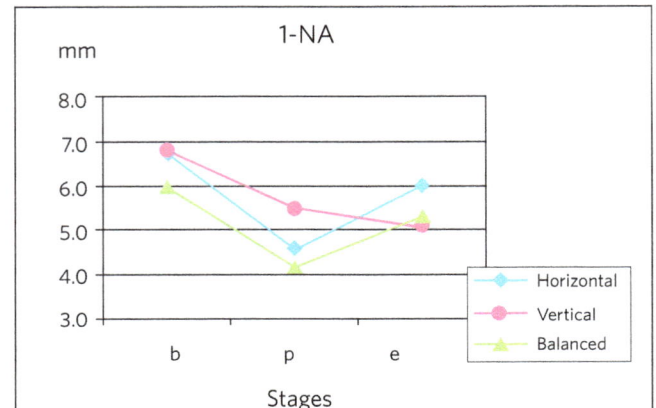

Figure 4 - Average behavior 1-NA at the beginning (b) and at the end (e) of treatment, mediated by the proposal (p).

ANB, 1-NB, P-NB and 1-NA cephalometric measurements were collected from the patients' files and the individualizations were done by Professors from the Course of Orthodontics, Londrina State University. After the analysis, the research was approved by the Ethics Committee under CEP opinion nº 042/08. The following inclusion factors were considered for sample selection.

Inclusion factors
   » Patients with Angle Class I and Class II malocclusion, treated with or without extractions.
   » Patients with no deleterious oral habits.
   » Cases that were well finished, both esthetically and functionally, with complete initial and final records.
   » Patients treated at the Orthodontics Specialization Course of the Londrina State University.

   » Lateral cephalometric radiographs taken with a Polomex-Siemens cephalometric device, model Orthopantomagraph 10E-0P10-EE60-Uel 73180, serial number 62249, Yoshida-Cephlo. expure, manufacturing/inclusion year 1992;

Since one of the criteria to estimate values during the individualization of each case consists of the evaluation of the growth pattern and that this pattern (dolichocephalic, mesocephalic and brachycephalic) exerts a greater influence on growth than the anterior-posterior relation (Class I and Class II), the sample was divided, according to the craniofacial growth in three groups:
   » Horizontal group (H): 11 female and 3 male.
   » Balanced group (E): 11 female and 14 male.
   » Vertical group (V): 32 female and 19 male.

The craniofacial growth pattern was established using SN.GoGn cephalometric measurements. Despite the existing controversy in the literature related to the reliability of the Sela-Nasio line, we opted for this measurement, mainly because it was advocated by Steiner[25,26,27,28] in his cephalometric analysis proposition.

The Craniofacial Growth Atlas, published by Martins et al[15] was used to divide the groups, since it offers the average values and their respective standard deviations from the selected measurement, and it was elaborated on a sample of Brazilians of Mediterranean descent. Since the corrective orthodontic treatment begins at around 12 years of age, the values for SN.GoGn were checked at that age, obtaining the measurements of 33.20 for the female genre and 34.30 for the male genre, and the limits for the balanced group of 28.20 to 38.20 for females and 30.30 to 38.60 for males. The horizontal group was classified from values below the inferior limits, and the vertical, above the superior limits.

Cephalometric growths were evaluated in the initial, proposed and final phases of the treatment. We also verified the differences between the final and the proposed phases to observe the behavior of the estimates, checking how higher or lower they were compared to the obtained values.

RESULTS AND DISCUSSION

Since Steiner's analysis is used all over the world and is considered an important tool for teaching and for the systemization of diagnosis and the elaboration of treatment plans, we tried, with this research, to establish a critical view of the way in which the analysis is being employed, as well as possible adjustments that the results of the research might suggest.

Predictability of the ANB angle

By observing the behavior of the initial and final ANB angle, we realized that it became smaller with age, more significantly in the horizontal group, and not in the vertical and balanced groups, whose final value was higher than the proposed value, which corroborates with the findings of Bishara,[3] Coura et al,[5] Silva et al[24] and the Craniofacial Growth Atlas.[15]

The proposed values for the initial and final ANB angles (Fig 1 and Table 1) were statistically different from the values obtained at the end of the treatment, with the exception of the balanced group. In reality, there was a

greater variation only in the horizontal group, different from the results found by Ortiz et al[18] whose final values were similar to the proposed estimates.

The horizontal group had the proposed value for the ANB angle higher than the final value from all the groups. This probably occurred due to the greater potential for mandibular growth, contributing to the reduction of this angle.

Results obtained by this research for the ANB angle corroborates with the findings of Farret[7] and Ortiz et al,[18] who utilized a similar methodology and obtained values that were very close to the proposed at the end of the treatment.

When comparing the three groups studied in relation to gender interference in the resulting values, results from the analysis of variance (ANOVA) showed no differences between them. This shows that the main effect, observed only in the horizontal group, is distributed equally between the male and female genders.

By comparing ANB angle averages at the initial and final phases with the proposed phase, we verify, through the paired t test, that there was a significant statistical difference between the proposed and the final stages of treatment (Table 1).

Rate of accuracy was reduced in the three groups, showing greater tendency to underestimate the reduction of the ANB angle, mainly in the horizontal group, which has greater growth potential (Table 2). Meanwhile, in the differences averages between the final and the proposed phases, the numeric values were clinically low.

From these results, it is possible to find the deficiency in the individualization of the estimates, mainly for the horizontal group, which leads to the need to avoid the underestimation of the mandibular growth potential with this age group and with both sexes. Based on these results, one can state that the ANB estimates have limitations and should not be taken as rigid parameters for the finishing of orthodontic treatment.

Predictability of the 1-NB measurement

The Holdaway principle, where the distances P-NB and 1-NB must be equal or vary within a 2 mm limit, was introduced by Steiner[26] in his analysis in 1959. This proportion was analyzed with young Brazilians, with normal occlusion and its use during diagnosis and treatment plan developments is indicated in literature.[7]

Silva and Martins[24] conducted a study with young Caucasian Brazilians with normal occlusion, demonstrating that the 1–NB measurement for this population is larger than the ideal values advocated by Steiner.[25,26,27,28]

In relation to the 1–NB measurement (Fig 2), results from this study shows that in the balanced and mainly in the horizontal group, a retrusion of the lower incisors is proposed, while in the horizontal group it was estimated that the lower incisors practically did not suffer any changes in relation to their angles of protrusion. At the end of the treatment, we observed retrusion in all groups, however, the proposed values during the elaboration of Steiner's analysis for the balanced and vertical groups were not reached. A similar behavior was observed by Farret,[7] who also verified a tendency to underestimate the values of the 1–NB measurement (averages obtained for 1–NB proposed 3.62 mm and final 4.98 mm), concluding that the use

of Steiner's analysis must be carried out with great caution and criteria for Brazilians with Class I occlusions, since the acceptable compromises underestimate the average position of the incisors.

Ramos et al,[22] and Hasund[11] emphasize the importance of taking into consideration the fact that the 1–NB measurement is larger in the cases where the growth pattern is divergent and smaller than a convergent growth pattern, during the elaboration of Steiner's analysis.

In the current evaluation, we verify a significant statistical difference between the proposed values and the ones obtained at the end of the treatment for the vertical and balanced groups (Table 3). We observed that these values were underestimated, just as in the studies of Farret[7] and Pinzan et al,[20] since the estimated P-NB for both groups did not present a significant difference in relation to the obtained value, and the value of 1–NB appeared higher for youths with a vertical growth pattern.[11,22]

Table 1 - Test result for the comparison between proposed values (p) and the values at the end of treatment (e) for the ANB angle.

Facial type	Initial average	Proposed average	Average after treatment	Difference e-p	p- value	Test
Horizontal	2.65	2.30	1.60	-0.70	2.9%	Student t test
Vertical	3.96	3.00	3.43	0.43	23.37%	Student t test
Balanced	3.93	2.82	2.96	0.14	54.68%	Student t test

Table 2 - Number and rate of accuracy (=) of the proposed value, of a larger final value (>), or smaller (<) than the estimates of the ANB measurement (e-p).

Groups	Accuracy =	Larger >	Smaller <	Total
Horizontal	6 (24%)	7 (28%)	12 (48%)	25
Balanced	9 (17%)	22 (43%)	20 (39%)	51
Vertical	3 (22%)	7 (50%)	4 (28%)	14

Table 3 - Comparison between proposed values (p) and the values at the end of treatment (e) for 1-NB.

Facial type	Initial average	Proposed average	Average after treatment	Difference e-p	p-value	Test
Horizontal	5.26	4.96	5.10	0.14	68.22%	Student t test
Vertical	8.46	6.79	7.11	0.32	85.55%	Wilcoxon
Balanced	6.41	5.14	6.27	1.13	0.01%	Wilcoxon

Table 4 - Number and rate of accuracy (=) for the proposed value, for a larger final value (>), or smaller (<) than the estimates of the 1-NB measurement (e-p).

Groups	Accuracy =	Larger >	Smaller <	Total
Balanced	6 (24%)	9 (36%)	10 (40%)	25
Balanced	9 (17%)	34 (66%)	8 (15%)	51
Vertical	3 (22%)	7 (50%)	4 (28%)	14

Table 5 - Comparison between the proposed values (p) and the values at the end of treatment (e) for P-NB.

Facial type	Initial average	Proposed average	Average after treatment	Difference e-p	p-value	Test
Horizontal	2.3	3.44	3.48	0.04	85.33%	Student t test
Vertical	1.10	2.11	2.18	0.07	82.10%	Student t test
Balanced	1.85	2.97	3.07	0.10	56.22%	Signs of posts

Table 6 - Number and accuracy rate (=) of the proposed value, of a larger final value (>) or smaller (<) than the estimates of the P-NB measurement e-p).

Groups	Accuracy =	Larger >	Smaller <	Total
Horizontal	3 (12%)	10 (40%)	12 (48%)	25
Balanced	8 (15%)	19 (37%)	24 (47%)	51
Vertical	3 (22%)	6 (42%)	5 (35%)	14

By evaluating the behavior of the 1-NB estimates considering the growth pattern and/or gender, we verified, in the balanced group, the same behavior for both genders. For the horizontal and vertical groups, we verified that, at the end of the orthodontic treatment, horizontal individuals of the female gender presented 1-NB larger than the proposed, horizontal individuals of the male gender presented 1-NB smaller than the proposed, vertical individuals of the female gender presented 1-NB smaller than proposed, and, finally, vertical individuals of the male gender presented 1-NB larger than the proposed. Thus, we have an inverted behavior between men and women, according to their facial type. Gender influence was also found by Pinzan,[20] but only in the vertical group.

The rate of accuracy was low for all facial types, where the margin of error for high values was higher in the balanced group, lower for the horizontal group and also higher for the vertical group (Table 4).

Since Steiner's acceptable compromise table underestimates the positioning of the lower incisors for young Caucasian Brazilians, we emphasize the need to individualize the values for this population.

Predictability of the P-NB measurement

The P-NB measurement was considered indispensable by Steiner[26] in his analysis, however, he did not specified the factors that subsidized his calculations, emphasizing the role represented by the clinical experience, pattern, growth potential and gender of the patient.

Holdaway's 1:1 proportion, with a tolerance limit of 3 mm, was verified in young Brazilians with normal occlusion, and, therefore, its use during the diagnostic and treatment plan elaborations is indicated in literature.[7,17]

By analyzing the P-NB measurement in all its stages, we verified, through Figure 3, that there was no difference between the proposed and the end values in all studied groups, which was also verified by Ramos et al.[2] However, they emphasize that the occurrence of individual variations in this region might have masked the P-NB's tendency to be smaller in the vertical group.

Bishara et al[2,3] described higher values for the P-NB in horizontal patients and lower in vertical ones, which is explained by Bishara,[2] and influenced by jaw rotation. Pinzan et al[19] found differences in their study for the proposed values in relation to the end-of-treatment values in the horizontal and balanced groups, whilst in the vertical group this difference was not noted. By comparing the averages of the P-NB in the initial and final stages with the proposed stage, we verified, through the paired "t" test, that there was no statistically significant difference between the proposed and final stages of treatment, determining a correct growth estimate in the anterior region of the chin[8] (Table 5). We observed no

Table 7 - Number and accuracy rate (=) of the proposed value, of a final larger value (>) or smaller (<) than the estimates of the 1-NA measurement (e-p).

Groups	Accuracy =	Larger >	Smaller <	Total
Horizontal	1 (4%)	17 (68%)	7 (28%)	25
Balanced	10 (19%)	10 (19%)	31 (60%)	51
Vertical	2 (14%)	6 (42%)	6 (42%)	14

Table 8 - Test result for the comparison between the proposed values (p) and the values at the end of the treatment (e) for 1-NA angle.

Facial Type	Initial average	Proposed average	Average after treatment	Difference e-p	p-value	Test
Horizontal	6.78	4.60	6.02	1.42	0.21%	Student *t* test
Vertical	6.82	5.51	5.07	-0.44	57.99%	Student *t* test
Balanced	5.97	4.19	5.31	1.12	< 0.01%	Signs of posts

difference between gender, since both presented measurements statistically similar to those proposed by the analyses of Steiner[25,26,27] and Pinzan.[20] The equivalence observed in this study is due, possibly, to the underestimation in the horizontals and the overestimation in the verticals, i.e., they have not suffered the influence of Steiner's[25,26,27] maxim "the more it has, the more it will have and vice versa" (Table 6)

Predictability of the 1-NA measurement

The value of the 1-NA measurement was underestimated at the time of the Steiner's individualization analysis on all three groups. As one can see in Table 7, the accuracy rate of the estimates was reduced. Values tend to overestimate the protrusion of the upper incisor in the horizontal and vertical groups, a result that agrees with those obtained by Silva[24] and the Craniofacial Growth Atlas,[15] confirming what would be a characteristic and/or preference of Brazilians for more protruding incisors. These results are also found in the limits of the average values found by Harris et al.[10]

The values obtained at the end of the treatment differ from the estimates in the horizontal and balanced groups, differently from the vertical group, where the values are closer to those projected by Steiner.[25] This result was also found in the work conducted by Farret[7] in his Class I sample, where values were very similar for all

groups (Fig 4). The average values for 1-NA, at the end of the treatment differ from the "ideal" value advocated by Steiner[25] in all facial types, differing also from the corresponding acceptable compromise for the ANB angle of 40, which would correspond to the 1-NA measurement equal to 2 mm since, in the present study, this measurement has the approximate value of 5 to 6 mm. In the study carried out by Kowalski,[13,14] they presented 1-NA equal to the value advocated by Steiner[25] (Table 8), even though they differed from the proposed ideal value.

The results of the analysis of variance (ANOVA) comparing the three studied groups as to the interference of the gender for the 1-NA measurement did not show a direct effect. In the horizontal group, female individuals present a significant difference between the proposed and the final measurements, which does not happen to males. In the vertical type, there was no difference, and in the balanced there was only a more accentuated behavior for males in relation to the difference between the proposed and the final measurement.

In the balanced patient group, the error margin for less was greater, in relation to the other groups, or, in other words, the predicted retraction of the upper incisors was greater than the obtained and than what was thought necessary in the proposal. This rigid vision of treatment can, determine unnecessary extractions causing straighter profiles, inconsistent with Brazilian esthetic standards.

CONCLUSION

Based on the results obtained and discussed, we were able to conclude that:

» There was no influence of gender on the behavior of measurements ANB, 1-NB, P-NB and 1-NA.

» The propositions made after Steiner's analysis elaboration differed significantly from the results obtained with the orthodontic treatment, with the exception of the variable P-NB.

» The proposed values for ANB were statistically different from the values obtained at the end of the treatment, with the exception of the balanced group, considering that the proposed value for

the horizontal group was underestimated in relation to the other groups.

» In relation to the 1-NB measurement, the proposed values during Steiner's analysis elaboration for the balanced and vertical groups were not reached.

» For the 1-NA measurement, the obtained values at the end of treatment differ from the estimates on all three analyzed groups. In the vertical group the final value was the one that came closer to the proposed one.

» The limitations of the measurement estimates for ANB, 1-NB, P-NB and 1-NA do not invalidate its use as long as they are used with restrictions.

REFERENCES

1. Anderson AA, Anderson AC, Hornbuckle AC, Hornbuckle K. Biological derivation or a range of cephalometric norms for children of African American descent (after Steiner). Am J Orthod Dentofacial Orthop. 2000;118(1):90-100.
2. Bishara SE. Facial and dental changes in adolescents and their clinical implications. Angle Orthod. 2000;70(6):471-83.
3. Bishara SE, Fahl JA, Peterson LC. Longitudinal changes in the ANB angle and Wits appraisal: clinical implications. Am J Orthod. 1983;84(2):133-9.
4. Broadbent BH. A new X-ray technique and its application to orthodontia. Angle Orthod. 1931;1(2):45-66.
5. Coura LC, Pinzan A, Freitas RM. Estudos cefalométrico longitudinal do complexo mandibular em pacientes adultos do sexo masculino tratados ortodonticamente com extração de quatro pré-molares. Ortodontia. 1997;30(1):19-30.
6. Downs WB. Variations in facial relationships: their significance in treatment and prognosis. Am J Orthod. 1948;34(10):812-40.
7. Farret MMB, Araújo MCM. Comportamento da análise de Steiner em casos tratados ortodonticamente. Ortodontia. 1981;14(3):164-72.
8. Fêo PS. Aumento da distância Pog-NB na adolescência. Estomatol Cult. 1970;4(1):5-14.
9. Gleis R, Brezniak N, Lieberman M. Israeli cephalometric standards compared to Downs and Steiner analyses. Angle Orthod. 1990; 60(1):35-40.
10. Harris JE, Kowalski CJ, Walker GF. Discrimination between normal and class II individual using Steiner's analysis. Angle Orthod. 1972;42(3):212-20.
11. Hasund A, Ulstein G. The position of the incisors in relation to the lines NA and NB in different facial types. Am J Orthod. 1970;57(1):1-14.
12. Hofrath H. Problems of standard and methods. In: Krogman WM, Sassouni V. A syllabus in roentgenographic cephalometry. 2nd ed. Philadelphia: College Offsets; 1957. cap. 1, p. 9-25.
13. Kowalski CJ, Walker GF. The use of incisal angles in the Steiner cephalometric analysis. Angle Orthod. 1972;42(2):87-95.
14. Kowalski CJ, Nasjleti CE, Walker GF. Differential diagnosis of adult male black and white populations. Angle Orthod. 1974;44(4):346-50.
15. Martins DR. Atlas de crescimento craniofacial. São Paulo: Ed. Santos; 1998.
16. Miura F, Inoue N, Suzuki K. Cephalometric standards for Japanese according to the Steiner analysis. Am J Orthod. 1965;51:288-95.

17. Oliveira JN, Martins DR. Estudo longitudinal e comparativo da variação do pogônio com os incisivos inferiores, em relação à linha NB, em adolescentes brasileiros, leucodermas, de 12 aos 18 anos de idade, com "oclusão normal". Ortodontia. 1978;11(2):99-107.
18. Ortiz MF, Pinzan A, Pinzan C, Martins DR. Previsibilidade das medidas ANB e 1-Na da análise cefalométrica de Steiner. Rev Dental Press Ortod Ortop Facial. 2005;10(1):79-87.
19. Pinzan A. Estudo comparativo da medida P-NB, em adolescentes leucodermas, brasileiras, de origem mediterrânea,com normal e más oclusões (Classe I e Classe II, divisão 1), tratadas ortodonticamente. Ortodontia. 1987;20(1-2):47-51.
20. Pinzan CRM, Pinzan A, Freitas MR, Henriques JFC, Almeida MR. Estudo da previsibilidade das medidas P-NB e 1-NB na elaboração da análise cefalométrica de Steiner. Rev Dental Press Ortod Ortop Facial. 2004;9(2):23-34.
21. Platou C, Zachrisson B. Incisor position in Scandinavian children with ideal occlusion: a comparison with the Ricketts and Steiner standards. Am J Orthod. 1983;83(4):341-51.
22. Ramos AL, Almeida RR, Pinzan A, Freitas MR. Influência da divergência facial no posicionamento dentário e das bases apicais, em jovens brasileiros com oclusão normal. Ortodontia. 1996;29(3):44-54.
23. Servoss JM. The acceptability of Steiner's acceptable compromises. Am J Orthod. 1960;46(11):834-47.
24. Silva LG, Martins DR. Determinação dos valores cefalométricos 1.NA, 1.NB, 1-NA, 1-NB para adolescentes brasileiros, leucodermas, com "oclusão normal" (estudo longitudinal e comparativo). Ortodontia. 1978;11:108-16.
25. Steiner CC. Cephalometrics for you and me. Am J Orthod. 1953;39(10):729-55.
26. Steiner CC. Cephalometrics clinical practice. Angle Orthod. 1959;29(1):8-29.
27. Steiner CC. The use os cephalometrics as an aid to planning and assessing orthodontic treatment. Am J Orthod. 1960;46(10):721-35.
28. Steiner CC. Cephalometrics as a clinical tool. In: Kraus BS, Riedel RA. Vistas in Orthodontics. Philadelphia: Lea & Fegiber; 1962. p. 131-61.
29. Uesato G, Kinoshita Z, Kawamoto T, Koyama I, Nakanishi Y. Steiner cephalometric norms for Japanese and Japanese-Americans. Am J Orthod. 1978;73(3):321-7.

12

Evaluation of a photographic method to measure dental angulation

Jordana Rodrigues Amorim[1], Diogo de Vasconcelos Macedo[2], David Normando[3]

Objective: To analyze the reliability and reproducibility of a simplified method for analysis of dental angulation using digital photos of plaster dental casts. **Methods:** Digital and standardized photographs of plaster casts were performed and posteriorly imported to an angle reading graphic program in order to have measurements obtained. Such procedures were repeated to evaluate the random error and to analyze reproducibility through intraclass correlation. The sample consisted of 12 individuals (six male and six female) with full permanent dentition orthodontically untreated. The analyses were bilaterally carried out, and generated 24 measurements. **Results:** The random error showed variation of 0.77 to 2.55 degrees for teeth angulation. The statistical analysis revealed that the method presents excellent reproducibility (p < 0.0001) for all teeth, except for the upper premolars. In spite of that, it is still considered statistically significant (p < 0.001). **Conclusion:** The proposed method presents enough reliability that justifies its use in the development of scientific research as well as in clinical practice.

Keywords: Dental crown. Dental photography. Evaluation.

[1] Student at the specialization course in Preventive Orthodontics, Hospital for Rehabilitation of Craniofacial Anomalies/USP.
[2] Degree in Dentistry, Federal University of Pará (UFPA).
[3] Adjunct professor, Federal University of Pará (UFPA).

» The authors report no commercial, proprietary or financial interest in the products or companies described in this article.

Jordana Rodrigues Amorim
Rua Prof. Gerson Rodrigues, 7-51 – Apt. 801 – Vila Universitária — Brazil
CEP: 17012-515 – E-mail: jordanamori@gmail.com

INTRODUCTION

Knowledge on mesiodistal angulation of dental crowns became more prominent after the study described by Andrews in 1972, regarding the "Six keys for an optimal occlusion,"[1] among which the second key states that a tooth correctly angulated in the arch is one of the criteria used to achieve functional occlusion. In this study, the angulations of the dental crowns were determined by measuring the angle formed between the buccal axis of the clinical crown with a line perpendicular to the occlusal plane, on the specimens previously cut out in the center of the clinical crown, using a plastic protractor.

Although undoubtedly important, Andrews' work was applied to only one sample of American individuals and on the reproduction of his methods, it was observed difficulty regarding the accuracy on the positioning of rulers and protractor, thus, generating doubts and high variance of results.[3] Moreover, the cut out of specimens mentioned in that method proves to be inconvenient due to the amount of work and clinical time that is spent, in addition to the discard of orthodontic models.

From the values obtained by Andrews' study, the means of angulations for each dental crown were established. It is possible, however, to assert that dental angulations do not always follow a constant pattern, so that there might be variability on angular values according to the individual characteristics of each patient, considering different cases of malocclusion. Thus, studies that engage in learning and evaluating the ideal mesiodistal positioning become undoubtedly relevant.

A device projected specifically to measure the angulations and inclinations of the dental crowns in plaster casts has been recently presented.[3] With the development of this device, which consists of an alteration in the original methods of Andrews, it was possible to establish mean values of angulation and inclinations of dental crowns for Brazilian individuals with normal occlusion. However, this methods involve a device that is not available in the market, thus, requiring customized production.

Computed tomography (CT) can be useful to assess dental inclinations and angulations,[4] allowing great progress to researches involving tooth positioning and, also, to the individualization of orthodontic treatment. However, since this method is relatively new and still needs further studies that prove

its efficiency and reliability, it must be used with reservations. Furthermore, the high costs of CT scans and the risks inherent to its radiation are some of the disadvantages of this technique.

Therefore, there is a need for methods of simple application that allow the orthodontist to identify and quantify, in a reliable manner, the mesiodistal positioning of the dental crowns, as well as the natural compensation existing in many patients with malocclusion. Thus, the objective of this study is to evaluate the reliability of a photographic method previously described, which, however, had been limited to analyzing canine angulation.[5,6] In the present study, this method was used to quickly and simply measure the angulations of all teeth anteriorly positioned in relation to the permanent first molar.

MATERIAL AND METHODS

This study was approved by the Institutional Review Board of the Institute of Health Sciences of the Federal University of Pará (ICS/UFPA), under protocol number 154-09 and by the National Committee of Ethics in Research (CONEP), under number 25000.066559/2010-11, report number 462/2010.

The sample comprised 12 individuals with permanent dentition and with natural normal occlusion, of which six were males and six females, with mean age of 13.7 years old. The angulations of the first molars, premolars, canines and incisors were bilaterally obtained, in both arches of the initial casts of the selected individuals, thus generating 24 measurements for each tooth, according to the method previously described.[5,6]

In this method,[5,6] the specimens were positioned on a glass plate, at a distance of 20 cm from the photographic lens. A black device with a mark in the center was placed in the background of each specimen, and used as reference to centralize the group of teeth that would be examined. The camera lens was placed against a red wax plate in order to optimize the direction of the lens (Fig 1). Five photographs were taken per arch: two lateral — one in each hemi arch — centralizing the second premolar to the mark in the background, to measure the angulation of the first molar and the premolars; two diagonal, having the line between the canine and the lateral as the central point for the bilateral measurement of these teeth; and one frontal for the measurement of the central incisors (Fig 2).

Ten photographs were taken per individual, totalizing 120 photographs which were then imported to a computer software (Paint Microsoft®, Microsoft Corporation, Redmond, USA) in order to have the occlusal plane drawn. Posteriorly, the images were imported to a graphical computer software (Image Tool® — www.imagetool.com, Image Tool Software, USA), in order to measure teeth angulation.

In both lateral and diagonal photographs, the line corresponding to the occlusal plane was traced from the incisal surface of the central incisors to the mesiobuccal cusp of the permanent first molar. On the frontal photographs, this line was traced touching the tip of the cusp of the canines, as proposed in previously published researches.[5,6]

Posteriorly, through Image Tool®, the long axis of the canine's clinical crown was traced and, from the intersection of these two lines (occlusal plane and long axis), the value of angulation of the clinical crown of the plaster cast was obtained (Fig 3). As for random error analysis, the hemi-arches of the initial plaster molds of all patients were photographed again after 7 days and all the aforementioned steps were repeated until new measurements of the dental angulation were obtained. The random error was calculated according to Dahlberg's formula . The analysis of reproducibility was performed by the test of intraclass correlation, both with a level of reliability of 95%.

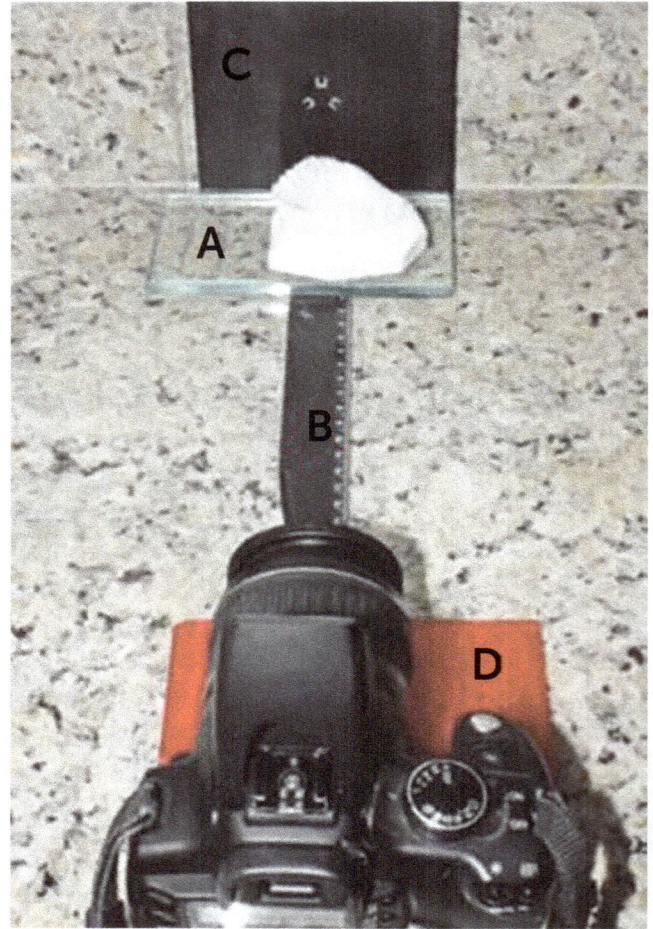

Figure 1 - Method used for standardization of the photographic takes of the plaster molds: A= 10-mm-thick glass plate; B= 20-cm millimeter ruler; C= black plastic plate with mark indicating the center of the object (the back of a CD-ROM case), D= red wax plate.

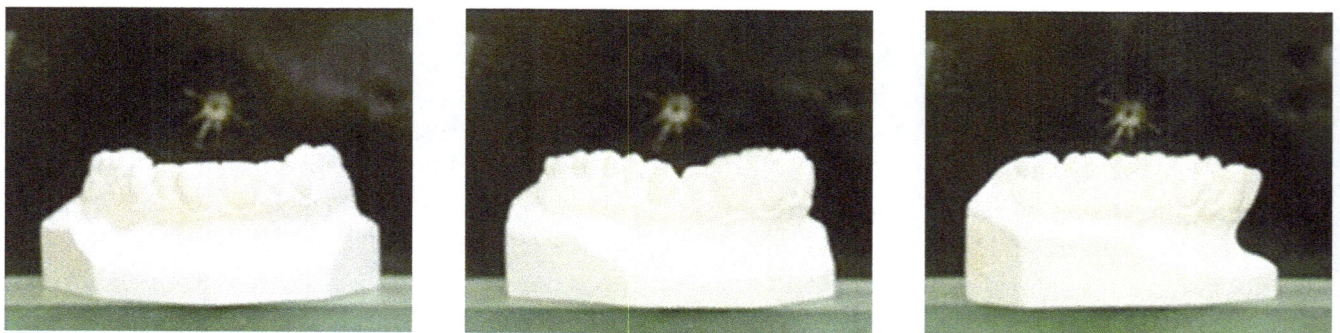

Figure 2 - Plaster molds used in the sampling.

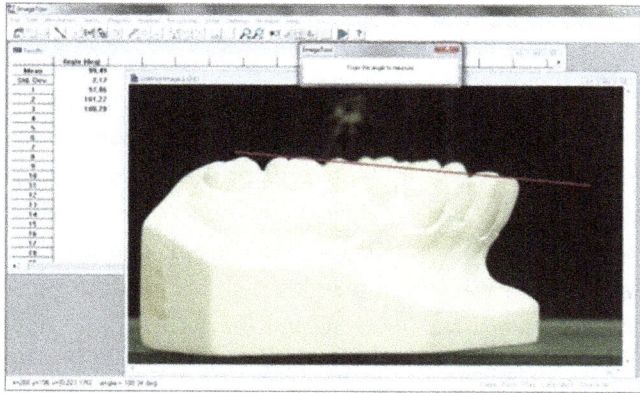

Figure 3 - Photograph of the plaster mold exported to the graphic software used to obtain the measurements of the dental angulations.

RESULTS

The results revealed a minor random error, less than one degree, except for the upper molars (2.55 degrees). With regard to the analysis of reproducibility (intraclass correlation), the statistical analysis revealed an excellent reproducibility of the method (p < 0.0001), except for the upper premolars, of which reproducibility was classified as being from regular to good (r = 0.65 and 0.71, p < 0.001) (Table 1). The results also revealed that the difference of the angulation means was relatively minor and less than one degree, except for the upper first molars (2.29 degrees) (Table 2).

Table 1 - Upper and lower teeth – Random error, method reproducibility (intraclass correlation) and analysis of normality of the distribution of values.

Tooth	Random error	Intraclass correlation (r)	p value	Reproducibility
U6	2.55	0.76	p < 0.0001	Excellent
U5	1.98	0.65	p = 0.0003	Regular to good
U4	2.35	0.71	p < 0.0001	Regular to good
U3	1.84	0.91	p < 0.0001	Excellent
U2	1.12	0.93	p < 0.0001	Excellent
U1	0.77	0.92	p < 0.0001	Excellent
L6	1.58	0.84	p < 0.0001	Excellent
L5	1.86	0.84	p < 0.0001	Excellent
L4	1.62	0.88	p < 0.0001	Excellent
L3	1.57	0.90	p < 0.0001	Excellent
L2	1.55	0.91	p < 0.0001	Excellent
L1	1.06	0.78	p < 0.0001	Excellent

Table 2 - Upper and lower teeth – Angulation means and difference means.

Teeth	Mean – T_1	Mean – T_2	Difference means
U6	89.69	91.98	-2.29
U5	90.02	89.99	0.03
U4	89.48	89.69	-0.22
U3	92.46	91.47	0.98
U2	100.2	99.6	0.6
U1	96.47	96.24	0.23
L6	95.56	95.92	-0.36
L5	92.82	93.15	-0.33
L4	88.61	88.94	-0.325
L3	94.57	93.52	1.06
L2	91.44	90.51	0.94
L1	89.93	89.77	0.16

DISCUSSION

The degree of reliability of measurements taken in specimens has not yet been properly evaluated, perhaps because, originally, it is considered a direct method. However, the changes used in the present study showed that the method used to measure the angulations of dental crowns is greatly reproducible, presenting a random error equal to or less than 2.55 degrees, in addition to being very simple and avoiding the need for detrition of the specimens.

Some methods have been described in the literature for the evaluation of teeth angulation, similarly to the method proposed by Andrews, which uses measurements directly taken on the specimens through a plastic protractor,[1] and others that involve advanced technological resources, such as the use of computed tomography.[4] Other methods also describe the use of devices specially developed for this purpose.[3,7,8] It is natural, however, that each one of the described methods present inherent difficulties, such as certain imprecision on the positioning of the measuring tool,[1] cut out and discard of the plaster molds,[1] high costs,[4] radiation risks[4] and devices that are not available in the market and, for this reason, have to be customized.[3,7,8]

With the technological progress, modern computer software allow reliable analysis of images at low costs. Thus, for the present study, a computed graphical program capable of accurately reading the teeth angulations from the standardized digital photographs of the plaster molds was used.

The method proposed presents differences in relation to Andrews' original proposal. First, the occlusal plane, that, in this study, was represented by a line that connected the incisal surface of the incisors to the tip of the mesiobuccal cusp of the first molar and, on the frontal photographs, a line that touched the tip of the cusp of the canines. This plane is not always parallel to Andrews' plane, especially in cases of malocclusion.

The values found by Andrews and described as normal were very important factors for the development of the Straight-Wire technique, which aimed to individualize the appliance according to patient's orthodontic needs.[2] This pre-programmed appliance uses brackets individually built for each tooth: to these brackets is conferred the information about the ideal mesiodistal and buccolingual position that each element must achieve by the end of the orthodontic treatment. However, the occlusal and skeletal characteristics of each patient are unique, which hinders the creation of a rigid protocol for the detailing of the cases. Since then, many orthodontists began to individualize brackets angulation according to their clinical experience, due to the morphological variations inherent to the dentofacial complex, being most of these modifications introduced without any scientific support.

What seems to be clinical evidence based on the experience of each professional, needs scientific evaluation that support or not the changes inserted on orthodontic appliances used with the objective of individualizing the cases. Methods of simple application, which allow the orthodontist to identify the presence of existing natural compensations, or even to reliably quantify them, would allow the clinician to extend the use of this concept in a scientifically adequate way.

The challenge of developing accessible methodological procedures is the main factor responsible for the lack of studies aimed at discovering the buccallingual and mesiodistal positioning of each dental element in the arch. Thus, a method that allows analysis of the dental angulation in a quick and simple way through materials easily available and software of free access represents a great resource to clinicians.

The method for analysis of the dental angulation described and tested in the present study had been previously used to compare the angulation of canines in individuals with Class I and III malocclusion,[5] as well as to analyze the correlation between the angulation of canines and the inclination of incisors.[6] In both studies, the random error and the systematic error were evaluated and yielded results based on which it can be concluded that the method is considered valid. However, both authors only applied and evaluated this method in anterior teeth and in lateral photographs. It is worth noting that no studies have been yet conducted to prove the reproducibility and reliability of the proposed method when applied to analyze the mesiodistal angulations of the crowns of all teeth anterior to the permanent first molar.

By using and testing the new method proposed in the present study, it is reasonable to conclude that the suggested method presents excellent reproducibility (P < 0.0001), agreeing with the results described by other authors,[5,6] except for the upper premolars that presented a reproducibility classified as being from regular to good (P < 0.001), but yet statistically significant.

The lowest reproducibility found in the measurements performed on upper premolars possibly occurred due to the shorter length of the clinical crown of these teeth, since these teeth present a shorter cervico-occlusal distance the more posterior they are. Once premolars do not present reference lines on the buccal surfaces, as molars do, in addition to being shorter teeth, it is possible to find greater variance on the marking of the long axis of the crown and consequent distortion on the obtained results.

CONCLUSION

Based on the analysis of the results of this study, it is reasonable to conclude that the method described herein presents enough reliability to justify its use both in clinical practice and as auxiliary means on the development of scientific research that focus on the evaluation of the angulations of dental crowns. Moreover, it presents excellent reproducibility, without any difference between the two measurements performed, and with random error relatively small, it achieves the initial proposal of reducing the time that is necessary to take the measurements. Furthermore, it is easy to be executed by the clinician and also allows the preservation of the plaster casts , important objects of orthodontic documentation of the patient.

REFERENCES

1. Andrews LF. The six keys to normal occlusion. Am J Orthod. 1972;62(3):296-309.

2. Andrews LF. Straight-Wire: the concept and appliance. San Diego: L.A. Well; 1989. p. 159.

3. Zanelato ACT, Maltagliati LA, Scanavini MA, Mandetta S. Método para mensuração das angulações e inclinações das coroas dentárias utilizando modelos de gesso. Rev Dental Press Ortod Ortop Facial. 2006;11(2):63-73.

4. Capelozza Filho L, Fattori L, Maltagliati LA. Um novo método para avaliar as inclinações dentárias utilizando a tomografia computadorizada. Rev Dental Press Ortod Ortop Facial. 2005;10(5):23-9.

5. Azevedo LR, Torres TB, Normando D. Angulação dos caninos em indivíduos portadores de má oclusão de Classe I e de Classe III: análise comparativa através de um novo método utilizando imagens digitalizadas. Dental Press J Orthod. 2010;15(5):109-17.

6. Ohashi ASC, Nascimento KCGD, Normando D. Análise da correlação entre a angulação (mesiodistal) dos caninos e a inclinação (vestibulolingual) dos incisivos. Dental Press J Orthod. 2011;16(3):79-86.

7. Ghahferokhi AE, Elias L, Jonssons S, Rolfe B, Richmond S. Critical assessment of a device to measure incisor crown inclination. Am J Orthod Dentofacial Orthop. 2002;121(2):185-91.

8. Richmond S, Klufas ML, Syawany M. Assessing incisor inclination: a non-invasive technique. Eur J Orthod. 1998;20(6):721-6.

13

Björk-Jarabak cephalometric analysis on CBCT synthesized cephalograms with different dentofacial sagittal skeletal patterns

Yalil Augusto Rodriguez-Cardenas[1], Luis Ernesto Arriola-Guillen[2], Carlos Flores-Mir[3]

Objective: The objective of this study was to evaluate the Björk and Jabarak cephalometric analysis generated from cone-beam computed tomography (CBCT) synthesized lateral cephalograms in adults with different sagittal skeletal patterns. **Methods:** The sample consisted of 46 CBCT synthesized cephalograms obtained from patients between 16 and 40 years old. A Björk and Jarabak cephalometric analysis among different sagittal skeletal classes was performed. Analysis of variance (ANOVA), multiple range test of Tukey, Kruskal-Wallis test, and independent t-test were used as appropriate. **Results:** In comparison to the standard values: Skeletal Class III had increased gonial and superior gonial angles (P < 0.001). This trend was also evident when sex was considered. For Class I males, the sella angle was decreased (P = 0.041), articular angle increased (P = 0.027) and gonial angle decreased (P = 0.002); whereas for Class III males, the gonial angle was increased (P = 0.012). For Class I females, the articular angle was increased (P = 0.029) and the gonial angle decreased (P = 0.004). Björk's sum and Björk and Jabarak polygon sum showed no significant differences. The facial biotype presented in the three sagittal classes was mainly hypodivergent and neutral. **Conclusions:** In this sample, skeletal Class III malocclusion was strongly differentiated from the other sagittal classes, specifically in the mandible, as calculated through Björk and Jarabak analysis.

Keywords: Cephalometry. Computed tomography scanners. Malocclusion.

[1] Specialist in Orthodontics, National University of Colombia. Specialist in Oral and Maxillofacial Radiology, Universidad Peruana Cayetano Heredia.

[2] Associate Professor, Department of Orthodontics, School of Dentistry, Universidad Científica del Sur–UCSUR and Universidad Nacional Mayor de San Marcos, UNMSM.

[3] Associate Professor and Head of the Department of Orthodontics, University of Alberta.

» The authors report no commercial, proprietary or financial interest in the products or companies described in this article.

Yalil Augusto Rodríguez-Cárdenas
Carrera 17 # 15 - 08 Of 201 - Duitama, Colombia
E-mail: yalilrodriguez@gmail.com

INTRODUCTION

The recent development of cone-beam computed tomography (CBCT) for craniofacial imaging has encouraged its use in Orthodontics by providing volumetric information that allows the development of three-dimensional models valuable for impacted teeth localization, TMJ visualization, among other applications.[1,2,3] It has also allowed the production of 2D high resolution imaging without magnification.[4] This latter aspect facilitates the use of CBCT synthesized cephalograms for orthodontic treatment planning. In this regard, three methods to simulate conventional two-dimensional cephalograms from CBCT images and volumetric data sets have been described:[5] Lateral scout radiograph taken initially to confirm patient's positioning, maximum intensity projection (MIP), and ray-sum technique.

Replacement of conventional 2D radiographs by their 3D counterpart appears to be a trend.[7] 3D volumetric imaging of the maxilla and mandible has been studied in various skeletal classifications.[8] Moreover, no statistical differences between cephalometric analyses performed on conventional and CBCT-generated cephalograms of patients has been shown several times.[9,11,12]

CBCT-synthesized cephalograms have been used to perform cephalometric analyses, comparing the three types of 2D images that can be produced (conventional, ray-sum, or MIP).[9] However, other authors have found better accuracy on ray-sum produced images, and reported it as a potential method to better simulate lateral cephalometric images from CBCT data sets.[10] The latter is described in more detail in a previous study.[6] In summary, the produced images can be thickened by increasing the number of adjacent voxels. This summation process is called "ray-sum", and can create an image that represents a specifically defined volume of the patient. By adding the intensity values of adjacent voxels along a particular section, its thickness increases and creates a thin plate of 5 to 10 mm, or thicker (more than 20 mm if desired), allowing the production of flat cephalograms without distortion, which can be exported and analyzed by means of cephalometric analysis programs.

Jarabak's cephalometric analysis,[13] based on a study by Björk,[14] has been used to compare facial variations of shape and size based on age, sex and race. Jarabak's cephalometric analysis mainly considers vertical inter-maxillary relationships and uses the cranial base as reference. The final response of Jarabak's polygon to different sagittal skeletal malocclusions, including facial biotypes as shown in non-growing young adults, is an issue that has not been studied yet. The purpose of this study is, therefore, to evaluate Björk and Jabarak cephalometric analysis on CBCT-generated cephalograms with different dentofacial sagittal skeletal patterns.

METHODS

The study was approved by local ethics committee. CBCT-synthesized lateral cephalograms from 46 subjects (24 men, 22 women) were randomly selected from an available database (Table 1). Sample size was calculated considering a gonial angle difference[15] of 3° between Class I and III malocclusion as clinically relevant, with an expected variance of 9°. With a one-sided significance level of 0.05 and a power of 80%, a minimum of 12 patients per group was required.

The final number of participants included was of 46 (15 for Class I, 15 for Class II, and 16 for Class III malocclusion subjects). Inclusion criteria were: CBCT with large field of view (FOV), and patients aged between 16 and 40 years (all subjects had complete craniofacial growth as determined by CVM 6).[16] Participants were in centric occlusion (maximum intercuspidation) during CBCT imaging, and no chin positioner was used to avoid possible alterations in jaw position. Exclusion criteria were: Patients with severe asymmetries, known craniofacial syndromes, under active orthodontic

Table 1 - Descriptive statistics of the sample by skeletal class and sex.

Skeletal Class	Sex	n	ANB	FMA
Class I	Male	8	3.19	25.74
	Female	7	2.86	27.46
Class II	Male	8	7.12	31.01
	Female	7	7.84	32.00
Class III	Male	8	-4.04	32.02
	Female	8	-4.58	27.07
Total		46		

treatment, with tooth loss (except for third molars) or with prior history of orthognatic surgery.

Imaging was performed with a Picasso Master 3D (Vatech, E-WOO Technology Co, Ltd, Republic of Korea). Device settings were set at 8 mA and 90 kV. Each field of view mode was 20 cm X 19 cm. The image was processed with EZImplant 3D software which allowed the generation of ray-sum type generated 2D lateral skull projection cephalometrics (Fig 1).

Cephalometric analysis

The cephalometric analysis was derived from Björk and Jarabak analysis[13] (Fig 2) and included: N-S-Ar (saddle angle), S-Ar-Go (articular angle), Ar-Go-Me (gonial angle), Ar-Go-N (upper gonial angle), N-Go-Me (lower gonial angle) plus the following linear measurements: S-Go (posterior facial height), and N-Me (anterior facial height) (Fig 1).

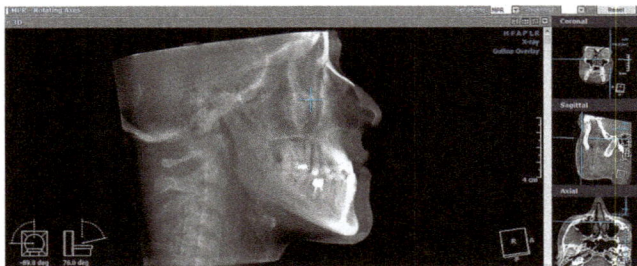

Figure 1 - Example of CBCT cephalogram used in this study.

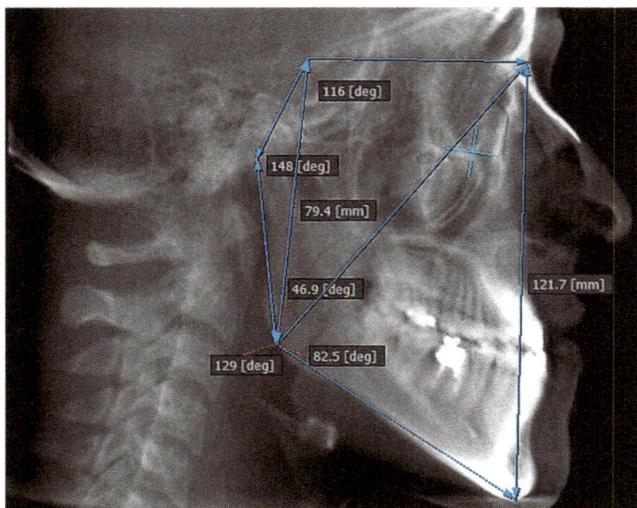

Figure 2 - Angular and linear parameters for Björk and Jarabak analysis used in this study.

Additionally, ANB angle was determined and analyzed for each participant. Participants were classified into three groups according to skeletal pattern: Skeletal Class I ($0° \leq$ ANB $<4°$), Class II (ANB $\geq 4°$), and Class III (ANB $<0°$). The definitions of points and angles used in this study were according to those described by Northway et al.[17]

Methods for error analysis

Cephalometric tracings were performed by an orthodontist previously calibrated for the Björk and Jarabak analysis and with 10 years of experience drawing cephalograms. Intraexaminer reliability was assessed with the intraclass correlation coefficient (ICC) which gave a result greater than 0.90 for all measurements (confidence intervals between 0.900 – 0.999). In addition, Dahlberg error was less than 1° (0.25 to 0.99) in angular measurements and less than 0.8 mm (0.5 to 0.8) in linear measurements. All cephalometric tracings were drawn twice with a one-week interval in between.

Statistical analysis

All statistical analyses were performed using SPSS v.19 for Windows (IBM SPSS, Chicago, Illinois, USA). Normal distribution was confirmed by Shapiro-Wilk tests. One-way analysis of variance (ANOVA) was performed to determine whether there were differences in angles across the sagittal malocclusion types, if normality and homogeneity of variance assumptions were satisfied; otherwise, the equivalent non-parametric Kruskal-Wallis test was used. In addition, analysis of variance (ANOVA) was performed to take into account the significant differences between males and females in terms of sagittal skeletal patterns. The post-hoc analysis was a Tukey HSD. For comparisons between sex, angular measurements and comparisons of Björk and Jarabak analysis, an independent t-test was used. Statistical significance was set at $P < 0.05$ for all tests.

RESULTS

Descriptive statistics for ANB angle, FMA angle, sex and the number of patients for each sagittal skeletal class are shown in Table 1. Class III skeletal had increased gonial and superior gonial angles ($P < 0.001$) during intergroup analysis (Table 2).

Table 2 - Evaluation of cephalometric Björk and Jarabak's measurements according to sagittal skeletal class.

Skeletal class	Cephalometric measurements	X	SD	Min	Max	S²	p (1,2,3)	Multiple comparison (p)
1. Class I	NSAr	122.27	6.32	114.00	134.00	39.92	0.07**	
	SArGo	148.27	8.81	132.00	161.00	77.64	0.054*	
	ArGoMe	122.87	4.05	117.00	129.00	16.41	0.001*	
	ArGcN	43.32	7.84	30.70	57.60	61.49	0.001*	
	MeGoN	76.48	4.89	65.20	83.30	23.87	0.124**	
	NMe	118.85	6.99	106.90	132.90	48.91	0.928**	
	SGo	80.99	5.47	72.70	91.50	29.97	0.152*	
2. Class II	NSAr	122.73	7.51	102.00	135.00	56.35		
	SArGo	149.20	8.92	138.00	167.00	79.60		
	ArGoMe	125.93	6.15	116.00	139.00	37.78		(I, III p = < 0.001) (II, III p = 0.018)***
	ArGcN	44.73	5.71	34.90	53.20	32.56		(I, III p = 0.001) (II, III p = 0.009)***
	MeGoN	79.32	6.49	72.60	91.30	42.08		
	NMe	119.39	6.74	105.70	127.90	45.42		
	SGo	78.35	4.59	72.10	88.40	21.10		
3. Class III	NSAr	121.63	6.02	113.00	133.00	36.25		
	SArGo	142.31	7.29	129.00	154.00	53.16		
	ArGoMe	132.81	8.89	119.00	146.00	79.10		
	ArGcN	51.32	3.49	43.30	56.60	12.20		
	MeGoN	81.89	6.20	74.00	92.50	38.47		
	NMe	120.09	9.36	109.20	135.00	87.55		
	SGo	76.84	7.18	66.00	88.90	51.54		

*ANOVA. ** Kruskal-Wallis. *** Tukey.

Table 3 - Comparison between the studied sella, articular and gonial angles and the Björk and Jabarak standard by skeletal class and sex.

Skeletal class	Sex	Angle	SD	Standard	SD	p	Mean difference	95% confidence interval Lower	Upper
				Sella angle					
Class I	Male	118.50	4.50	123	5	0.041	-4.42	-8.9	-0.26
	Female	125.50	6.07	123	5	0.282	2.50	-2.58	7.58
Class II	Male	123.10	11.02	123	5	0.974	0.14	-10.05	10.34
	Female	122.37	2.87	123	5	0.558	-0.62	-3.03	1.78
Class III	Male	121.80	4.54	123	5	0.507	-1.12	-4.93	2.68
	Female	121.30	7.53	123	5	0.561	-1.62	-7.93	4.68
				Articular angle					
Class I	Male	151.40	7.63	143	6	0.027	8.42	1.37	15.49
	Female	145.50	9.30	143	6	0.472	2.50	-5.28	10.28
Class II	Male	147.10	9.82	143	6	0.307	4.14	-4.94	13.23
	Female	151.00	8.28	143	6	0.029	8.00	1.08	14.92
Class III	Male	137.80	6.89	143	6	0.074	-5.12	-10.89	0.64
	Female	146.70	4.62	143	6	0.055	3.75	-0.11	7.61
				Gonial angle					
Class I	Male	122.80	3.48	130	7	0.002	-7.14	-10.37	-3.92
	Female	122.80	4.73	130	7	0.004	-7.12	-11.08	-3.17
Class II	Male	125.80	7.69	130	7	0.204	-4.14	-11.26	2.97
	Female	126.00	4.98	130	7	0.058	-4.00	-8.17	0.17
Class III	Male	138.80	7.51	130	7	0.012	8.87	2.60	15.15
	Female	126.70	5.39	130	7	0.132	-3.25	-7.76	1.26

Independent t-test.

Table 4 - Comparison between the sum (Björk) studied and the standard by skeletal class and sex.

Skeletal class	Sex	Sum (Björk) Studied	SD	Sum (Björk) Standard	SD	p	Mean difference	95% confidence interval	
								Lower	Upper
Class I	Male	392.70	5.20	396	6	0.074	-3.14	-6.70	0.42
	Female	393.80	6.70	396	6	0.263	-2.12	-6.26	2.01
Class II	Male	396.00	9.51	396	6	0.331	0.14	-6.05	6.33
	Female	399.00	5.37	396	6	0.957	3.37	-4.26	11.01
Class III	Male	398.40	4.80	396	6	0.274	2.62	-2.60	7.85
	Female	394.70	5.84	396	6	0.309	-1.12	-3.55	1.30

Independent t-test.

Table 5 - Characteristics of Björk and Jabarak facial height ratio by sex and skeletal class.

Class	Female	Facial type	Male	Facial type
I	67.30°	CCW – HIPO	69.04°	CCW–HIPO
II	64.62°	NEUTRO	66.74°	CCW– HIPO
III	63.62°	NEUTRO	64.28°	NEUTRO

CCW-HYPO: Counterclockwise rotation hypodivergent.

In comparison to published standards:

For Class I males, the sella angle was decreased (P = 0.041), articular angle increased (P = 0.027) and gonial angle decreased (P = 0.002); whereas for Class III males, the gonial angle was increased (P = 0.012). For Class I females, the articular angle was increased (P = 0.029) and the gonial angle decreased (P = 0.004) (Table 3).

Björk's sum and Björk and Jabarak polygon sum showed no significant differences among the different sagittal patterns. (Table 4)

For this sample, the facial biotype presented in the three sagittal classes was mainly hypodivergent and neutral (Table 5).

DISCUSSION

Lateral cephalometric analyses have been extensively used to develop guidelines that aid in orthodontic diagnosis and treatment planning. CBCT images allow clinicians to reformat volumetric 3D data set to conventional 2D by simulating plane projections such as a synthesized lateral cephalometric view. Several studies have been conducted to assess the accuracy of cephalometric measurements using CBCT images;[18,19] however, no previous study has analyzed Björk and Jarabak's cephalometric analysis in a young adult non-growing population. The sample of this study comprised non-growing patients,

which was confirmed by Bacceti's analysis, revealing that all patients were on CS6. Thus, age was not a variable and there was no bias. Björk and Jabarak analysis provides extensive information about the facial biotype of a patient through only a few cephalometric measurements. Previous researchers have emphasized the need to expand available norms for adult populations.[20,21,22]

A few published studies have specifically used significant parts or all of Björk and Jabarak analysis. All of them were conducted only on growing individuals with different facial biotypes. Chung et al[23] reported the longitudinal craniofacial growth changes in untreated skeletal Class I subjects with low, average, and high MP-SN angles. They found that the SNA and SNB angles increased with age in all groups. Moreover, Alexander et al[24] reported cephalometric growth changes in untreated Class III malocclusions by using semi-longitudinal cephalometric records. They found that the length of the anterior skull base increases with age less than 1 mm per year for women and around 1 mm for men. This increase is similar to Class I subjects; however, the longitudinal nature of this study is not accurate, because the sample comparisons between age groups were not performed on the same initial study group.

Reyes et al[25] provided an estimate of facial growth in Class III malocclusion and found that the sella angle is smaller in Class III than in subjects with normal occlusion in both males and females. A report by Kuramae et al[26] found that cephalometric measurements calculated for black Brazilian patients were similar to Jarabak's standards, except for S-N mean value for female patients, which was significantly lower than the established Jarabak's standard. The application of Björk and Jarabak analysis in all mentioned studies reinforces its relevance in the current context of orthodontic diagnosis, but no reports highlight findings on an adult population.

Because subjects at the same chronological age may have different skeletal maturation levels, evaluation of non-growing subjects may be important to determine specific characteristics of a given skeletal class. Dibbets[27] stated that differences in mandibular size between Angle classes emerge later during development, and therefore, these differences are more likely to be found in adult samples. Kerr and Hirst,[28] in a longitudinal study, found that the craniofacial characteristics of subjects with normal and postnormal occlusions became more defined with advancing age. These studies evaluated growing subjects at various ages, but none considered non-growing adults.

Regarding the present results, the significant differences found for sex in Class I malocclusion cases correspond to the sella angle. The behavior of this angle is strongly linked to the behavior of facial height. If the angle is small, the condyle is projected downward and slightly forward reflecting an increase in posterior and anterior facial height. This same characteristic was also observed for facial height on the skeletal Class III group. This result is consistent with the findings by Baccetti et al[29] who studied a population between 3 and 57 years old. They found that Class III malocclusion is associated with a significant degree of sexual dimorphism in craniofacial parameters, especially from the age of 13 onward. In women, the sella angle turned out to be broader than in men, causing backward projection of the condyle and generating a slightly retrognathic profile reflected in the associated convex facial pattern. This sex characteristic was also reported by Pecora et al.[21] The significant differences found in our study according to sex in Class III patients on the articular angle level do not coincide with the findings by Baccetti et al[29] who found no sex differences at this angle, the so-called "cranial bending angle", neither sex differences in Class II. This result is consistent with findings by Chung and Wong[30] who studied Class II growing patients and found that skeletal changes in angular measurements were similar in male and female groups. However, linear measurements showed significant differences. Our results suggest that the behavior of the saddle angle affects facial height, and it is also reflected in the dentofacial skeletal pattern.

In our study, the facial growth pattern of Class III patients was strongly differentiated from other skeletal classes. There were significant differences found in the gonial and superior gonial angles on Class III subjects compared with Class I and II subjects. The development of Class III is multifactorial and complex, being derived from different combinations of dental and skeletal factors, changes in magnitude, direction, and timing of craniofacial growth. The findings of this study indicate a specific characterization of adult Class III subjects in which the behavior of their facial growth tends to be hyperdivergent, derived from the opening of the gonial angle and upper gonial angle and the projection of the symphysis of the chin forward. Other known factors that contribute to this condition are size, position and shape of the maxilla, mandible, skull base, teeth and glenoid fossa.

The sum of the sella, articular, and gonial angles according to Björk is one of the parameters that define the type of growth in a subject. The estimated value is $396 \pm 6°$, for an individual with neutral growth.[31] Variations on this estimate can cause hyper or hypodivergent facial growth tendencies. In our study, the behavior of the polygon sum (Björk) showed no significant differences in relation to the published standard for the three sagittal skeletal classes. This reveals that despite differences between the various angles between skeletal classes, the result of growth was similar in this sample. In addition, an increased angle in one sagittal skeletal class can be compensated with the decrease of another angle on the same group. Saltaji et al[32] evaluated the association between vertical facial morphology and overjet in untreated Class II subjects. They performed an analysis of the performance criteria of the sum (Björk) and facial proportions, and found a strong relationship between overjet, the sum (Björk), gonial angle and lower gonial angle. Their findings are in agreement with our results. Furthermore, findings such as the behavior of the lower gonial angle in Class III subjects are interesting. This angle has a strong tendency to increase in this sagittal skeletal pattern with respect to the other sagittal skeletal classes. This difference reinforces the vertical and hyperdivergent pattern of this sagittal skeletal class.

Also, similar findings were reported for the sella angle when skeletal Class I and Class III were compared in men. This angle is also called "angle of the cranial base" and there is no consensus if the articular or the basion point should be used. Proff et al[33] found a statistically significant reduction in this angle, with a mean of 17.7 ± 3.05° in Class III subjects. Guyer et al[34] also reported an acute cranial base angle compared with skeletal Class I subjects in subjects growing up to 15 years. In the present study, there were almost no changes in this angle. No statistically significant differences were found, with skeletal Class III patients reporting the lowest values. The role of the cranial base is still controversial, and some authors argue that the cranial base in skeletal Class III subjects did not differ morphologically from the one in a Class I normal profile.[35]

The present study can shed some additional light on our understanding on how the sum of Björk and Jarabak's polygon behaves in different sagittal skeletal relations. According to the proportion calculation between the posterior facial height (S-Go) and the anterior facial height (N-Me), one subject can be considered hyperdivergent if this ratio is 59% or less, hypodivergent if it is 65% or more and neutral if proportion is between 60 to 64%.[13] Our sample of Class I male and female adults had an hypodivergent biotype. Class II women had a neutral biotype, while Class II men were hypodivergent. In Class III,

there were no sex differences and the facial biotype was neutral. Therefore, in our sample, there was a tendency to develop hypodivergent growth pattern in the three sagittal skeletal classes with a mandibular rotation in counterclockwise direction. According to these findings, the study population can be characterized not only by the three facial biotypes defined by Björk, since almost all of them are classified as hypodivergent or neutral facial growth, and the most extreme vertical cases were classified as neutral. In this regard, the verticality criteria in the facial subject context can be highlighted. Also, this issue is not considered by the ANB in the classic sagittal skeletal classification.

The deep vertical orientation described on Class III subjects was demonstrated with the gonial angles in a downward and backward direction on Björk and Jabarak analysis. This finding may be of paramount importance as it adds clinical information to other studies on Class III patients.

CONCLUSIONS

Björk and Jabarak cephalometric analysis on CBCT synthesized cephalograms with different dentofacial sagittal skeletal patterns showed a downward and backward direction at the gonial and superior gonial angle on Class III sagittal malocclusion subjects.

REFERENCES

1. Cevidanes LH, Heymann G, Cornelis MA, DeClerck HJ, Tulloch C. Superimposition of 3-dimensional cone-beam computed tomography models of growing patients. Am J Orthod Dentofacial Orthop. 2009;136(1):94-9.

2. Cevidanes LH, Figueiredo Oliveira AE, Grauer D, Styner M, Proffit WR.Clinical application of 3D imaging for assessment of treatment outcomes. Semin Orthod. 2011;17(1):72-80.

3. Tai K, Hotokezaka H, Hyun Park J, Tai H, Miyajima K, Choi M, et al. Preliminary cone-beam computed tomography study evaluating dental and skeletal changes after treatment with a mandibular Schwartz appliance. Am J Orthod Dentofacial Orthop. 2010;138(3):262-11.

4. Ludlow JB, Davies-Ludlow LE, Brooks SL. Dosimetry of two extraoral direct digital imaging devices: NewTom cone beam CT and Orthophos Plus DS panoramic unit. Dentomaxillofac Radiol. 2003;32(4):229-34.

5. Farman AG, Scarfe WC. Development of imaging selection criteria and procedures should precede cephalometric assessment with cone-beam computed tomography. Am J Orthod Dentofacial Orthop. 2006;130(2):257-65.

6. Farman AG, Scarfe WC.The Basics of maxillofacial cone beam computed tomography. Semin Orthod. 2009;(15):2-13.

7. Huang J, Bumann A, Mah J. Three-dimensional radiographic analysis in orthodontics. J Clin Orthod. 2005;39(7):421-8.

8. Deguchi T Sr, Katashiba S, Inami T, Foong KW, Huak CY. Morphologic quantification of the maxilla and the mandible with cone-beam computed tomography. Am J Orthod Dentofacial Orthop. 2010;137(2):218-22.

9. Cattaneo PM, Bloch CB, Calmar D, Hjortshoj M, Melsen B. Comparison between conventional and cone-beam computed tomography-generated cephalograms. Am J Orthod Dentofacial Orthop. 2008;134(6):798-802.

10. Moshiri M, Scarfe WC, Hilgers ML, Scheetz JP, Silveira AM, Farman AG. Accuracy of linear measurements from imaging plate and lateral cephalometric images derived from cone-beam computed tomography. Am J Orthod Dentofacial Orthop. 2007;132(4):550-60.

11. Kumar V, Ludlow JB, Mol A, Cevidanes L. Comparison of conventional and cone beam CT synthesized cephalograms. Dentomaxillofac Radiol. 2007;36(5):263-9.

12. Kumar V, Ludlow J, Soares Cevidanes LH, Mol A. In vivo comparison of conventional and cone beam CT synthesized cephalograms. Angle Orthod. 2008;78(5):873-9.

13. Jarabak JR, Fizzel JA. Technique and treatment with lightwire appliances. 2a ed. St Louis: CV Mosby; 1972.

14. Bjork A. Prediction of mandibular growth rotation. Am J Orthod. 1969;55(6):585-99.

15. Burstone CJ, James RB, Legan H, Murphy GA, Norton LA. Cephalometrics for orthognathic surgery. J Oral Surg. 1978;36(4):269-77.

16. Baccetti T, Franchi L, McNamara JA Jr. The cervical vertebral maturation method: some need for clarification. Am J Orthod Dentofacial Orthop. 2003;123(1):19A-20A.

17. Northway RO Jr, Alexander RG, Riolo ML. A cephalometric evaluation of the old Milwaukee brace and the modified Milwaukee brace in relation to the normal growing child. Am J Orthod. 1974;65(4):341-63.

18. Oz U, Orhan K, Abe N. Comparison of linear and angular measurements using two-dimensional conventional methods and three-dimensional cone beam CT images reconstructed from a volumetric rendering program in vivo. Dentomaxillofac Radiol. 2011;40(8):492-500.

19. Ghoneima A, Albarakati S, Baysal A, Uysal T, Kula K. Measurements from conventional, digital and CT-derived cephalograms: a comparative study. Aust Orthod J. 2012;28(2):232-9.

20. Franchi L, Baccetti T, McNamara JA Jr. Cephalometric floating norms for North American adults. Angle Orthod. 1998;68(6):497-502.

21. Pecora NG, Baccetti T, McNamara JA Jr. The aging craniofacial complex: a longitudinal cephalometric study from late adolescence to late adulthood. Am J Orthod Dentofacial Orthop. 2008;134(4):496-505.

22. West KS, McNamara JA Jr. Changes in the craniofacial complex from adolescence to midadulthood: a cephalometric study. Am J Orthod Dentofacial Orthop. 1999;115(5):521-32.

23. Chung CH, Mongiovi VD.Craniofacial growth in untreated skeletal Class I subjects with low, average, and high MP-SN angles: a longitudinal study. Am J Orthod Dentofacial Orthop. 2003;124(5):670-8.

24. Alexander AE, McNamara JA Jr, Franchi L, Baccetti T. Semilongitudinal cephalometric study of craniofacial growth in untreated Class III malocclusion. Am J Orthod Dentofacial Orthop. 2009;135(6):700.e1-14; discussion 700-1.

25. Reyes BC, Baccetti T, McNamara JA Jr.An estimate of craniofacial growth in Class III malocclusion. Angle Orthod. 2006;76(4):577-84.

26. Kuramae M, Magnani MB, Boeck EM, Lucato AS. Jarabak 's cephalometric analysis of Brazilian black patients. Braz Dent J. 2007;18(3):258-62.

27. Dibbets JM. Morphological associations between the Angle classes. Eur J Orthod. 1996;18(2):111-8.

28. Kerr WJS, Hirst D. Craniofacial characteristics of subjects with normal and postnormal occlusions. Am J Orthod Dentofacial Orthop. 1987;92(3):207-12.

29. Baccetti T, Reyes BC, McNamara JA Jr. Gender differences in Class III malocclusion. Angle Orthod. 2005;75(4):510-20.

30. Chun-Hsi Chung, Wallace W.Craniofacial growth in untreated skeletal Class II subjects: a longitudinal study. Am J Orthod Dentofacial Orthop. 2002;122(6):619-26.

31. Bjork A.Variations in the growth pattern of the human mandible: longitudinal radiographic study by the implant method. J Dent Res. 1963;42(1 Pt 2):400-11.

32. Saltaji H, Flores-Mir C, Major PW, Youssef M. The relationship between vertical facial morphology and overjet in untreated Class II subjects. Angle Orthod. 2012;82(3):432-40.

33. Proff P, Will F, Bokan I, Fanghanel J, Gedrange T. Cranial base features in skeletal Class III patients. Angle Orthod. 2008;78(3):433-9.

34. Guyer EC, Ellis E III, McNamara JA Jr, Behrents RG. Components of class III malocclusion in juveniles and adolescents. Angle Orthod. 1986;56(1):7-30.

35. Anderson D, Popovich F. Relation of cranial base flexure to cranial form and mandibular position. Am J Phys Anthropol. 1983;61(2):181-7.

14

Comparison of the changes of alveolar bone thickness in maxillary incisor area in extraction and non-extraction cases: Computerized tomography evaluation

Paulo Roberto Barroso Picanço[1], Fabricio Pinelli Valarelli[2], Rodrigo Hermont Cançado[2],
Karina Maria Salvatore de Freitas[3], Gracemia Vasconcelos Picanço[1]

Objective: To compare, through computed tomography, alveolar bone thickness changes at the maxillary incisors area during orthodontic treatment with and without tooth extraction. **Methods:** Twelve patients were evaluated. They were divided into 2 groups: G1 - 6 patients treated with extraction of right and left maxillary first premolars, with mean initial age of 15.83 years and mean treatment length of 2.53 years; G2 - 6 patients treated without extraction, with mean initial age of 18.26 years and mean treatment length of 2.39 years. Computed tomographies, lateral cephalograms and periapical radiographs were used at the beginning of the treatment (T_1) and 18 months after the treatment had started (T_2). Extraction space closure occurred in the extraction cases. Intragroup and intergroup comparisons were performed by dependent and independent t test, respectively. **Results:** In G1, the central incisor was retracted and uprighted, while in G2 this tooth showed vestibularization. Additionally, G1 presented a higher increase of labial alveolar bone thickness at the cervical third in comparison with G2. The incidence of root resorption did not present significant differences between groups. **Conclusion:** There were no changes in alveolar bone thickness when extraction and nonextraction cases were compared, except for the labial alveolar bone thickness at the cervical third of maxillary incisors.

Keywords: Alveolar ridge. Tooth movement. Tooth extraction. Tomography.

[1] MSc in Orthodontics, Uningá. Professor, Paulo Picanço Center of
  Orthodontics.
[2] Adjunct Professor, Uningá.
[3] Post-Doc in Orthodontics, University of Toronto. Professora, Uningá.

» The authors report no commercial, proprietary or financial interest in the products or companies described in this article.

Fabrício Valarelli
Rua Manoel Pereira Rolla, 12-75, apto 503 – Bauru/SP – CEP: 17012-190
E-mail: fabriciovalarelli@uol.com.br

INTRODUCTION

Orthodontic movement can be quick or slow, depending on the physical characteristics of the applied force, the size and the biological response of the periodontal ligament.[1] According to Vardimon, Oren and Ben-Bassat,[2] there is an axiom in orthodontics that says: "tooth movement leaves marks on the bone", however, this fact is not always favorable. In vertical direction, during tooth extrusion, the changes in the underlying bone tissue may not follow tooth displacement, leading to an increase in clinical length of the tooth crown, oftentimes undesirable. In transverse and anteroposterior directions, bone dehiscence and fenestration have been reported when the incisors are either protruded or retracted.[3,4] According to Handelman,[5] labial and lingual/palatal bone cortical plates at incisors' apexes may represent anatomical limits to orthodontic tooth movement. The literature has speculated that protrusion and vestibularization of the maxillary incisors may produce labial bone cortical dehiscence while teeth retraction affects the palatal bone plate, although this would be reversible only if the teeth returned to their original position.[6]

Designing the limits of tooth movement before beginning the orthodontic treatment may be extremely beneficial, especially in situations in which skeletal discrepancy is severe or the maxilla and/or mandible can accommodate, in a limited way, the repositioning of the teeth after orthodontic movement.[5,7]

To detect bone levels, the following methods may be used: periapical radiographs, lateral cephalograms and panoramic radiographs. Notwithstanding, bidimensional radiographs reveal some limitations, such as image superimposition and distortions as well as the inability of measuring bone thickness in panoramic and periapical radiographs.[7,8] Taking these factors into account, computed tomography (CT) has been considered of paramount importance for diagnosing initial bone levels as well as bone level changes during orthodontic treatment.[9,10]

The aim of this study was to compare, through computed tomography, the alveolar bone thickness changes at the maxillary incisors area during orthodontic treatment with or without maxillary premolar extractions.

MATERIAL AND METHODS
Sample

Twelve patients of both genders were selected in the orthodontic clinic Paulo Picanço. Inclusion criteria were: 1) permanent dentition; 2) absence of systemic disease that may alter bone metabolism; 3) nonsmoker; 4) patients who are not using steroid-based drugs; 5) absence of chronic kidney disease; 6) if female, patients who do not present low level of estrogen; 7) presence of all six maxillary anterior teeth; 8) patients who have not undergone tooth trauma, alveolar bone fracture or luxation in maxillary incisors; 9) patients who do not present a prosthetic crown on maxillary incisors; 10) absence of alveolar cleft in the maxillary anterior area.

The sample was divided into two groups: G1 – 6 patients (5 male; 1 female) with mean initial age of 15.83 ± 4.87 years, presenting Class II malocclusion, treated with 2 maxillary premolar extractions during a mean period of 2.53 ± 0.49 years; G2 – 6 patients (5 male; 1 female), with mean initial age of 18.26 ± 6.42 years, 3 showing Class I and 3 Class II malocclusion, treated without extractions during a mean treatment period of 2.39 ± 0.66 years.

Patients were treated by post-graduation students oriented by the same professor, following the same diagnosis pattern, treatment planning and orthodontic mechanics (Edgewise, 0.018 x 0.025-in brackets – Morelli – Sorocaba, SP, Brazil).

Methods

Computed tomographies were performed at the beginning of the orthodontic treatment (T_1) and 18 months after the treatment had started, (T_2). The exams confirmed extraction space closure. Additionally, periapical radiographs were performed at T_1 and T_2 using the parallelism technique in order to evaluate external root resorption of the maxillary incisors. Lateral cephalograms were performed to evaluate anteroposterior and vertical changes as well as the inclination of these teeth.

For cephalograms and tomographs evaluation, image digitalization and measurement processing, Dolphin Imaging Premium 10.5 software (Dolphin Imaging & Management Solutions, Chatsworth, CA, USA) was used.

UL (labial) and UP (palatal) variables were obtained from the long axis of the maxillary incisor and a point of reference (zero point) marked at the enamel-cementum junction (ECJ). From this point of reference, three lines were traced towards apical direction, with a 3 mm interval, up to the most external limit of the labial (UL) and palatal (UP) alveolar bone, perpendicularly to the tooth long axis (Fig 1).

On the lateral cephalograms, the following variables were analyzed: 1-PTV incisal, 1-PTV apical, FMA, PFH/AFH, Wits, 1.NA, H-11 and UL+UP.

The degree on initial and final root resorption was analysed through periapical radiographs, based on the scores of Levander and Malmgren's score system:[11] 0 – lack of root resorption; 1 – presence of apical irregularities; 2 – presence of root resorption up to 2 mm; 3 – presence of root resorption from 2 mm to one third of the root original length; 4 – presence of root resorption greater than one third of the original length of the root. Root length was obtained from measuring the distance from root apex to ECJ, following the incisor long axis (Fig 2).

Method error

To determine intraexaminer error, both lateral cephalograms and tomographies were reevaluated in 6 randomly selected patients after a month interval. Systematic error was determined by dependent t test while casual error was determined by the Dahlberg's formula. Kappa test was used to establish root resorption score error.

Statistical analysis

The following statistical tests were employed: difference between two means for carrying out the sample calculation, chi-square test for intergroup comparison concerning the malocclusion type; independent t test for intergroup age and treatment period comparison; dependent t test for intragroup initial and final stages comparison; independent t test for intergroup initial and final stages as well as treatment changes comparison. All tests were performed with Statistica software (Statistica for Windows, version 7.0, Statsoft, 2005). The results were considered significant at $p < 0.05$.

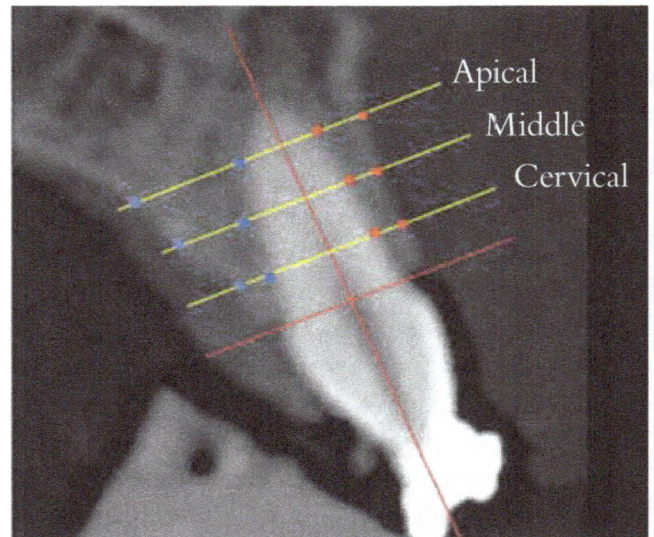

Figure 1 - Alveolar bone thickness assessment evaluated through computed tomography.

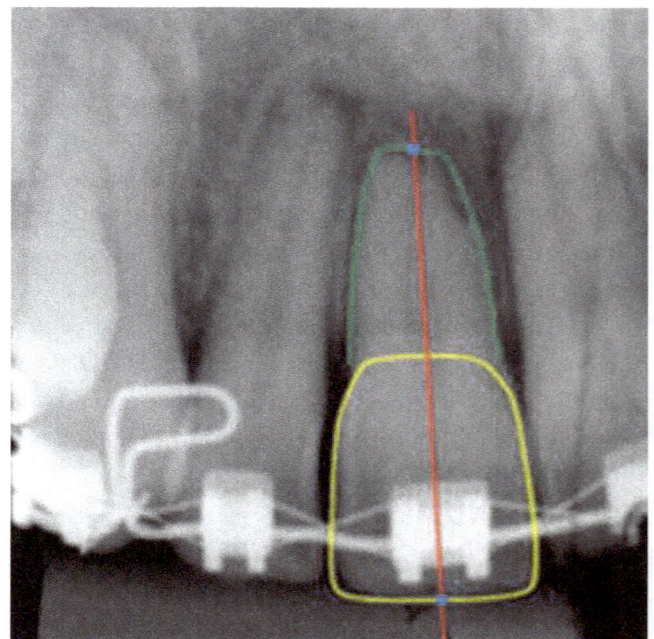

Crown-root ratio
Example: Degree 4

Crown = 11 mm

11 ------- 100%
10 ------ X

X = 1000 ÷ 11/100

X= 0.9

Ratio = 1:09

Figure 2 - Crown-root ratio and maxillary central incisor length assessment.

RESULTS

The 1-PTV apical variable showed the greatest casual error (1.57 mm). Systematic error occurred only for the following variables: 1-PTV incisal and UP middle. Kappa coefficient demonstrated a concordance percentage of 90%.

There were differences in the distribution of the malocclusion type between groups (Table 1). The groups were compatible regarding gender, initial and final ages as well as treatment period (Table 2).

At the initial stage (T_1), only 1-PTV apical showed statistically significant difference between groups, indicating that in G1 the maxillary incisor was more protruded than in G2 (Table 3).

The comparison between G1 (treated with two maxillary premolar extractions) stages (T_1 and T_2) demonstrated that there was a decrease in the crown-root ratio and in the central incisor length, a retraction of these teeth both in apical (1-PTV apical) and incisal (1-PTV incisal) measurements, a decrease in anteroposterior discrepancy (ANB), an increase of the UL cervical (labial cervical third) measurement and decrease of the UP cervical (palatal cervical third) and UP middle (palatal middle third) measurements (Table 4).

In G2 (treated without extractions), the comparison between T_1 and T_2 demonstrated that there was a decrease in the crown-root ratio, in the central incisor length, in FMA angle, in the relation between posterior and anterior face height, vestibularization of the maxillary incisors (1.NA) and a decrease in the UP middle measurement as well (Table 5).

At T_2, there was statistically significant difference between the groups in two variables: 1-PTV incisal and UL cervical. The difference in 1-PTV incisal indicated that, at the end of the treatment, central incisors in G1 were more retruded than in G2 while the difference in UL cervical showed higher bone thickness at this area in G1 than in G2 (Table 6).

With regard to treatment changes (T_2-T_1), the 1-PTV incisal, 1-PTV apical and 1.NA measurements were statistically significant different between groups, revealing that G1 showed maxillary incisor's retraction and uprighting while G2 exhibited this tooth protrusion and vestibularization (Table 7). Additionally, UL cervical measurement was also significantly different between groups indicating an increase of labial bone thickness in G1 when compared to G2 (Table 7).

With regard to root resorption degree, there were no significant differences between groups at any of the evaluated periods (Table 8).

DISCUSSION

Handelman[5] claims that a thin tooth alveolus or an inappropriate alveolar cavity for the amount of desirable tooth movement must be considered as a risk for

Table 1 - Intergroup comparison of malocclusion type (chi-square test).

Group	Class I	Class II	Total
1	0	6	6
2	3	3	6
Total	3	9	12
$\chi^2 = 4.00$; GL= 1; p = 0.045*			

*Statistically significant difference (P<0.05).

Table 2 - Intergroup comparison of initial and final ages as well as treatment period (independent t tests).

Variables (years)	G1 Extraction of #14 and #24 teeth (n = 6)	G2 Without extractions (n = 6)	p
	Mean ± SD	Mean ± SD	
Initial age	15.83 ± 4.87	18.26 ± 6.42	0.477
Final age	18.36 ± 4.84	20.65 ± 6.45	0.502
Treatment period	2.53 ± 0.49	2.39 ± 0.66	0.682

Table 3 - Intergroup comparison of variables studied during the initial stage (T_1) (independent t tests).

Variables	G1 Extraction of #14 and #24 teeth n = 6	G2 Without extraction n = 6	p
	Mean ± SD	Mean ± SD	
Crown-root ratio (mm)	1.44 ± 0.20	1.52 ± 0.16	0.444
Length 11 (mm)	24.92 ± 1.91	25.48 ± 2.17	0.643
1-PTV incisal(mm)	63.78 ± 6.35	55.65 ± 6.65	0.055
1-PTV apical (mm)	51.71 ± 4.57	36.66 ± 5.04	0.000*
FMA (degrees)	23.81 ± 5.11	25.22 ± 5.02	0.640
PFH/AFH (mm)	0.63 ± 0.07	0.70 ± 0.06	0.153
ANB (degrees)	4.10 ± 1.71	3.29 ± 2.98	0.580
Wits (mm)	-0.20 ± 4.57	-0.26 ± 5.12	0.982
1.NA (degrees)	27.96 ± 10.67	21.06 ± 6.32	0.202
H-11 (mm)	20.51 ± 1.98	18.05 ± 3.56	0.169
UA+UP (mm)	18.11 ± 8.95	13.46 ± 3.75	0.267
UA cerv (mm)	0.84 ± 0.52	0.67 ± 0.41	0.539
UP cerv (mm)	1.68 ± 0.91	1.20 ± 0.49	0.283
UA middle (mm)	0.61 ± 0.28	0.47 ± 0.30	0.398
UP middle (mm)	2.77 ± 1.64	2.01 ± 0.62	0.315
UA apical (mm)	1.31 ± 0.84	0.99 ± 0.36	0.408
UP apical (mm)	4.24 ± 2.45	3.03 ± 1.38	0.318

*Statistically significant difference (P < 0.05).

Table 4 - Comparison between initial (T₁) and final (T₂) stages of group 1, with premolar extractions (dependent t tests).

Variables	Initial stage (T₁) n = 6 Mean ± SD	Final stage (T₂) n = 6 Mean ± SD	Changes T₂-T₁	p
Crown-root ratio (mm)	1:1.44 ± 0.20	1:1.32 ± 0.25	-0.12	0.009*
Length. 11 (mm)	24.92 ± 1.91	23.65 ± 2.12	-1.27	0.013*
1-PTV incisal (mm)	63.78 ± 6.35	52.45 ± 4.18	-11.33	0.003*
1-PTV apical (mm)	51.71 ± 4.57	43.30 ± 5.17	-8.41	0.013*
FMA (degrees)	23.81 ± 5.11	23.28 ± 5.13	-0.53	0.458
PFH/AFH (mm)	0.63 ± 0.07	0.64 ± 0.08	0.01	0.258
ANB (degrees)	4.10 ± 1.71	2.61 ± 1.38	-1.49	0.006*
Wits (mm)	-0.20 ± 4.57	-0.50 ± 5.05	-0.30	0.752
1.NA (degrees)	27.96 ± 10.67	20.99 ± 4.08	-6.97	0.136
H-11 (mm)	20.51 ± 1.98	19.09 ± 2.09	-1.42	0.399
UA+UP (mm)	18.11 ± 8.95	13.53 ± 3.18	-4.58	0.133
UA cerv (mm)	0.84 ± 0.52	1.48 ± 0.40	0.64	0.025*
UP cerv (mm)	1.68 ± 0.91	0.28 ± 0.69	-1.40	0.001*
UA middle (mm)	0.61 ± 0.28	1.77 ± 1.43	1.16	0.077
UP middle (mm)	2.77 ± 1.64	1.15 ± 0.96	-1.62	0.005*
UA apical (mm)	1.31 ± 0.84	3.27 ± 3.44	1.96	0.170
UP apical (mm)	4.24 ± 2.45	2.69 ± 2.09	-1.55	0.200

*Statistically significant difference (P<0.05).

Table 5 - Comparison between initial (T₁) and final (T₂) stages of group 2, without extractions (dependent t tests).

Variables	Initial stage (T₁) n = 6 Mean ± SD	Final stage (T₂) n = 6 Mean ± SD	Changes T₂-T₁	p
Crown-root ratio (mm)	1.52 ± 0.16	1.43 ± 0.14	-0.09	0.013*
Length 11 (mm)	25.48 ± 2.17	24.59 ± 1.86	-0.89	0.005*
1-PTV incisal (mm)	55.65 ± 6.65	63.26 ± 6.00	7.61	0.142
1-PTV apical (mm)	36.66 ± 5.04	41.80 ± 4.04	5.14	0.138
FMA (degrees)	25.22 ± 5.02	23.16 ± 4.60	-2.06	0.015*
PFH/AFH (mm)	0.70 ± 0.06	0.72 ± 0.07	0.02	0.034*
ANB (degrees)	3.29 ± 2.98	2.82 ± 2.34	-0.47	0.482
Wits (mm)	-0.26 ± 5.12	-0.28 ± 5.51	0.02	0.986
1.NA (degrees)	21.06 ± 6.32	24.63 ± 6.61	3.57	0.007*
H-11 (mm)	18.05 ± 3.56	19.90 ± 3.27	1.85	0.267
UA+UP (mm)	13.46 ± 3.75	14.35 ± 4.89	0.89	0.662
UA cerv (mm)	0.67 ± 0.41	0.61 ± 0.57	-0.06	0.762
UP cerv (mm)	1.20 ± 0.49	0.53 ± 0.59	-0.67	0.132
UA middle (mm)	0.47 ± 0.30	0.63 ± 0.61	0.16	0.658
UP middle (mm)	2.01 ± 0.62	1.21 ± 0.81	-0.80	0.049*
UA apical (mm)	0.99 ± 0.36	0.99 ± 0.78	0.00	0.995
UP apical (mm)	3.03 ± 1.38	2.47 ± 1.28	-0.56	0.406

*Statistically significant difference (P<0.05).

Table 6 - Intergroup comparison of the studied variables at the final stage (T₂) (independent t tests).

Variables	G1 Extraction of #14 and #24 teeth n = 6 Mean ± SD	G2 Without extraction n = 6 Mean ± SD	p
Crown-root ratio (mm)	1.32 ± 0.25	1.43 ± 0.14	0.343
Length 11 (mm)	23.65 ± 2.12	24.59 ± 1.86	0.434
1-PTV incisal (mm)	52.45 ± 4.18	63.26 ± 6.00	0.004*
1-PTV apical (mm)	43.30 ± 5.17	41.80 ± 4.04	0.586
FMA (degrees)	23.28 ± 5.13	23.16 ± 4.60	0.968
PFH/AFH (mm)	0.64 ± 0.08	0.72 ± 0.07	0.133
ANB (degrees)	2.61 ± 1.38	2.82 ± 2.34	0.855
Wits (mm)	-0.50 ± 5.05	-0.28 ± 5.51	0.944
1.NA (degrees)	20.99 ± 4.08	24.63 ± 6.61	0.277
H-11 (mm)	19.09 ± 2.09	19.90 ± 3.27	0.621
UA+UP (mm)	13.53 ± 3.18	14.35 ± 4.89	0.738
UA cerv (mm)	1.48 ± 0.40	0.61 ± 0.57	0.012*
UP cerv (mm)	0.28 ± 0.69	0.53 ± 0.59	0.515
UA middle (mm)	1.77 ± 1.43	0.63 ± 0.61	0.103
UP middle (mm)	1.15 ± 0.96	1.21 ± 0.81	0.907
UA apical (mm)	3.27 ± 3.44	0.99 ± 0.78	0.146
UP apical (mm)	2.69 ± 2.09	2.47 ± 1.28	0.828

*Statistically significant difference (P < 0.05).

Table 7 - Intergroup comparison of the studied variables concerning treatment changes (T₂-T₁) (independent t tests).

Variables	G1 Extraction of #14 and #24 teeth n = 6 Mean ± SD	G2 Without extraction n = 6 Mean ± SD	p
Crown-root ratio (mm)	-0.12 ± 0.07	-0.08 ± 0.05	0.402
Length 11 (mm)	-1.26 ± 0.82	-0.89 ± 0.46	0.359
1-PTV incisal (mm)	-11.33 ± 5.44	7.61 ± 10.73	0.003*
1-PTV apical (mm)	-8.40 ± 5.48	5.13 ± 7.15	0.004*
FMA (degrees)	-0.53 ± 1.62	-2.05 ± 1.40	0.113
PFH/AFH (mm)	0.00 ± 0.01	0.02 ± 0.01	0.209
ANB (degrees)	-1.48 ± 0.82	-0.47 ± 1.52	0.182
Wits (mm)	-0.29 ± 2.18	-0.01 ± 2.23	0.830
1.NA (degrees)	-6.97 ± 9.62	3.57 ± 2.04	0.025*
H-11 (mm)	-1.42 ± 3.79	1.85 ± 3.63	0.157
UA+UP (mm)	-4.58 ± 6.27	0.88 ± 4.66	0.117
UA cerv (mm)	0.63 ± 0.49	-0.06 ± 0.47	0.031*
UP cerv (mm)	-1.39 ± 0.51	-0.66 ± 0.90	0.113
UA middle (mm)	1.15 ± 1.27	0.16 ± 0.86	0.145
UP middle (mm)	-1.62 ± 0.86	-0.80 ± 0.76	0.111
UA apical (mm)	1.95 ± 2.98	0.00 ± 0.74	0.151
UP apical (mm)	-1.54 ± 2.57	-0.56 ± 1.51	0.436

*Statistically significant difference (P < 0.05).

Table 8 - Intergroup comparison of external root resorption (ERR) variable at initial and final stages as well as treatment changes (Mann-Whitney).

Variable	G1 Extractions of #14 and #24 teeth n = 6	G2 Without extractions n = 6	p
	Mean ± SD	Mean ± SD	
ERR T_1	0,16 ± 0,40	0,16 ± 0,40	1,000
ERR T_2	1,50 ± 1,04	1,00 ± 0,00	0,336
ERR T_{2-1}	1,33 ± 0,81	0,83 ± 0,40	0,240

the occurrence of unfavorable sequelae to orthodontic movement, especially fenestration, bone dehiscence and root resorption. This information can influence the patient's treatment planning which, prior to orthodontic treatment, can be diagnosed as unfavorable to great teeth movement. The tridimensional analysis provided by computed tomography is of great importance for an accurate assessment of craniofacial morphology because through this examination, it is possible to obtain more reliable information on the dimensions and levels of facial bone tissues when compared to traditional bidimensional examinations. Moreover, CT is considered as a noninvasive, fast, high-accurate diagnosis method.[7,12,13]

It is important to underline the difficulty and the merit of obtaining a sample comprising 12 patients not only examined with lateral cephalograms, computed tomographies and periapical radiographs at the beginning of the treatment and after 18 months, but also who meet the aforementioned inclusion criteria of this study methodology. As the study was accomplished using CT, which is difficult to be obtained due to the cost and the ethical question concerning radiation exposure, the sample of 12 patients,, is considered acceptable.

Methods

Measurements were performed on the maxillary central incisor because this is the tooth that shows more resorption during orthodontic movement.[14,15] Periapical radiograph was the examination chosen to evaluate root resorption because it presents less distortion and more details when compared to panoramic radiograph and lateral cephalograms.[11]

Lateral cephalograms were used to obtain standard cephalometric measurements as well as to measure the alveolar thickness at the apical area of the right maxillary central incisor from a linear distance traced parallel to the palatal plane extending from labial to palatal cortical plate.[5]

Computed tomography was performed by two different radiology centers, by the same examiner in each one of them. CTs were obtained during T_1 (the beginning of the orthodontic treatment) and T_2 (after tooth extraction space closure). CT scans were used to evaluate bone thickness at the cervical, middle and apical thirds of the root of the right maxillary central incisor, tracing three lines parallel to the ECJ plane at a 3 mm interval. These measurements aimed to identify lack of bone tissue which may indicate fenestration or bone dehiscence. Fenestration is the lack of bone tissue in a restricted area of the tooth root[16] while dehiscence occurs when the lack of bone involves the alveolar bone ridge.[16]

Results

The results demonstrate that there was no difference between genders, i.e., the intergroup comparison showed compatibility regarding the number of males and females in each group. Additionally, there was no difference concerning the variables "age" and "treatment period". Considering the variable "malocclusion type", the samples were not compatible at the beginning of the treatment. G1 exhibited 3 patients with Class II malocclusion which did not influence the results of this study because the objective was to evaluate the changes in bone thickness at incisors area during the retraction of the anterior teeth, i.e., the importance was in performing or not the retraction of the anterior teeth regardless of the malocclusion type.

Regarding the variables studied during T_1, only 1-PTV demonstrated statistically significant difference. This occurred because G2 presented less protrusion of maxillary anterior teeth when compared to G1. This result was already expected, since great dentoalveolar protrusion of G1 patients probably influenced the decision to perform teeth extraction in this group. Premolar extractions have been frequently employed aiming to reduce dentoalveolar protrusion.[17]

During treatment, G1 (with extractions) underwent changes in the crown-root ratio, maxillary incisor length, 1-PTV incisal, 1-PTV apical and in the maxillomandibular relationship. These changes were expected due to premolar extractions and space closure caused by retraction of the maxillary anterior teeth.[18] Alveolar bone thickness at the labial cervical third (UL cervical) significantly increased. Bone thickness decreased at the palatal cervical and middle thirds (UP cervical and UP middle).

As Handelman[5] reported, tooth movement can alter the distance between alveolar cortical plates in relation to the roots of the orthodontically moved teeth, i.e., the antero-posterior movement of the incisors can lead to bone loss in the direction of the movement.[19]

The changes occurring in G2 (without extractions), during the treatment phase, were significant in the following variables: crown-root ratio, incisor length, FMA, PFH-AFH, 1.NA, and UP middle. Similarly to G1, there were significant root resorptions in the studied teeth due to tooth movement during treatment.[20,21] The maxillary incisors presented significant vestibulariza-tion. This occurred for two main reasons: the incisors alignment that were slightly crowded and the Curve of Spee flatting during treatment.

At the final stage (T_2), the results of the studied variables indicated a statistically significant difference in two variables: 1-PTV incisal and UL cervical. At this stage, 1-PTV incisal of G2 was greater than 1-PTV incisal of G1, indicating that in G2, the maxillary central incisors were more protruded at the end of the treatment than those of G1. This occurred due to the sum of the statistically significant retraction (1-PTV incisal and 1-PTV apical) suffered by the incisors of G1 and the vestibu-larization (1.NA) suffered by the incisors of G2 during the treatment period (Tables 4 and 5). UL cervical also presented a statistically significant difference between Groups at T_2. The maxillary incisors of G1 presented a statistically significant decrease of the labial alveolar bone thickness at the cervical third in relation to the maxillary incisors of G2. This effect occurred because G1 (with extractions) underwent maxillary incisors re-traction during treatment and G2 (without extractions) presented only vestibularization of these teeth.

The intergroup comparison concerning the variables changes occurring as a result of the treatment (Table 7) demonstrates that 1-PTV incisal and 1-PTV apical ex-hibited statistically significant differences. With regard to the 1-PTV incisal, the group with extractions pre-sented a maxillary incisor retraction of 11.33 mm while the group without extractions presented a protraction of 7.61 mm. In respect to 1-PTV apical, the group with extractions presented a maxillary incisor retrac-tion of 8.40 mm while the group without extractions presented a protraction of 5.13 mm. The sum of these changes resulted in the statistically differences showed by these variables in relation to these groups of study.

Such differences have already been proved by several previous studies comparing dentoskeletal changes be-tween extraction and nonextraction cases.[22,23,24]

The inclination of the incisors evaluated by the variable 1.NA also underwent a statistically signifi-cant difference between groups. While in G1 the inci-sors showed a palatal change of 6.97°, in G2, without extractions, the incisors were vestibularized in 3.57°. This result was expected, since G1 presented retraction of maxillary incisors during the extraction space closure and G2 had these teeth vestibularized by the alignment and leveling of the teeth that presented mild crowding and overbite, as described above.

According to Lupi, Handelman and Sadowsky,[25] both the treatment carried out with extractions and the amount of force used for orthodontic movement may influence alveolar bone loss. These authors also claim that bone de-hiscence and fenestration have been reported when the in-cisors are protracted or retracted; maxillary incisor protrac-tion produces a dehiscence in labial alveolar bone while its retraction affects the palatal alveolar ridge.[25]

The change in UL cervical also showed a significant difference between groups. In G1, labial bone thickness at the cervical area presented an increase of 0.67 mm while in G2 bone thickness decreased 0.06 mm. These changes were also expected due to the same aforemen-tioned reasons. The other variables analyzed on CT scans, aiming to assess the alveolar bone thickness at other root areas, did not undergo any significant chang-es between groups, therefore demonstrating strong evi-dence that the alveolar cortical plates could be submit-ted to re-anatomization, modifying their shape and po-sition.[2,26] These results do not agree with the hypothesis of Hadelman regarding the limitation of tooth move-ment by alveolar cortical plates,[5] showing that alveolar bone remodeling is possible during tooth movement induced by biological forces.[2,26]

External root resorption

External root resorption is one of the consequences caused by orthodontic movement. This study evalu-ated the degree of external root resorption through the scores proposed by Levander and Malmgren in 1988.[11] According to Cheng et al[27] one of the biological factors influencing inflammatory root resorption during orth-odontic movement is the root morphology, moreover, age, gender, metabolism velocity and tooth anomaly, factors which the clinician cannot control, also influence inflammatory root resorption during orthodontic movement. Factors related to the treatment are: amount of movement, treatment time and the magnitude of the applied force.[28,29]

This study did not find statistically significant differences in root resorption between the groups, however, it is not advisable to affirm that these resorptions did not occur or were not clinically important. According to some authors, patients submitted to retraction of anterior teeth through lingual root torque presenting low bone thickness, i.e., small alveolar width, clinically demonstrate a decrease in alveolar bone thickness and a greater tendency towards external root resorption.[2,30]

CONCLUSIONS

There were no changes in alveolar bone thickness when extractions and nonextraction cases were compared, except for labial alveolar bone thickness at the cervical third of the maxillary incisors.

REFERENCES

1. Krishnan V, Davidovitch Z. Cellular, molecular, and tissue-level reactions to orthodontic force. Am J Orthod Dentofacial Orthop. 2006;129(4):469-e1-32.
2. Vardimon AD, Oren E, Ben-Bassat Y. Cortical bone remodeling/tooth movement ratio during maxillary incisor retraction with tip versus torque movements. Am J Orthod Dentofacial Orthop. 1998;114(5):520-9.
3. Artun J, Krogstad O. Periodontal status of mandibular incisors following excessive proclination. A study in adults with surgically treated mandibular prognathism. Am J Orthod Dentofacial Orthop. 1987;91(3):225-32.
4. Yared KF, Zenobio EG, Pacheco W. Periodontal status of mandibular central incisors after orthodontic proclination in adults. Am J Orthod Dentofacial Orthop. 2006;130(1):6 e1-8.
5. Handelman CS. The anterior alveolus: its importance in limiting orthodontic treatment and its influence on the occurrence of iatrogenic sequelae. Angle Orthod. 1996;66(2):95-109; discussion 109-10.
6. Karring T, Nyman S, Thilander B, Magnusson I. Bone regeneration in orthodontically produced alveolar bone dehiscences. J Periodontal Res. 1982 May;17(3):309-15.
7. Garcia R, Claro C, Chagas R, Almeida G. Espessura do processo alveolar da região anterior da maxila e mandíbula em pacientes com discrepância óssea ântero-posterior. Rev Dental Press Ortod Ortop Facial. 2005;10(5):137-48.
8. Kim HJ, Yun HS, Park HD, Kim DH, Park YC. Soft-tissue and cortical-bone thickness at orthodontic implant sites. Am J Orthod Dentofacial Orthop. 2006;130(2):177-82.
9. Capelozza Filho L, Fattori L, Maltagliati LA. Um novo método para avaliar as inclinações dentárias utilizando a tomografia computadorizada. Rev Dental Press Ortod Ortop Facial. 2005;10(5):23-9.
10. De Vos W, Casselman J, Swennen GR. Cone-beam computerized tomography (CBCT) imaging of the oral and maxillofacial region: a systematic review of the literature. Int J Oral Maxillofac Surg. 2009;38(6):609-25.
11. Levander E, Malmgren O. Evaluation of the risk of root resorption during orthodontic treatment: a study of upper incisors. Eur J Orthod. 1988;10(1):30-8.
12. Consolaro A. Tomografia volumétrica (Odontológica) versus helicoidal (Médica) no planejamento ortodôntico e no diagnóstico das reabsorções dentárias. Rev Clín Ortod Dental Press. 2007;6(4):108-11.
13. Rodrigues AF, Vitral RWF. Aplicações da tomografia computadorizada na Odontologia. Pesq Bras Odontoped Clín Integrada. 2007;7:317-24.
14. Parker RJ, Harris EF. Directions of orthodontic tooth movements associated with external apical root resorption of the maxillary central incisor. Am J Orthod Dentofacial Orthop. 1998;114(6):677-83.
15. Janson G, De Luca Canto G, Martins D, Henriques J, De Freitas M. A radiographic comparison of apical root resorption after orthodontic treatment with 3 different fixed appliance techniques. Am J Orthod Dentofacial Orthop. 2000;118(3):262-73.
16. Carranza F, Newman M, Takei H. Periodontia clínica. 9a ed. Rio de Janeiro: Guanabara Koogan; 2002.
17. Baumrind S, Korn EL, Boyd RL, Maxwell R. The decision to extract: part II. Analysis of clinicians stated reasons for extraction. Am J Orthod Dentofacial Orthop. 1996;109(4):393-402.

18. Luppanapornlarp S, Johnston LE Jr. The effects of premolar-extraction: a long-term comparison of outcomes in "clear-cut" extraction and nonextraction Class II patients. Angle Orthod. 1993;63(4):257-72.
19. Wehrbein H, Bauer W, Diedrich P. Mandibular incisors, alveolar bone, and symphysis after orthodontic treatment. A retrospective study. Am J Orthod Dentofacial Orthop. 1996;110(3):239-46.
20. Consolaro A. Reabsorção dentária na movimentação ortodôntica. In: Reabsorções dentárias nas especialidades clínicas. 1a ed. Maringá: Dental Press; 2002. p. 259-89.
21. Marques LS, Ramos-Jorge ML, Rey AC, Armond MC, Ruellas AC. Severe root resorption in orthodontic patients treated with the edgewise method: prevalence and predictive factors. Am J Orthod Dentofacial Orthop. 2010;137(3):384-8.
22. Basciftci FA, Usumez S. Effects of extraction and nonextraction treatment on Class I and Class II subjects. Angle Orthod. 2003;73(1):36-42.
23. Kocadereli I. Changes in soft tissue profile after orthodontic treatment with and without extractions. Am J Orthod Dentofacial Orthop. 2002;122(1):67-72.
24. Rains MD, Nanda R. Soft-tissue changes associated with maxillary incisor retraction. Am J Orthod. 1982;81(6):481-8.
25. Lupi JE, Handelman CS, Sadowsky C. Prevalence and severity of apical root resorption and alveolar bone loss in orthodontically treated adults. Am J Orthod Dentofacial Orthop. 1996;109(1):28-37.
26. Meikle MC. The dentomaxillary complex and overjet correction in Class II, division 1 malocclusion: objectives of skeletal and alveolar remodeling. Am J Orthod. 1980;77(2):184-97.
27. Cheng LL, Turk T, Elekdag-Turk S, Jones AS, Petocz P, Darendeliler MA. Physical properties of root cementum: Part 13. Repair of root resorption 4 and 8 weeks after the application of continuous light and heavy forces for 4 weeks: a microcomputed-tomography study. Am J Orthod Dentofacial Orthop. 2009;136(3):320 e1-10; discussion -1.
28. Brezniak N, Wasserstein A. Orthodontically induced inflammatory root resorption. Part I: The basic science aspects. Angle Orthod. 2002;72(2):175-9.
29. Mirabella AD, Artun J. Risk factors for apical root resorption of maxillary anterior teeth in adult orthodontic patients. Am J Orthod Dentofacial Orthop. 1995;108(1):48-55.
30. Horiuchi A, Hotokezaka H, Kobayashi K. Correlation between cortical plate proximity and apical root resorption. Am J Orthod Dentofacial Orthop. 1998;114(3):311-8.

15

Immediate periodontal bone plate changes induced by rapid maxillary expansion in the early mixed dentition: CT findings

Daniela Gamba Garib[1], Maria Helena Ocké Menezes[2], Omar Gabriel da Silva Filho[3], Patricia Bittencourt Dutra dos Santos[4]

Objective: This study aimed at evaluating buccal and lingual bone plate changes caused by rapid maxillary expansion (RME) in the mixed dentition by means of computed tomography (CT). **Methods:** The sample comprised spiral CT exams taken from 22 mixed dentition patients from 6 to 9 years of age (mean age of 8.1 years) presenting constricted maxillary arch treated with Haas-type expanders. Patients were submitted to spiral CT scan before expansion and after the screw activation period with a 30-day interval between T1 and T2. Multiplanar reconstruction was used to measure buccal and lingual bone plate thickness and buccal bone crest level of maxillary posterior deciduous and permanent teeth. Changes induced by expansion were evaluated using paired t test (p < 0.05). **Results:** Thickness of buccal and lingual bone plates of posterior teeth remained unchanged during the expansion period, except for deciduous second molars which showed a slight reduction in bone thickness at the distal region of its buccal aspect. Buccal bone dehiscences were not observed in the supporting teeth after expansion. **Conclusion:** RME performed in mixed dentition did not produce immediate undesirable effects on periodontal bone tissues.

Keywords: Palatal expansion technique. Periodontium. Spiral computed tomography.

[1] Full professor, School of Dentistry — University of São Paulo/Bauru.(FOB-USP).
[2] MSc in Orthodontics, University São Paulo, UNICID.
[3] MSc in Orthodontics, São Paulo State University (UNESP).
[4] PhD resident in Applied Dental Sciences (FOB-USP).

» The authors report no commercial, proprietary or financial interest in the products or companies described in this article.

Daniela Gamba Garib
Faculdade de Odontologia de Bauru – Al. Octávio Pinheiro de Brisola 9-75
CEP: 17.012-901 – Bauru/SP – Brazil — E-mail: dgarib@uol.com.br

INTRODUCTION

During rapid maxillary expansion, orthopedic effect is produced by midpalatal suture splitting. Additionally, a dental effect characterized by buccal movement of supporting teeth is also produced.[19-22,27,33] As a result, maxillary posterior teeth are buccally displaced by an association of inclination and translation. The literature evinces that buccal tooth movement is associated with the occurrence of bone dehiscences. Engelking and Zachrisson,[15] Steiner et al,[28] Thilander et al[29] and Wennströn et al[32] conducted animal investigations and demonstrated that buccal tooth movement with mild forces increases the distance between the cementoenamel junction and the buccal alveolar crest. Wehrbein et al[31] reached a similar conclusion when conducting a cadaver study. Buccolingual tooth movement seems to occur through the alveolar bone and not along the bone. It leads to bone dehiscences in the short-term[15,28,29,31,32] and to gingival recession in the long-term.[1-4]

Recent studies conducted with CT have shown apical migration of buccal alveolar crest of posterior teeth after RME is performed in permanent dentition patients.[18,25] By means of CT methodology, Garib et al[18] assessed a sample of eight female adolescents before RME and after the removal of the expander following a 3-month retention period. The authors concluded that RME induced bone dehiscences on the buccal aspect of supporting teeth (first premolars and first molars), especially in subjects who initially presented thinner buccal bone plate. Rungcharassaeng et al[25] found similar results in a sample of thirty consecutive RME patients with a mean age of 13.8 years. Their findings included buccal bone loss in both horizontal and vertical dimensions for all posterior teeth after expansion, and displayed a significant correlation with age, amount of expansion and initial buccal bone thickness. Ballanti et al[8] observed, at the end of the active expansion phase, a significant decrease of buccal bone plate thickness of permanent maxillary first molars in a sample of 17 prepubertal patients with a mean age of 11.2 years. However, a tendency for partial recovery was found six months after expansion.

Buccal bone changes produced by rapid maxillary expansion in the permanent dentition raise the question about the periodontal effects of RME performed in the early phases of mixed dentition. During deciduous and early mixed dentitions, RME produces greater orthopedic effects[14,23] and transfers anchorage to deciduous molars and canines. A classic implant study showed that, in adolescents, skeletal effects corresponded to 35% of expansion, whereas dental effects accounted for 65%.[23] On the other hand, in young children, the proportion between skeletal and dental effects was 1:1. Baccetti et al[5] also observed that RME performed before the peak of skeletal maturation produced more skeletal effects than RME performed after the peak. Thus, the periodontal changes related to the orthodontic effect of RME in the early phases of mixed dentition deserve to be differentiated from those observed in late mixed dentition or even in permanent dentition. Therefore, the aim of this study was to investigate, by means of spiral CT, the periodontal bone changes of RME in early mixed dentition using deciduous teeth as anchorage.

MATERIAL AND METHODS

This study was approved by the School of Dentistry — University of São Paulo/Bauru Institutional Review Board. The sample comprised spiral CT exams taken from 22 orthodontic patients (10 males and 12 females) with mean initial age of 8.1 years (ranging from 6 to 9 years). The exams had been taken for a previous study,[13] in 2002, before CBCT was introduced in Brazil. In selecting the sample, the following inclusion criteria were applied: patients in early mixed dentition, and the presence of constricted maxillary arch with or without posterior crossbites. In the examined sample, all subjects were in the early transitional phase, as described by Van der Linden,[30] and either at stage CS1 or CS2 at the time of treatment.[6] In other words, patients were treated before or at the beginning of the pubertal growth spurt.

Maxillary expansion was performed with Haas-type expanders anchored exclusively on deciduous teeth (Fig 1). For all patients, maxillary deciduous second molars functioned as supporting teeth and received bands, whereas maxillary deciduous canines were bonded to a "C" shape anterior extension wire (Fig 1). The expansion screw was activated at two-quarter turns in the morning and two-quarter turns in the evening for approximately 8 days, reaching a mean opening of 7 mm.

All patients were submitted to computed tomography imaging before expansion and after the active expansion phase, with a mean interval of 30 days in between. A spiral computed tomography machine model Xvision EX (Toshiba Corporation Medical Systems Company,

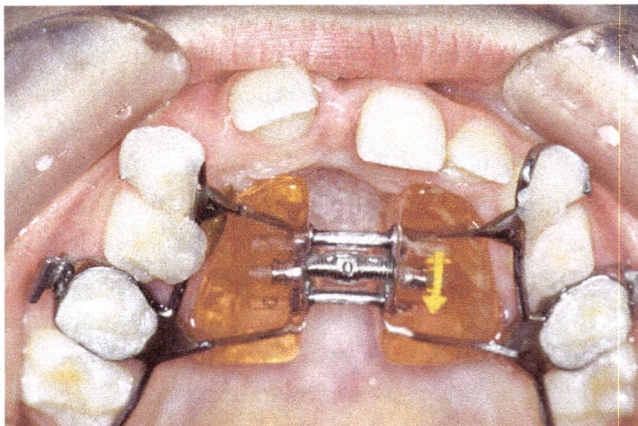

Figure 1 - Haas-type expander used in this study.

Otawara-Shi, Japan) was used at 120 kV and 100 mA, with a scanning time of one second per section. A FC 30 scanning filter, field of view (FOV) of 12.6 x 12.6 cm and matrix of 512 x 512 pixels was used. Window width was 2400 HU with a center of 1300 HU.

For standardization of head positioning in all three planes, the perpendicular light beam resource provided by the machine was used; thereby, allowing comparison of images obtained before and after expansion.[18, 19] For that purpose, patients were positioned with Camper's plane perpendicular to the ground, while the longitudinal light beam passed through the center of the glabella and the filtrum, and the transverse light beam passed through the lateral eye canthus. Teeth were kept apart in order

to avoid imaging the mandibular dental arch. One-millimeter thick axial sections were performed parallel to the palatal plane, including the dentoalveolar and basal areas of the maxilla, up to the lower third of the nasal cavity. The imaged area encompassed 36 to 40 mm, totalizing 36 to 40 sections. This protocol results in images with a spacial resolution that ranges from 0.2 to 0.5 mm.[17]

Data were transferred to a network computer workstation (Silicon Graphics, Toshiba Corporation Medical Systems Company, Otawara-Shi, Japan), using Alatoview software (Toshiba Corporation Medical Systems Company, Otawara-Shi, Japan) on which 2D reformatted images were generated and measured by the computerized method. The Allatoview software generates a very small ball size pointer for linear measurements.

Measurement of alveolar bone plate thickness of maxillary posterior teeth at the buccal and lingual aspects was conducted on two axial sections parallel to the palatal plane, one at the level of right maxillary permanent first molar furcation and another at the level of right maxillary deciduous second molar furcation (Figs 2 and 3). Measurements of alveolar bone thickness were performed on magnified images (4x), before and after expansion. Whenever tooth rotations were present, bone plate thickness was measured at the area where the root was closer to the external contour of the alveolar ridge.

Evaluation of the buccal alveolar bone crest level of maxillary posterior teeth was conducted by means

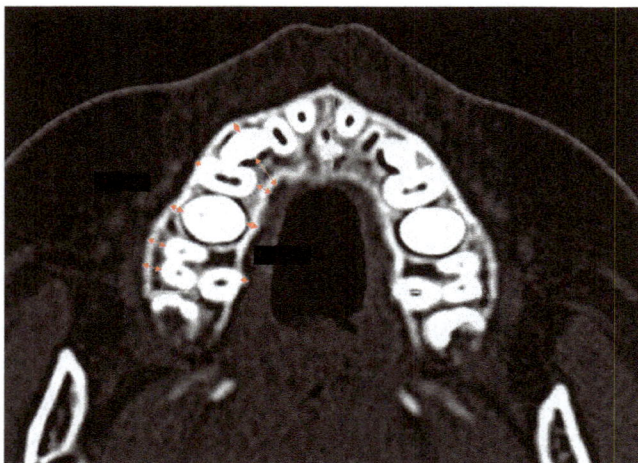

Figure 2 - Measurements of buccal and lingual bone plate thickness (BBPT and LBPT) of permanent erupted and non-erupted posterior teeth were performed in the axial section, parallel to the palatal plane, passing at the level of right maxillary permanent first molar furcation.

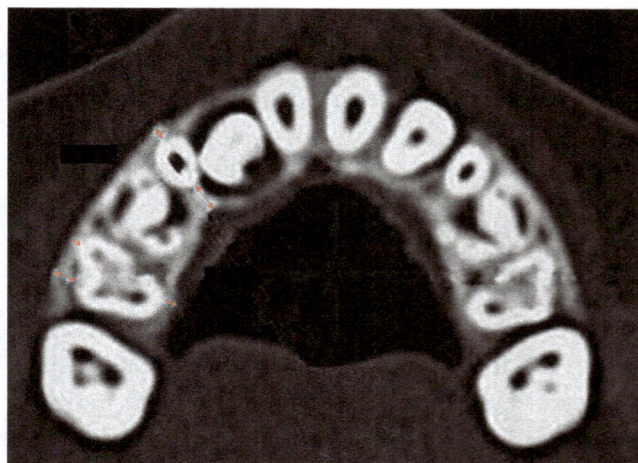

Figure 3 - Measurements of buccal and lingual bone plate thickness (BBPT and LBPT) of deciduous posterior teeth were performed in the axial section, parallel to the palatal plane, passing at the level of right maxillary deciduous second molar furcation.

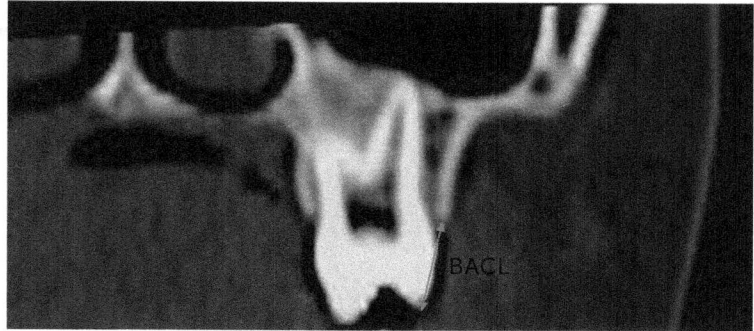

Figure 4 - Measurement of maxillary posterior teeth buccal alveolar crest level. BACL: buccal alveolar crest level measured from the buccal cusp tip to the buccal alveolar crest.

of orthoradially reformatted images perpendicular to the contour of the dental arch (cross sections), passing through the center of the buccal aspect of the deciduous canines, deciduous first molar and through the center, mesial and distal areas of the buccal aspect of deciduous second molars and permanent first molars. Figure 4 illustrates the linear variable obtained on each of these eight images both before and after expansion.

Statistical analyses

All measurements were performed twice within a monthly interval by the same calibrated examiner. Statistical analysis was performed taking into account the mean of these two measurements. Each tooth category corresponded to the mean of right and left side teeth. Mean and standard deviation of each variable were calculated before and after expansion, and so were the changes between these stages. An exploratory test revealed normal distribution of data. Therefore, dependent t-tests were used to compare inter-phase changes. Sample size calculation (with an alfa value of 0.05 and statistical power of 90%) revealed that a sample size of 23 was more than enough. Results were regarded as significant for p < 0.05.

Systemic and casual errors

Casual and systematic errors were calculated by comparing the first and second measurements with Dahlberg's formula and dependent t-test respectively, at a significance level of 5%.

RESULTS

The results of the error of the method are shown in Table 1. Two out of 22 variables had a statistically significant systematic error (LBPT of the permanent first molars and BABCL at the center of deciduous second molars — as shown in Figures 2 and 4). Casual errors ranged from 0.11 (BBPT at the distal region of permanent first molars) to 0.52 (BBPT at the mesial region of permanent first molars).

Buccal and lingual bone plate thickness (BBPT and LBPT)

Table 2 shows that buccal bone plate thickness of supporting teeth was not significantly changed by RME. Additionally, no changes were observed in the buccal bone plate thickness of tooth germs and permanent first molars (Table 2). The only exceptions were the buccal bone plate of first premolar germ which showed a statistically significant decrease (mean of 0.18 mm), and the buccal bone plate of deciduous second molar which showed a statistically significant decrease at the distal region (mean of 0.3 mm).

No changes were observed for the lingual bone plate thickness of deciduous and permanent teeth (Table 2).

Buccal alveolar bone crest level (BABCL)

No statistically significant changes were observed in the level of buccal alveolar bone crest of supporting teeth (deciduous canines and deciduous second molars) and permanent first molars (Table 3).

Table 1 - Systematic and casual errors (dependent t-tests and Dalhberg's formula).

Variables	First Mean ± SD	Second Mean ± SD	t	p	Dalhberg
Buccal bone plate thickness (BBPT)					
Permanent canine germ	1.54 ± 0.60	1.52 ± 0.59	0.260	0.798	0.21
1st premolar germ	0.97 ± 0.46	0.95 ± 0.42	0.356	0.727	0.12
2nd premolar germ	2.10 ± 1.01	2.15 ± 1.17	-0.612	0.549	0.25
Deciduous canine	1.13 ± 0.64	1.15 ± 0.68	0.74	0.463	0.12
Deciduous 2nd molar/mesial	1.11 ± 0.58	1.14 ± 0.59	0.91	0.367	0.12
Deciduous 2nd molar/distal	1.72 ± 0.70	1.75 ± 0.67	0.95	0.349	0.15
Permanent 1st molar/mesial	2.96 ± 1.21	2.77 ± 1.21	1.121	0.277	0.52
Permanent 1st molar/distal	2.92 ± 0.88	2.87 ± 0.90	1.334	0.200	0.11
Lingual bone plate thickness (LBPT)					
Permanent canine germ	5.60 ± 2.03	5.72 ± 2.07	-1.170	0.259	0.30
1st premolar germ	3.09 ± 0.97	3.03 ± 1.05	0.637	0.534	0.29
2nd premolar germ	2.71 ± 1.05	2.74 ± 1.02	-0.421	0.680	0.16
Deciduous canine	4.73 ± 1.58	4.79 ± 1.61	1.955	0.057	0.16
Deciduous 2nd molar	1.16 ± 0.55	1.18 ± 0.55	0.64	0.527	0.11
Permanent 1st molar	1.41 ± 0.57	1.30 ± 0.61	3.082	0.007*	0.13
Buccal alveolar crest level (BACL)					
Deciduous canine	9.14 ± 2.02	9.28 ± 2.12	-0.690	0.512	0.39
Deciduous 1st molar	7.66 ± 1.16	7.67 ± 1.18	-0.031	0.976	0.27
Deciduous 2nd molar/mesial	7.72 ± 1.40	7.72 ± 1.44	-0.026	0.980	0.35
Deciduous 2nd molar/center	7.80 ± 0.45	7.98 ± 0.40	-2.545	0.020 *	0.24
Deciduous 2nd molar/distal	8.10 ± 0.58	8.03 ± 0.62	1.108	0.284	0.18
Permanent 1st molar/mesial	8.39 ± 1.24	8.50 ± 1.08	-1.130	0.275	0.29
Permanent 1st molar/center	7.64 ± 1.02	7.71 ± 1.21	-0.725	0.479	0.27
Permanent 1st molar/distal	7.79 ± 0.88	7.79 ± 0.90	0.000	1.000	0.22

*Statistically significant at $P < 0.05$

Table 2 - Buccal and lingual bone plate thickness expansion changes (Paired t test).

Variables	n	Pre-expansion Mean ± SD		Postexpansion Mean ± SD		Changes	t	p
Buccal bone plate thickness (BBPT)								
Permanent canine germ	23	1.32	0.55	1.31	0.71	-0.01	0.109	0.914
1st Premolar germ	17	0.92	0.41	1.10	0.37	-0.18	-3.318	0.004*
2nd Premolar Germ								
Canine	20	2.33	1.08	2.28	1.14	-0.05	0.572	0.574
Deciduous canine	20	1.20	0.82	1.03	0.38	-0.17	0.913	0.373
Deciduous 2nd molar/mesial	19	1.14	0.50	1.06	0.63	-0.09	0.785	0.443
Deciduous 2nd molar/distal	19	1.89	0.69	1.59	0.68	-0.30	2.494	0.023 *
Permanent 1st molar/mesial	22	3.21	1.20	2.90	1.32	-0.31	1.478	0.154
Permanent 1st molar/distal	22	3.01	0.75	2.95	0.81	-0.05	0.823	0.420
Lingual bone plate thickness (LBPT)								
Permanent canine germ	19	5.81	2.07	5.47	1.98	-0.34	1.627	0.121
1st premolar germ	17	3.46	1.30	3.36	1.15	-0.10	0.580	0.570
2nd premolar germ	18	2.81	1.14	2.85	1.02	0.04	-0.331	0.744
Deciduous canine	21	4.77	1.72	4.81	1.54	0.04	-0.200	0.844
Deciduous 2nd molar	17	1.26	0.53	1.19	0.55	-0.07	0.714	0.486
Permanent 1st molar	20	1.34	0.59	1.42	0.66	0.08	-1.128	0.273

*Statistically significant at $P < 0.05$

Table 3 - Buccal alveolar crest level (BACL) expansion changes (Paired t test).

Variables	n	Pre-expansion Mean ± SD	Postexpansion Mean ± SD	Change	t	p
Deciduous canine	17	9.02 ± 2.67	8.01 ± 3.55	-1.01	0.934	0.364
Deciduous 1st molar	20	7.32 ± 2.06	7.31 ± 2.07	-0.01	0.088	0.931
Deciduous 2nd molar/mesial	18	7.82 ± 0.67	7.60 ± 1.19	-0.22	0.863	0.400
Deciduous 2nd molar/center	22	7.73 ± 0.57	8.03 ± 0.77	0.30	-1.810	0.085
Deciduous 2nd molar/cistal	20	7.82 ± 1.25	8.30 ± 0.93	0.48	-1.714	0.103
Permanent 1st molar/mesial	20	8.31 ± 1.19	8.27 ± 0.80	-0.04	0.190	0.851
Permanent 1st molar/center	21	7.68 ± 0.96	7.59 ± 1.10	-0.09	0.474	0.640
Permanent 1st molar/distal	19	7.91 ± 0.92	7.81 ± 0.84	-0.10	0.495	0.627

*Statistically significant at P < 0.05

DISCUSSION

Spiral CT proves valuable in assessing alveolar bone thickness and level . Fuhrmann et al[16] demonstrated that buccal and lingual bone plates can be identified in spiral CT images provided that they are at least 0.5 mm thick. On the other hand, when the periodontal ligament space is apparent, CT identifies even thinner buccal and lingual bone plates (0.2 mm). Measurements taken with spiral CT showed high accuracy and precision.[10,11] While periapical radiographs underestimate horizontal alveolar bone defects in 0.6 to 2.2 mm, spiral CT overestimate them in 0.2 mm.[17] Moreover, previous studies measuring alveolar bone plate thickness and level in spiral CT showed high reproducibility and no-significant errors.[8,18,24]

This study assessed the changes in alveolar bone thickness and level at the region of maxillary posterior teeth after RME was performed during early mixed dentition. The comparison between initial and post expansion CT images was possible due to standardization of head positioning during the exam associated with selection of standardized image sections for measurements. Molar furcation was used as reference to obtain standardized axial sections before and after expansion. This region is relatively stable, since — in reference to the palatal plane — posterior tooth extrusion is very small during RME and may be compensated by tooth buccal tipping.[9]

With regard to changes in buccal bone plate thickness of supporting teeth, deciduous canines, which received a bonded C wire extension, did not reveal reduction in BBPT after expansion (Table 2). Conversely, deciduous second molars, which received bands, showed statistically significant reduction in buccal bone plate thickness at the distal region after expansion, while the mesial aspect of buccal bone plate remained stable (Table 2).

The mean decrease in thickness of the distal aspect of buccal bone plate of deciduous second molars was 0.3 mm. Although statistically significant, this reduction was of lesser magnitude than the reduction in BBPT observed for permanent first molars when RME is performed in permanent dentition.[18,25]

RME performed in mixed dentition and anchored exclusively in deciduous teeth produces permanent first molar expansion of one-half the amount of screw expansion, following the orthopedic effect of basal bones.[12] In this study, palatal wire extension was used at permanent first molars and probably produced further orthodontic effect in this region. However, results revealed that buccal bone plate of permanent first molars did not undergo any changes (Table 2). Previous studies assessing changes in buccal bone plate thickness of posterior teeth after rapid maxillary expansion were performed in permanent dentition[18,25] or in late mixed and permanent dentitions.[8] In these previous studies, only permanent teeth were analyzed.[8] Garib et al[18] reported a significant decrease in buccal bone plate thickness of banded supporting teeth (first premolars and permanent first molars) that ranged from 0.6 to 0.9 mm, three months after expansion. Rungcharassaeng et al[25] corroborated the findings by Garib et al[18] and showed a significant decrease in buccal bone plate thickness of first premolars, second premolars and permanent first molars, with an average of 1.1 mm, 0.8 mm and 1.2 mm, respectively, three months after expansion. Ballanti et al[8] assessed a sample of young patients aged between 8 to 14 years old, and reported a significant decrease in buccal bone plate thickness of supporting maxillary permanent first molars immediately after the active phase of RME. The mean decrease was less than 0.5 mm and tended to recover six months after expansion.

The effects of RME on mixed dentition are similar to the effects observed in permanent dentition, including an orthopedic effect represented by midpalatal suture split and an orthodontic effect represented by buccal movement of posterior teeth.[13,14] The V shaped maxillary split observed after RME, in both occlusal and frontal planes during permanent dentition, is also observed during mixed dentition.[13,14] However, maxillary halves separation is greater in mixed dentition and corresponds to 50% of screw activation, while in permanent dentition it corresponds to approximately 30% of screw activation.[23] Consequently, the amount of orthodontic effect decreases in mixed dentition in comparison to permanent dentition. Considering that periodontal bone changes are related to tooth movement in the alveolar ridge, it would be expected that RME during the mixed dentition causes less changes in buccal bone plate thickness, as confirmed in this study.

Lingual bone plate thickness (LBPT) of supporting teeth and permanent first molars did not change after RME (Table 2). A previous study performed in permanent dentition reported an increase in lingual bone thickness of posterior teeth after RME, thereby reflecting the buccal movement of these teeth.[18] This increase had a mean value of 0.7 to 1.4 mm, three months after expansion.[18] The absence of changes in lingual bone plate thickness in mixed dentition observed in this study can be explained by the smaller amount of orthodontic effects caused by RME during childhood.[5,23] Furtheremore, the relatively short interval between the first and second CT exam might have influenced the results. A previous study assessing patients in permanent and late mixed dentitions reported that lingual bone plate thickness of permanent first molars did not immediately change after the active phase of expansion; however, an increase was observed 6 months after RME.[8]

All patients comprising the sample had maxillary permanent canines and premolars unerupted when RME was performed. Thus, one of the goals of the present study was to observe the behavior of posterior tooth germs during expansion. Results showed that buccolingual position of posterior tooth germs is not affected by RME. Thickness of buccal and lingual bone plates of posterior tooth germs remained unchanged from T1 to T2 (Table 2).

Only the buccal bone plate of first premolars germs demonstrated a small decrease. Such decrease might be related to tooth eruption, although the mean decrease of 0.18 mm is not clinically relevant. It is interesting to note that a favorable side effect of RME in early mixed dentition consists in facilitating eruption of palatally displaced maxillary permanent canines.[7] This aspect can be regarded as a "bonus" of early expansion therapy at the maxillary arch.

The level of buccal alveolar crest of posterior teeth showed a slight reduction in the distal region of deciduous second molars, only; although changes were not statistically significant (Table 3). Results indicated that bone dehiscences did not occur immediately after RME in the early mixed dentition. In permanent dentition, Garib et al[18] found that banded teeth showed a significant reduction in buccal alveolar crest level, with a mean loss of 7 mm in the first premolar and 3.5 mm at the mesial aspect of first molars. Rungcharassaeng et al[25] observed significant vertical bone losses at the buccal aspect of all supporting teeth after RME in permanent dentition. The mean change in buccal crest level of first premolars, second premolars and first molars was 4.4, 1.3 and 2.9 mm, respectively.[25] Therefore, RME performed in early mixed dentition seems to preserve the integrity of buccal bone plate more than RME performed in permanent dentition. The possible explanation is that the reduced orthodontic effect of RME on mixed dentition in comparison to permanent dentition[5,23] is not enough for moving posterior teeth throughout the alveolar bone.

Evidence provided by current investigation suggests that early mixed dentition proves adequate to accomplish orthopedic expansion. In addition to good stability[26] and greater orthopedic effect,[5,23] RME performed in early mixed dentition may avoid collateral buccal bone changes that predispose gingival recession in the long-term.

CONCLUSION

RME performed in early mixed dentition did not produce immediate undesirable effects on alveolar bone morphology of maxillary posterior teeth, mainly in terms of bone dehiscences and decrease in buccal bone plate thickness.

REFERENCES

1. Andlin-Sobocki A, Bodin L. Dimensional alterations of the gingiva related to changes of facial/lingual tooth position in permanent anterior teeth of children. A 2-year longitudinal study. J Clin Periodontol. 1993;20(3):219-24.

2. Andlin-Sobocki A, Persson M. The association between spontaneous reversal of gingival recession in mandibular incisors and dentofacial changes in children. A 3-year longitudinal study. Eur J Orthod. 1994;16(3):229-39.

3. Artun J, Grobety D. Periodontal status of mandibular incisors after pronounced orthodontic advancement during adolescence: a follow-up evaluation. Am J Orthod Dentofacial Orthop. 2001;119(1):2-10.

4. Artun J, Krogstad O. Periodontal status of mandibular incisors following excessive proclination. A study in adults with surgically treated mandibular prognathism. Am J Orthod Dentofacial Orthop. 1987;91(3):225-32.

5. Baccetti T, Franchi L, Cameron CG, McNamara JA Jr. Treatment timing for rapid maxillary expansion. Angle Orthod. 2001;71(5):343-50.

6. Baccetti T, Franchi L, McNamara JA Jr. An improved version of the cervical vertebral maturation (CVM) method for the assessment of mandibular growth. Angle Orthod. 2002;72(4):316-23.

7. Baccetti T, Mucedero M, Leonardi M, Cozza P. Interceptive treatment of palatal impaction of maxillary canines with rapid maxillary expansion: a randomized clinical trial. Am J Orthod Dentofacial Orthop. 2009;136(5):657-61.

8. Ballanti F, Lione R, Fanucci E, Franchi L, Baccetti T, Cozza P. Immediate and post-retention effects of rapid maxillary expansion investigated by computed tomography in growing patients. Angle Orthod. 2009;79(1):24-9.

9. Byrum AG Jr. Evaluation of anterior-posterior and vertical skeletal change vs. dental change in rapid palatal expansion cases as studied by lateral cephalograms. Am J Orthod. 1971;60(4):419.

10. Cavalcanti MG, Yang J, Ruprecht A, Vannier MW. Accurate linear measurements in the anterior maxilla using orthoradially reformatted spiral computed tomography. Dentomaxillofac Radiol. 1999;28(3):137-40.

11. Cavalcanti MG, Yang J, Ruprecht A, Vannier MW. Validation of spiral computed tomography for dental implants. Dentomaxillofac Radiol. 1998;27(6):329-33.

12. Cozzani M, Rosa M, Cozzani P, Siciliani G. Deciduous dentition-anchored rapid maxillary expansion in crossbite and non-crossbite mixed dentition patients: reaction of the permanent first molar. Prog Orthod. 2003;4:15-22.

13. Silva Filho OG, Lara TS, Almeida AM, Silva HC. Evaluation of the midpalatal suture during rapid palatal expansion in children: a CT study. J Clin Pediatr Dent. 2005;29(3):231-8.

14. Silva Filho OG, Montes LA, Torelly LF. Rapid maxillary expansion in the deciduous and mixed dentition evaluated through posteroanterior cephalometric analysis. Am J Orthod Dentofacial Orthop. 1995;107(3):268-75.

15. Engelking G, Zachrisson BU. Effects of incisor repositioning on monkey periodontium after expansion through the cortical plate. Am J Orthod. 1982;82(1):23-32.

16. Fuhrmann RA, Bucker A, Diedrich PR. Assessment of alveolar bone loss with high resolution computed tomography. J Periodontal Res. 1995;30(4):258-63.

17. Fuhrmann RA, Wehrbein H, Langen HJ, Diedrich PR. Assessment of the dentate alveolar process with high resolution computed tomography. Dentomaxillofac Radiol. 1995;24(1) 50-4.

18. Garib DG, Henriques JF, Janson G, Freitas MR, Fernandes AY. Periodontal effects of rapid maxillary expansion with tooth-tissue-borne and tooth-borne expanders: a computed tomography evaluation. Am J Orthod Dentofacial Orthop. 2006;129(6):749-58.

19. Garib DG, Henriques JF, Janson G, Freitas MR, Coelho RA. Rapid maxillary expansion--tooth tissue-borne versus tooth-borne expanders: a computed tomography evaluation of dentoskeletal effects. Angle Orthod. 2005;75(4):548-57.

20. Haas AJ. Palatal expansion: just the beginning of dentofacial orthopedics. Am J Orthod. 1970;57(3):219-55.

21. Haas AJ. Rapid expansion of the maxillary dental arch and nasal cavity by opening the midpalatal suture. Angle Orthod. 1963;31(2):73-90.

22. Haas AJ. The treatment of maxillary deficiency by opening the midpalatal suture. Angle Orthod. 1965;35(3):200-17.

23. Krebs A. Midpalatal suture expansion studies by the implant method over a seven-year period. Rep Congr Eur Orthod Soc. 1964;40:131-42.

24. Loubele M, Van Assche N, Carpentier K, Maes F, Jacobs R, van Steenberghe D, et al. Comparative localized linear accuracy of small-field cone-beam CT and multislice CT for alveolar bone measurements. Oral Surg Oral Med Oral Pathol Oral Radiol Endod. 2008;105(4):512-8.

25. Rungcharassaeng K, Caruso JM, Kan JY, Kim J, Taylor G. Factors affecting buccal bone changes of maxillary posterior teeth after rapid maxillary expansion. Am J Orthod Dentofacial Orthop. 2007;132(4):428.e1-8.

26. Spillane LM, McNamara JA Jr. Maxillary adaptation to expansion in the mixed dentition. Semin Orthod. 1995;1(3):176-87.

27. Starnbach H, Bayne D, Cleall J, Subtelny JD. Facioskeletal and dental changes resulting from rapid maxillary expansion. Angle Orthod. 1966;36(2):152-64.

28. Steiner GG, Pearson JK, Ainamo J. Changes of the marginal periodontium as a result of labial tooth movement in monkeys. J Periodontol. 1981;52(6):314-20.

29. Thilander B, Nyman S, Karring T, Magnusson I. Bone regeneration in alveolar bone dehiscences related to orthodontic tooth movements. Eur J Orthod. 1983;5(2):105-14.

30. Van der Linden FPGM. Development of the dentition. Chicago: Quintessence; 1983.

31. Wehrbein H, Fuhrmann RA, Diedrich PR. Periodontal conditions after facial root tipping and palatal root torque of incisors. Am J Orthod Dentofacial Orthop. 1994;106(5):455-62.

32. Wennstrom JL, Lindhe J, Sinclair F, Thilander B. Some periodontal tissue reactions to orthodontic tooth movement in monkeys. J Clin Periodontol. 1987;14(3):121-9.

33. Wertz RA. Skeletal and dental changes accompanying rapid midpalatal suture opening. Am J Orthod. 1970;58(1):41-66.

16

Facial height in Japanese-Brazilian descendants with normal occlusion

Fabiano Paiva Vieira[1], Arnaldo Pinzan[2], Guilherme Janson[3], Thais Maria Freire Fernandes[4], Renata Carvalho Sathler[5], Rafael Pinelli Henriques[6]

Objective: The aim of this study was to determine the standards of facial height in 30 young (14-year-old) Japanese-Brazilian descendants with normal occlusion, and assess whether sexual dimorphism is evident. **Methods:** The cephalometric measurements used followed the analyses by Wylie-Johnson, Siriwat-Jarabak, Gebeck, Merrifield and Horn. **Results:** Results showed dimorphism for total anterior facial height (TAFH), lower anterior facial height (LAFH), anterior facial height (AFH), total posterior facial height (TPFH) and upper posterior facial height (UPFH) measurements. **Conclusions:** The standards of facial heights in young Japanese-Brazilian descendants with normal occlusion were observed. Sexual dimorphism was identified in five out of thirteen evaluated variables at this age range.

Keywords: Orthodontics. Ethnic groups. Vertical dimension.

[1] Professor, Federal Institute of Paraná.
[2] Associate professor, Department of Pediatric Dentistry, Orthodontics and Collective Health, School of Dentistry — University of São Paulo/Bauru.
[3] Full professor, Department of Pediatric Dentistry, Orthodontics and Collective Health, School of Dentistry — University of São Paulo/Bauru.
[4] Professor, University of Northern Paraná (UNOPAR).
[5] Professor, Hospital for Rehabilitation of Craniofacial Anomalies/USP.
[6] Professor, Central-West College Pinelli Henriques.

Fabiano Paiva Vieira
Rua João XXIII, 600 – Jd. Dom Bosco – CEP: 86060-370,
Londrina/PR — Brazil
E-mail: fpvieir@hotmail.com.

INTRODUCTION

Within the context of contemporary Orthodontics, making accurate diagnosis and prognosis determines whether a clinician can provide patients with the best cost-benefit treatment. Based on principles of effectiveness and efficiency, only one or two treatment alternatives best fit patient's esthetic, functional and psychological needs.[1] Therefore, clinicians must use all possible resources to achieve this ideal goal on orthodontic practice.

Cephalometry is a valuable auxiliary diagnostic tool as it allows the relationship among bone structures, dental tissue and soft tissue to be determined by means of lateral radiographs,[6] thereby facilitating complete assessment of malocclusion in different space dimensions, including anterior-posterior[25] and vertical.[30] Analyzing malocclusion this way allows understanding of how and in what direction and manner each element of the stomatognathic system contributes to its conformation. For this reason,the use of cephalometric analysis is rendered necessary in the anterior-posterior and vertical directions, and so it is to analyze the influence of vertical changes in the severity of malocclusion in anterior-posterior direction.[23]

Vertical facial changes influence mandibular position and rotation, either clockwise or counterclockwise, thereby contributing to the development of deep or open bite. Thus, orthodontic treatment should induce desirable changes and minimize inevitable undesirable ones.[22]

To assess vertical facial changes, new cephalometric analyses were developed,[24] and the present study uses measurements employed by Wylie and Johnson,[30] Siriwat and Jarabak,[24] Gebeck,[8] Merrifield[17] as well as Horn,[9] all of which assess anterior and posterior facial height, facial ratios and facial height index, measurements which were used in previous studies.[5,26] In these studies, cephalometric standards from different racial and ethnic groups and with miscegenation were determined and compared, showing the need for individualization, which has also been reported in worldwide literature.[5,7,13,18,26]

The studies found in the literature were devoted to certain groups, such as Caucasians or Mongoloids, but not to the result of their miscegenation. For this reason, explaining the need for individualization and understanding of cephalometric characteristics of different miscegenation patterns is important.

To this end, the following were assessed: Specific cephalometric patterns of anterior and posterior facial heights; facial ratios and facial height index[9] for young Japanese-Brazilian descendants with normal occlusion using variables in the vertical direction of the face. The presence of sexual dimorphism was also assessed.

MATERIAL AND METHODS

A total of 30 lateral cephalometric radiographs of young Japanese-Brazilian descendants (15 males and 15 females with an average age of 14 years) with normal occlusion, selected from elementary and high schools located in the city of Bauru, were assessed. The selected patients had the following characteristics: Japanese-Brazilian descendent of parents and/or grandparents from Japan, except for the island of Okinawa, and Caucasian Brazilian parents (Portuguese, Spanish or Italian ancestry); aged between 11.91 to 16.61 years; with normal occlusion; and no history of previous orthodontic treatment.

All patients had permanent teeth in occlusion, except for third molars. Additionally, they had normal molar relationship, mild or absent crowding, no crossbite, normal overbite and overjet, no differences between mandibular positions in centric relation and maximum intercuspation, and well-balanced faces.

Cephalometric radiographs were obtained according to the standards recommended by the Department of Radiology, School of Dentistry/University of São Paulo, Bauru. Radiographic image magnification (using a Siemens equipment) was of 9.8%, corrected during measurements of radiographs so as to increase accuracy of the method employed.

Preparation of cephalograms

Anatomical tracing was carried out according to the recommendations described by Interlandi[11] and Vion;[28] the average of anatomical structures was used when two radiographic images of the same structure were identified. The following anatomical structures were assessed (Fig 1): Sella turcica, clivus, external cortex of the frontal bone and nasal bones; mean of pterygomaxillary fissure; mean of inferior borders of orbits; average of external auditory meatus; maxilla, mandible, teeth (upper and lower central incisors and first molars) and soft tissue profile.

After performing the anatomical tracing, landmarks were identified and then digitized by the digitizing tablet AccuGrid XNT, model A30TL.F (Numonics Corporation, Montgomeryville, PA, USA). Data were processed using Dentofacial Planner Software, version 7.02 (Dentofacial Planner Software Inc.,Toronto, Ontario, Canada) installed in a PC with 700MHz Intel Pentium III processor.

Cephalometric landmarks, lines and planes

After the anatomical tracing was prepared, cephalometric landmarks were located according to Miyashita:[19] S (Sella), N (Nasion), ANS (Anterior Nasal Spine), PNS (Posterior Nasal Spine), Me (Menton), Go (Gonion) and Ar (Articulare) (Fig 1). After locating the cephalometric landmarks that are independent of guidance tracing, plans and lines were drawn, and Ar' and ANS' points were constructed according to Wylie and Johnson[30] as well as Siriwat and Jarabak[24] (Fig 1).

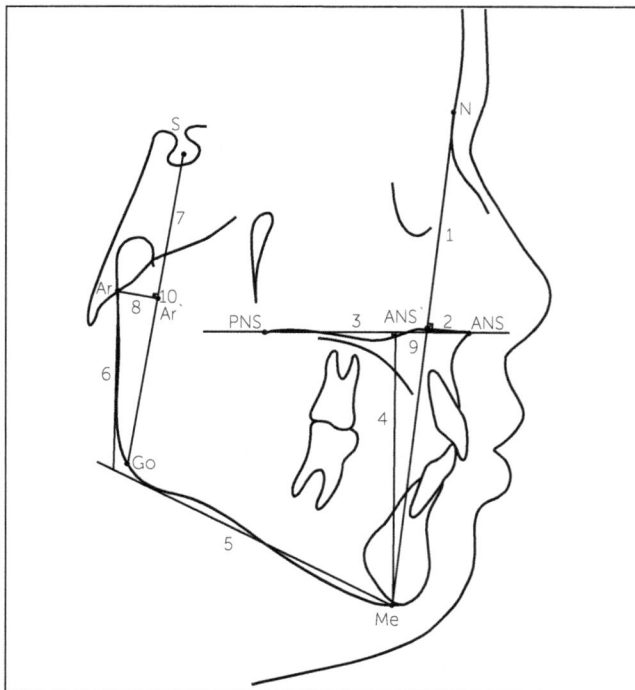

Figure 1 - Cephalometric landmarks, lines and planes.

1) N - Me line: The line formed by the union of Nasion (N) and Menton (Me).

2) ANS perp. line: The perpendicular line formed by the union of Anterior Nasal Spine (ANS) and N - Me line.

3) Palatal Plane (PP): The line formed by the union of Anterior Nasal Spine (ANS) and Posterior Nasal Spine (PNS).

4) Me - PP line: The line perpendicular to the Palatal Plane (PP) connecting this plan to the Menton (Me).

5) Mandibular Plane (MP): A line which bisects the distance between the left and right mandibular lower borders and connects anteriorly with Menton (Me).

6) Ar - MP line: The line connecting the Articulare (Ar) point to the Mandibular Plane (MP), touching the posterior border of the mandible branch.

7) S - Go line: The line formed by the union of Sella (S) and Gonion (Go).

8) Ar perp. line: The line formed by the projection of the Articulare (Ar) and perpendicular to S - Go line.

9) ANS' point (ANS projection point): Point formed by the intersection of ANS perp. line and N - Me line.

10) Ar' point (Ar projection point): the point formed by the intersection of Ar perp. line and S - Go line.

Cephalometric measurements in vertical direction

The measures taken according to the analysis by Wylie-Johnson[30] are shown in Figure 2.

1) Total Anterior Facial Height (TAFH): Linear distance between Nasion (N) and Menton (Me).

2) Upper Anterior Facial Height (UAFH): Linear distance between points N and ANS', measured in N - Me line.

3) Lower Anterior Facial Height (LAFH): Linear distance between ANS' and Me, measured in N - Me line.

4) Ratio of Upper Anterior Facial Height and Total Anterior Facial Height (UAFH/TAFH).

5) Ratio of Lower Anterior Facial Height and Total Anterior Facial Height (LAFH/TAFH).

The measures used according to the Siriwat and Jarabak[24] analysis are shown in Figure 3.

1) Total Posterior Facial Height (TPFH): Linear distance between Sella (S) and Gonion (Go).

2) Upper Posterior Facial Height (UPFH): Linear distance between S and Ar' (perpendicular projection of Ar), measured in S-Go line.

3) Lower Posterior Facial Height (LPFH): Linear distance between Ar' and Go, measured in S-Go line.

4) UPFH/TPFH — Ratio of Upper Posterior Facial Height and Total Posterior Facial Height.

5) LPFH/TPFH — Ratio of Lower Posterior Facial Height and Total Posterior Facial Height.

The measures used according to the Gebeck[8] and Merrifield[17] analysis and also used to determine the Facial Height Index of Horn[9], are shown in Figure 4.

1) Anterior Facial Height (AFH): Perpendicular linear distance between Palatal Plane and Me, measured in Me - PP line.

2) Posterior Facial Height (PFH): Linear distance between Ar and the Mandibular Plane (Go-Me), tangent to the mandibular ramus.

3) Facial Height Index (FHI): Ratio of PFH and AFH, multiplied by 100 (FHI = PFH/AFH x 100)

STATISTICAL METHOD
Descriptive and comparative analyses

Means and standard deviation were used to describe the sample of Japanese-Brazilian descendants. To investigate the existence of sexual dimorphism, t-test with significance level set at 0.05 was applied due to normal distribution of variables in the Kolmogorov-Smirnov test. All statistical analyses were performed using Statistica software (Statistica for Windows 6.0, Statsoft, Tulsa, OK).

Method error

Cephalometric tracings and measurements of 50% of the sample were remade by the same examiner a month after obtaining the initial cephalograms.

Systematic and casual errors were independently assessed for each cephalometric variable, as recommended by Houston.[10] Systematic error was calculated by dependent t-test for paired samples. Casual error was calculated by Dahlberg's formula[4] using the standard deviation of differences between repetitions.

RESULTS

Results are divided and presented in tables for didactics purposes and to favor visualization and understanding.

CASUAL AND SYSTEMATIC ERROR

Casual error was determined by Dahlberg's formula,[4] whereas systematic error was assessed by dependent t-test.[10] Statistical analysis carried out to assess intra-examiner error revealed no systematic errors. Casual errors, however, were minimal, since measurements were linear and most of them had a value lower than 1 mm. Only two variables, TAFH and UAFH, yielded slightly higher causal error values: 1.44 mm and 1.25 mm, respectively.

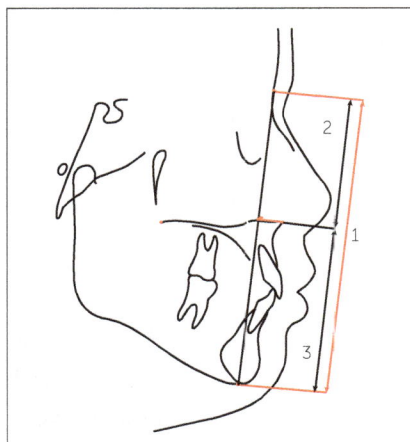

Figure 2 - Measurements assessed, according to Wylie and Johnson analysis.[20]

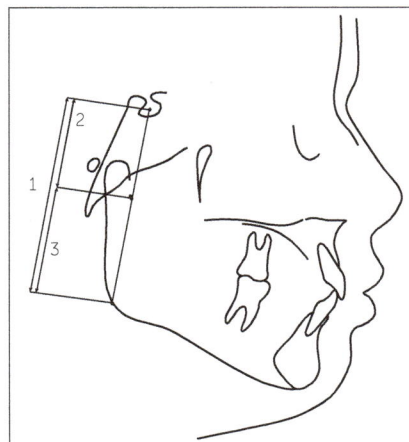

Figure 3 - Measurements assessed, according to Siriwat and Jarabak analysis.[24]

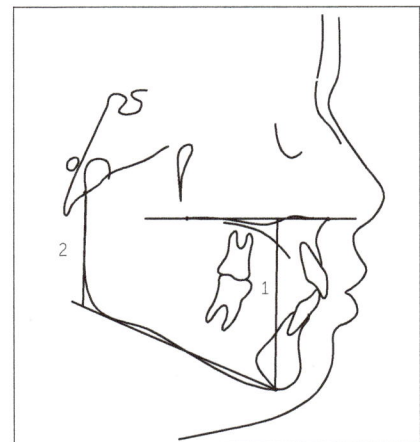

Figure 4 - Measurements assessed, according to Gebeck, Merrifield and Horn analysis.[8,9,17]

CHARACTERIZATION OF THE SAMPLE

The sample comprised 30 Japanese-Brazilian descendants, 15 males and 15 females, with mean age of 14 years old — 14.78 years for males and 13.22 years for females, representing an age difference of 1.56 years of which significance was tested and confirmed by independent t-test set at 5% significance level. Characterization of vertical facial growth pattern by means of SN.GoGn variable showed an average of 33.08 degrees (33.02 for males and 33.15 for females), with no statistically significant difference.

SAMPLE COMPARATIVE AND DESCRIPTIVE ANALYSES

Descriptive analysis determined the number of research subjects, means, standard deviations as well as minimum and maximum values of the population necessary for a confidence interval of 95% for each variable considered in the current study (Table 1).

Sexual dimorphism was assessed by means of independent t-test set at 5% significance level. Average male and female data with respective standard deviations and P-values are presented in Table 2.

DISCUSSION

Facial vertical pattern affects facial harmony and attractiveness. In this context, orthodontic treatment can favor or disfavor balance by implementing facial changes in the vertical direction of which

Table 1 - Descriptive analysis of Japanese-Brazilian descendent sample.

Variable	n	Mean ± SD	Min-Max values for a Confidence interval of 95%
TAFH	30	122.82 ± 7.54	120.00 – 125.63
UAFH	30	52.52 ± 4.08	50.99 – 54.04
LAFH	30	70.29 ± 4.81	68.49 – 72.09
UAFH/TAFH	30	42.76 ± 1.90	42.05 – 43.47
LAFH/TAFH	30	57.23 ± 1.90	56.52 – 57.94
TPFH	30	81.60 ± 5.47	79.56 – 83.64
UPFH	30	34.47 ± 3.58	33.13 – 35.81
LPFH	30	47.13 ± 3.89	45.67 – 48.58
UPFH/TPFH	30	42.23 ± 3.08	41.07 – 43.48
LPFH/TPFH	30	57.77 ± 3.08	56.61 – 58.92
AFH	30	69.45 ± 4.81	67.65 – 71.24
PFH	30	50.33 ± 4.03	48.83 – 51.84
FHI	30	72.65 ± 6.20	70.33 – 74.97

Table 2 - Comparative analysis of male and female Japanese-Brazilian descendents.

Variable	Mean ± SD Female (n = 15)	Mean ± SD Male (n = 15)	P
TAFH	119.74 ± 4.20	125.90 ± 8.93	0.022*
UAFH	51.64 ± 3.66	53.40 ± 4.41	0.243
LAFH	68.10 ± 2.86	72.49 ± 5.42	0.009*
UAFH/TAFH	43.10 ± 2.15	42.42 ± 1.62	0.337
LAFH/TAFH	56.89 ± 2.15	57.57 ± 1.62	0.337
TPFH	78.85 ± 3.91	84.36 ± 5.51	0.003*
UPFH	32.70 ± 2.45	36.24 ± 3.71	0.004*
LPFH	46.14 ± 3.00	48.12 ± 4.50	0.168
UPFH/TPFH	41.48 ± 2.35	42.98 ± 3.60	0.190
LPFH/TPFH	58.51 ± 2.35	57.02 ± 3.61	0.192
AFH	67.38 ± 2.75	71.52 ± 5.58	0.015*
PFH	49.51 ± 3.29	51.16 ± 4.62	0.270
FHI	73.48 ± 4.28	71.82 ± 7.74	0.473

* Significant for P < 0.05.

even lay people are aware of.[21] Therefore, clinicians should have an individualized reference[23] to conduct orthodontic treatment in order to induce the desired changes and minimize undesirable, inevitable ones.[2]

This study should be viewed as primarily descriptive. It aims at demonstrating how the values of young Japanese-Brazilian descendants are incomparable to values previously established for Caucasian and Mongoloid subjects. It also aims at analyzing sexual dimorphism for each variable. Thus, the values determined for the variables analyzed herein should be compared to other results previously reported in the literature with a view to further investigate this topic.

This discussion of results is divided into anterior facial height and its ratios, posterior facial height and its ratios, and Facial Height Index (Horn[9]). Each of these sections was divided into sub-sections so as to favor interpretation of results.

ANTERIOR FACIAL HEIGHTS
TAFH — Total anterior facial height

TAFH for Japanese-Brazilian descendants had an average value of 125.90 mm for males and 119.74 mm for females. Statistically significant difference, with significance level set at 5%, was identified between these values, thereby indicating sexual dimorphism with greater vertical development for males.

This may have been caused by age difference between males and females. However, there is a chronological gap between growth and development of males and females in the phase of adolescence, including the vertical development of the face. Additionally, females in general have their pubertal growth spurt at an earlier age than males. Therefore, growth will likely be more balanced between males and females in this condition, with a mean age difference of 1.56 years during adolescence, particularly because females represented the group with the lower average age. Similar findings were also reported in other studies.[14,26]

The values determined for Japanese-Brazilian descendants are close to the highest values found in the literature for Caucasians, but were even closer to values found for Mongoloids. Ishii et al[12] conducted a study in which significant differences were found between Japanese Mongoloid and British Caucasian groups for both males and females, with the Mongoloid group presenting the highest values. Takahashi[26] also found significant differences between Caucasian and Mongoloid racial groups, particularly for males, with the largest values found in the Mongoloid group. However, for females, no significant differences were found among racial groups. Additionally, the female Mongoloid group had higher values of TAFH.

Although the values found in the literature showed great variability for the TAFH variable, in general, the values reported in this study were very close to those found in the literature for Japanese[12] and their descendents[26] within a similar age range. Disagreement among some values found in the literature[12,14,23,24,26] explains the large variation among them (Fig 5).

UAFH — Upper anterior facial height

Young Japanese-Brazilian descendants showed an average UAFH value of 52.52 mm (53.40 mm for males and 51.64 mm for females) with no statistically significant difference at 0.05 significance level between them. Thus, sexual dimorphism was not evident, thereby implying that upper facial height does not contribute to dimorphism found in TAFH.

Results showed no differences between males and females, confirming the findings by Domiti et al[5] and Locks.[15] However, other authors, such as Jones and Meredith[14] as well as Ursi et al[27] found a higher value

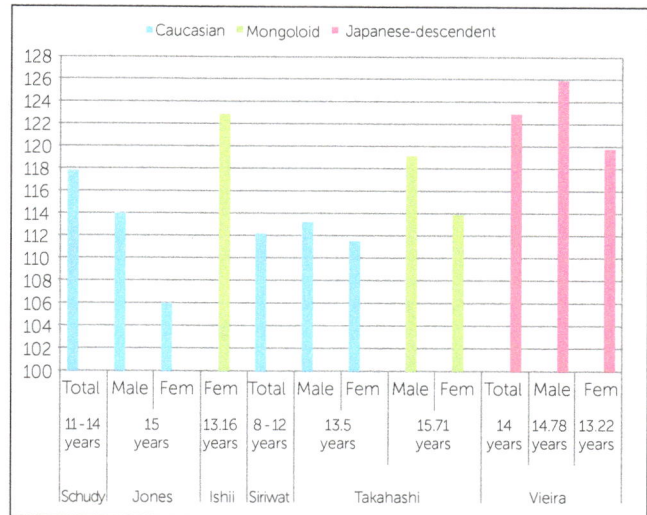

Figure 5 - TAFH means.

for the upper anterior facial height for males. Additionally, Takahashi[26] found a higher value for the Mongoloid group, but not for the Caucasian one.

The values for young Japanese-Brazilian descendants are between those found in the literature for Caucasians,[6,27] but once more are closer to those reported by Takahashi[26] for the Mongoloid group.

Ishii et al[13] showed that the upper anterior facial height was significantly higher in the Japanese Mongoloid group in comparison to the British Caucasian group. Takahashi[26] found a significant difference comparing Caucasian and Mongoloid racial groups for males, but not for females. He also observed higher values for the Mongoloid group when comparing males and females of both races.

Figure 6 shows the values found in the literature for UAFH.[5,14,23,26,27,29]

LAFH — Lower anterior facial height

The mean LAFH values for young Japanese-Brazilian descendants are 70.29 mm, 72.49 mm for males and 68.1 mm for females. Values were statistically different for males and females, thereby featuring sexual dimorphism and confirming the findings by other authors such as Lock[15] and Miyajima.[18] However, Domiti et al[5] and Takahashi[26] found no differences between males and females for either one of the two racial groups. Ursi et al[27] identified differences between males and females older than 16 years

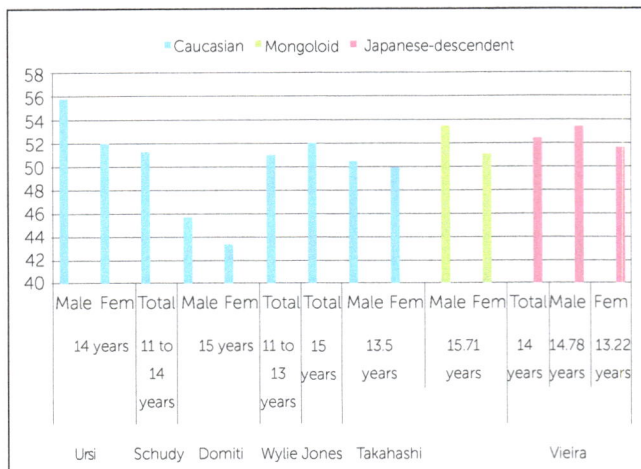

Figure 6 - Means of UAFH.

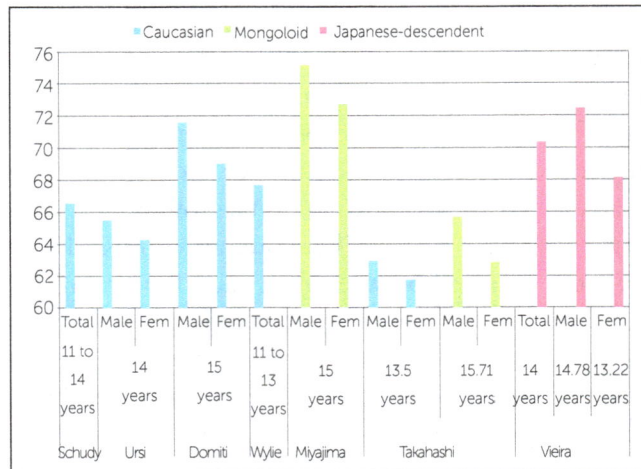

Figure 7 - Means of LAFH.

with LAFH values higher for males at this age. Sexual dimorphism in the Japanese-Brazilian descendent sample leads us to the conclusion that lower anterior facial height contributed significantly to the dimorphism found in TAFH.

The values determined for the young Japanese-Brazilian descendants are closely related to the highest values found in the literature for Caucasians[6] and Mongoloids.[18]

Ishii et al[13] reported that Japanese Mongoloid individuals have LAFH values significantly higher than British Caucasian individuals, although Takahashi[26] found significant differences between Caucasian and Mongoloid racial groups, only for males, thereby demonstrating greater LAFH values in the Mongoloid group for both males and females.

Figure 7 shows the values found in the literature[5,18,23,26,27,29] with a large variation for LAFH values.

UAFH/TAFH ratio

Young Japanese-Brazilian descendants showed an average UAFH/TAFH ratio of 42.76%, being 43.10% for females and 42.42% for males, with no statistically significant difference between these values, at 0.05 significance level. Consequently, no sexual dimorphism was evident, corroborating the findings by Wylie and Johnson,[30] as well as Takahashi[26] — who did not find a statistically significant

difference between males and females for both study groups at 0.05 significance level.

The values determined for young Japanese-Brazilian descendants are closer to the minimum value found by Locks[16] for Caucasians (42%).

Takahashi[26] also found no significant differences when comparing Caucasian and Mongoloid males and females, thus showing a balance in this ratio.

Figure 8 shows the comparison among values found in the literature.[3,14,16,26,30]

LAFH/TAFH ratio

Young Japanese-Brazilian descendents showed an average UAFH/TAFH ratio of 57.23%, being 56.89% for females and 57.57% for males, with no statistically significant difference between these values, at a 0.05 significance level. Consequently, no sexual dimorphism was evident, corroborating the findings by Takahashi[26] who found no statistically significant difference between males and females for both study groups.

The values determined for young Japanese-Brazilian descendants are close to the highest values found in the literature for Caucasians.[16,23]

Takahashi[26] also found no significant differences when comparing Caucasian and Mongoloid males and females, thus showing a balance in this ratio.

Figure 9 shows the values found in the literature for LAFH/TAFH.[3,14,16,23,26,30]

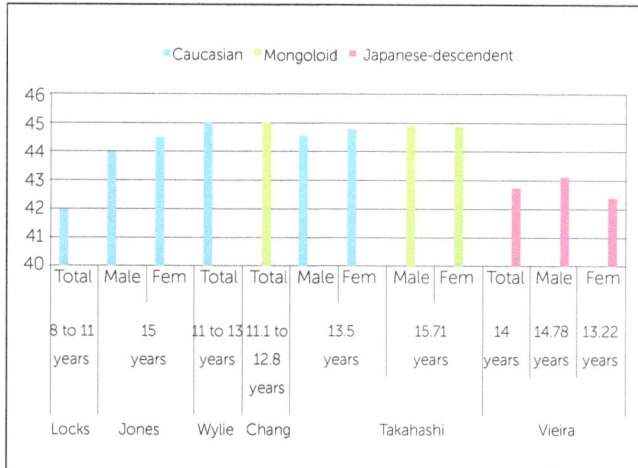

Figure 8 - Means of UAFH - TAFH.

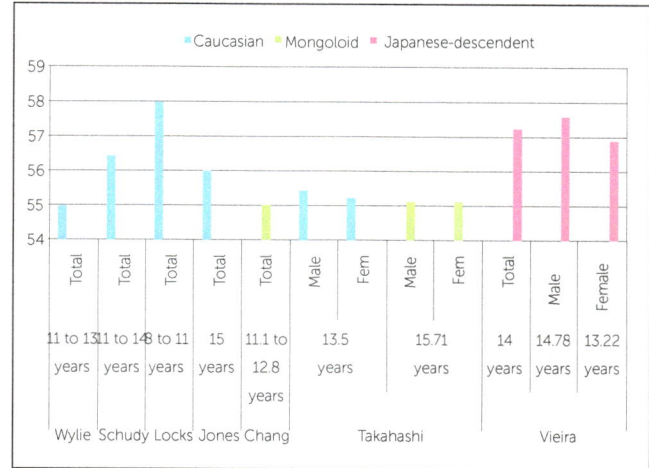

Figure 9 - Means of LAFH - TAFH.

POSTERIOR FACIAL HEIGHTS
TPFH — Total posterior facial height

Young Japanese-Brazilian descendants showed an average TPFH of 81.60 mm, being 84.36 mm for males and 78.85 mm for females, with a statistically significant difference at a 0.05 level, thereby indicating sexual dimorphism with greater development of male posterior facial height. As discussed regarding TAFH dimorphism, it can be inferred that this is not a simple reflection of age difference between males and females. In addition, a similar condition was reported by Takahashi[26] for the Mongoloid group, although Chang et al[3] did not find this difference.

The values determined for young Japanese-Brazilian descendants are closer to the values found by Takahashi[26] for the Mongoloid group. This author also found significant differences when comparing Caucasian and Mongoloid males and females, and reported that the Mongoloid group had higher values[26].

The values reported in the literature for TPFH[23,24,26] are shown in Figure 10.

UPFH — Upper posterior facial height

The mean UPFH value of young Japanese-Brazilian descendants was 34.47 mm, being 36.24 mm for males and 32.70 mm for females. Values were statistically different for males and females with significance level set at 0.05. Thus, sexual dimorphism

was characterized with high values for male posterior facial height. The upper portion of the posterior facial height can be inferred to contribute significantly to the dimorphism found in TPFH. Takahashi[26] also reported the presence of sexual dimorphism for both Caucasian and Mongoloid groups, in addition to a greater vertical development of male upper posterior facial height for both groups.

Takahashi[26] also identified significant differences when comparing Caucasian and Mongoloid racial groups, for males and females, with higher values for Mongoloids. These findings differed from those by Ishii et al[13] who found no difference between Japanese Mongoloid and British Caucasian.

Comparison between values found in this study and by Takahashi[26] indicate greater proximity between the values of young Japanese-Brazilian descendants and Mongoloids, with higher values for the first group, as presented in Figure 11. This finding can neither be attributed to differences in methodology, which was the same, nor to mean age difference, since the mean age of the Mongoloid group was greater (15.71 years) in Takahashi's study[26]. However, this finding may be due to the use of a different sample, with a slightly more vertical pattern of young Japanese-Brazilian descendants, or because of race miscegenation that generates a new biological and genetic conformation.

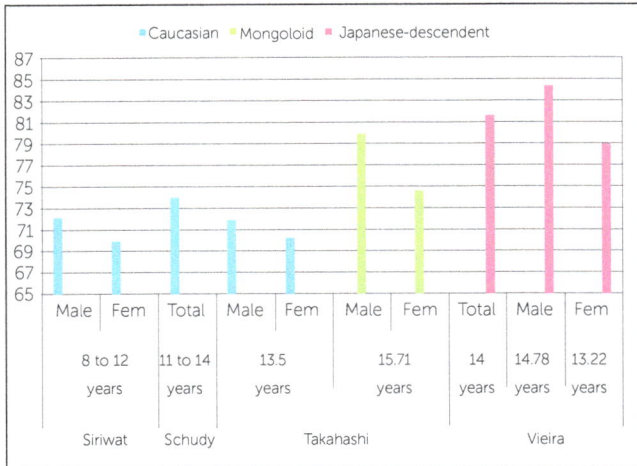

Figure 10 - Means of TPFH.

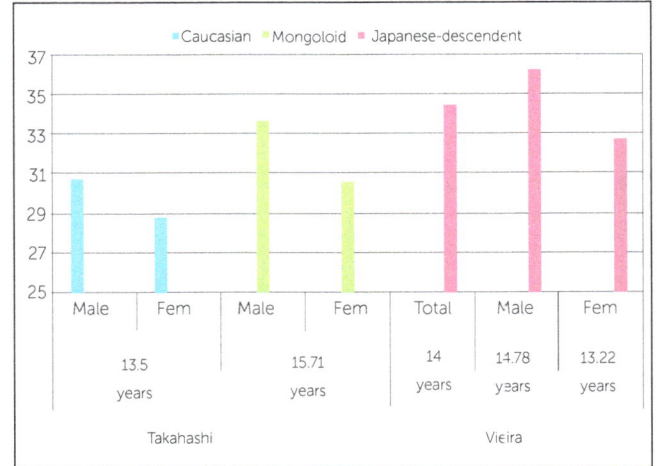

Figure 11 - Means of UPFH.

LPFH — Lower posterior facial height

Young Japanese-Brazilian descendants showed an average LPFH value of 47.13 mm, being 48.12 mm for males and 46.14 mm for females. No sexual dimorphism was evident, thereby corroborating the results by Takahashi[26] f r both groups.

Lack of dimorphism in LPFH values of young Japanese-Brazilian descendants inferred that LPFH does not contribute to the dimorphism found in TPFH.

Takahashi[26] identified significant differences when comparing Mongoloid and Caucasian males and females, with the Mongoloid group showing higher values. The values of young Japanese-Brazilian descendants are closer to the maximum values obtained with Caucasians,[23] and even closer to the values reported for Mongoloids.[12,26] This condition is well characterized in F igure 12.

UPFH/TPFH ratio

Young Japanese-Brazilian descendants showed an average UPFH/TPFH ratio of 42.23%, being 42.98% for males and 41.48% for females, with no statistically significant difference at a 0.05 significance level. Therefore, no sexual dimorphism was observed. This result corroborates the findings by Takahashi[26] for the Mongoloid group, although this author reported sexual dimorphism with higher UPFH/TPFH ratios for males in the Caucasian group.

Takahashi[26] found no significant difference when comparing Caucasian and Mongoloid males and females. The values for young Japanese-Brazilian descendants are close to those reported by Takahashi,[26] as shown in Figure 13, despite age difference and the use of a different sample with its own racial miscegenation. The cause may be stability of values for this variable after a certain age and a small variation between different races and their miscegenations.

LPFH/TPFH ratio

Young Japanese-Brazilian descendants showed an average LPFH/TPFH value of 57.77%, being 57.02% for males and 58.51% for females. The lack of dimorphism in these results corroborates Takahashi[26] for the Mongoloid group, although this author reported sexual dimorphism in the Caucasian group with higher LPFH/TPFH values for females.

Takahashi[26] found no significant differences when comparing Mongoloid and Caucasian males and females. The values for young Japanese-Brazilian descendants are close to those reported by Takahashi[26] for the two groups, as shown in Figure 14.

Determining the facial height index (FHI)

Horn[9] proposed a variable to track patient's vertical dimension during treatment. The proposed index is calculated by dividing the posterior facial height (PFH, the distance in millimeters from point

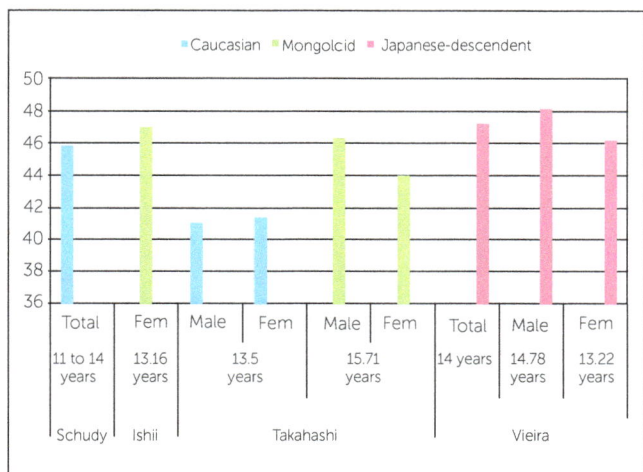

Figure 12 - Means of LPFH.

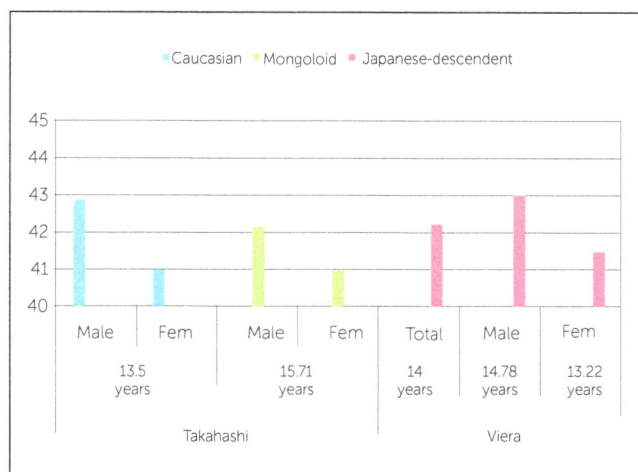

Figure 13 - Means of UPFH - TPFH.

Ar to the mandibular plane) and the anterior facial height (AFH) (the distance in millimeters from the palatal plane to the point Me). According to the author, the use of the facial height index[9] is an additional aid in the diagnosis of excess or reduced vertical dimension, allowing observation of vertical dimension during treatment and adjustment of orthodontic mechanics to offset any unfavorable trend.

AFH — Anterior facial height

The mean AFH value of young Japanese-Brazilian descendants was 69.45 mm, being 71.52 mm for males and 67.38 mm for females. Sexual dimorphism was identified, with larger vertical development of the male group. This result appears to be consistent with LAFH and TAFH values and also corroborates the findings by Takahashi[26] in the Mongoloid group, with more vertical development of the anterior facial height of males, although the same author reported the absence of dimorphism in the Caucasian group.

The values determined for young Japanese-Brazilian descendants are closer to the maximum values found in the literature for Caucasians,[9,17] and closer to the values reported by Takahashi[26] for the Mongoloid group. The variation in AFH found in the literature is shown in Figure 15.

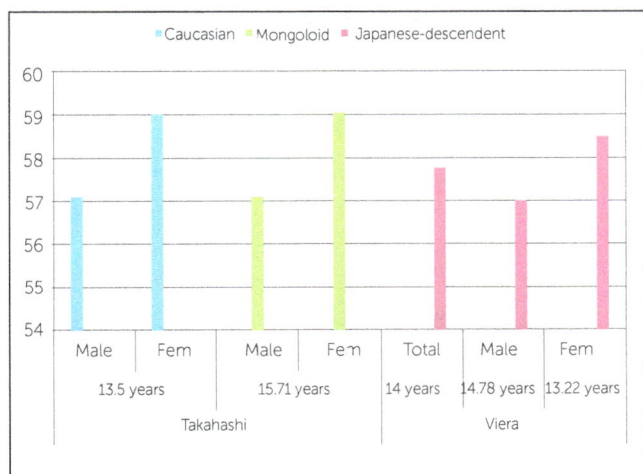

Figure 14 - Means of LPFH - TPFH.

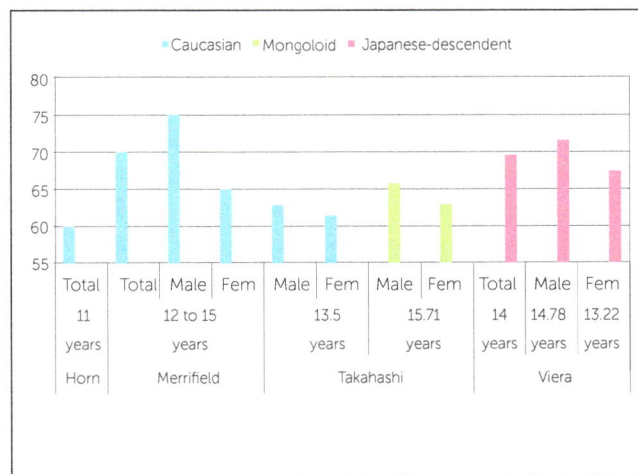

Figure 15 - Means of AFH.

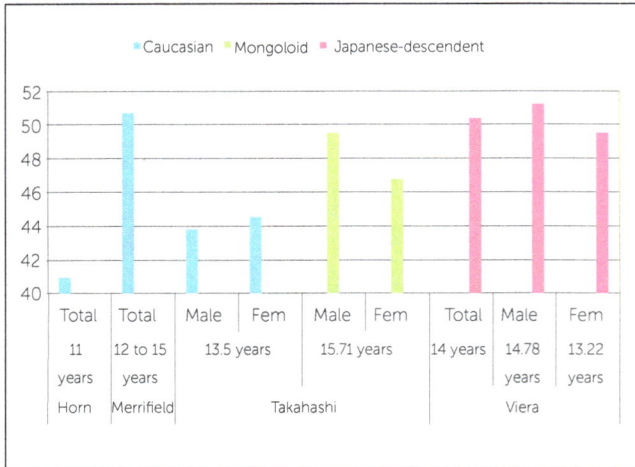

Figure 16 - Means of PFH.

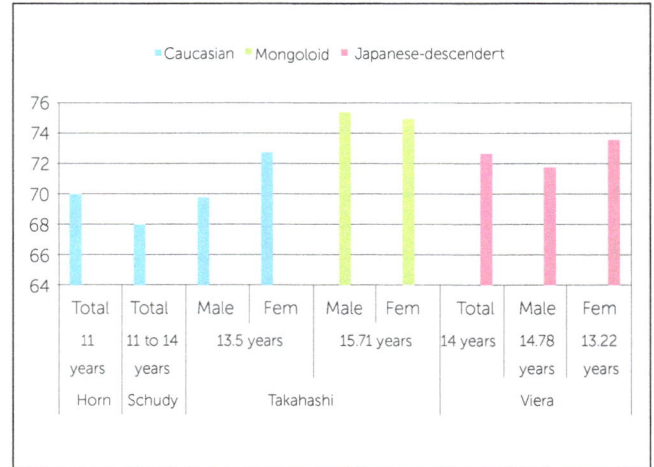

Figure 17 - Means of FHI.

Takahashi[26] identified significant differences when comparing Caucasian and Mongoloid males, and found no significant differences among racial groups for females. The same author also reported that, with regard to both males and females, Mongoloids had higher values than Caucasians.

PFH — Posterior facial height

The mean PFH value of young Japanese-Brazilian descendants was 50.33 mm, being 51.16 mm for males and 49.51 mm for females. No sexual dimorphism was found with these results, similar to what was observed in Takahashi's[26] study for both Mongoloid and Caucasian groups.

The values determined for young Japanese-Brazilian descendants are close to those found in the literature for Caucasians[17] and even closer to those reported for the Mongoloid group.[26] Takahashi[26] also reported significant difference when comparing Caucasian and Mongoloid males and females. The variation in PFH values found in the literature[9,17] is shown in Figure 16.

FHI — Facial Height Index (Horn[9])

The mean FHI value for Japanese-Brazilian descendants (Horn[9]) was 72.65%, being 71.82% for males and 73.48% for females. No sexual dimorphism was found, thereby corroborating the results by

Takahashi[26] for the Mongoloid group, although this author reported sexual dimorphism in the Caucasian group.

A small variation in FHI values was observed in the literature,[9,23,26] as shown in Figure 17. For this variable, the results of the present study were similar to those reported by Takahashi[26] for Caucasians and Mongoloids. He also reported significant differences between Caucasian males, but not for females.

Results for young Japanese-Brazilian descendants showed, in general, that the values of variables and the analysis of sexual dimorphism — particularly when compared with those reported by Takahashi[26] — suggested a closer relationship between the values of Japanese-Brazilian descendants and the Mongoloid group for all variables except for the ratios UAFH/TAFH, LAFH/TAFH, UPFH/TPFH, and LPFH/TPFH as well as FHI. Thus, further comparison between young Japanese-Brazilian descendants, Caucasians and Mongoloids should be performed in a study with the specific objective of precisely establishing the relationship between these groups.

Moreover, the analysis of sexual dimorphism of young Japanese-Brazilian descendants suggests a more vertical pattern for males, characterized by higher values in the variables TAFH, LAFH, AFH, TPFH and UPFH. However, the variables denoting vertical facial ratio do not show the same trend.

CLINICAL CONSIDERATIONS

Vertical facial changes influence mandibular position and rotation, either clockwise or counterclockwise,[22,23] thereby contributing to the development of deep bite or open bite, and potentially increasing the severity of anterior-posterior malocclusion. Thus, orthodontic treatment should induce desirable alterations and minimize the undesirable ones when the latter are inevitable.[2]

Therefore, malocclusion should be analyzed completely and in all different dimensions of space so as to favor understanding of how and in what direction each element of the stomatognathic system contributes to the conformation of malocclusion, which is necessary for cephalometric analysis of anterior-posterior and vertical directions, as well as analysis of the influence of vertical changes in the severity of antero-posterior malocclusion.[23]

However, the literature indicates that malocclusion analysis requires full assessment so as to individualize cephalometric norms regarding patient's sex, age and race.[20] Thus, cephalometric standards from different ethnic and racial groups and miscegenations were determined and compared, and the need for individualization for each specific group was demonstrated[5,7,18,20,26] to better understand and assess the cephalometric characteristics of different groups and miscegenations with respect to orthodontic diagnosis and planning. Thus, the present study provides the clinician with a more specific reference in the vertical direction of the face, particularly for young Japanese-Brazilian descendants with normal occlusion.

Moreover, as a topic for future research, the values of Japanese-Brazilian descendants should be compared with those of other subjects, particularly Mongoloid and Caucasian Brazilians.

CONCLUSIONS

Based on the sample and methods employed herein, values are presented to establish a cephalometric pattern of anterior and posterior facial heights and its ratios, as well as the facial height index (Horn[9]) for young Japanese-Brazilian descendants with normal occlusion. Results revealed the presence of sexual dimorphism in the following cephalometric measurements: TAFH, LAFH, AFH, TPFH and UPFH.

REFERENCES

1. Ackerman M. Evidence-based orthodontics for the 21st century. J Am Dent Assoc. 2004;135(2):162-7.

2. Ahn JG, Schneider BJ. Cephalometric appraisal of posttreatment vertical changes in adult orthodontic patients. Am J Orthod Dentofacial Orthop. 2000;118(4):378-84.

3. Chang HP, Kinoshita Z, Kawamoto T. A study of the growth changes in facial configuration. Eur J Orthod. 1993;15(6):493-501.

4. Dahlberg G. Statistical methods for medical and biological students. New York: Interscience; 1940.

5. Domiti SS, Daruge E, Cruz VF. Variability of the nasion-subnasal, subnasal-gnathion, and bizygomatic distances of individuals of 6, 7, 11, and 15 years of age and their importance in the determination of the vertical dimension. Aust Dent J. 1976;21(3):269-71.

6. Downs WB. The role of cephalometrics in orthodontic case analysis and diagnosis. Am J Orthod. 1952;38(3):162-82.

7. Freitas LM, Pinzan A, Janson G, Freitas KM, Freitas MR, Henriques JF. Facial height comparison in young white and black Brazilian subjects with normal occlusion. Am J Orthod Dentofacial Orthop. 2007;131(6):706.e1-6.

8. Gebeck TR. Analysis: concepts and values. Part I. J Charles H Tweed Int Found. 1989;17:19-48.

9. Horn AJ. Facial height index. Am J Orthod Dentofacial Orthop. 1992;102(2):180-6.

10. Houston WJB. The analysis of errors in orthodontic measurements. Am J Orthod. 1983;83(5):382-90.

11. Interlandi S. O cefalograma padrão do curso de pós-graduação de Ortodontia da Faculdade de Odontologia da USP. Rev Fac Odont Bauru. 1968;6(1):63-74.

12. Ishii N, Deguchi T, Hunt NP. Craniofacial morphology of Japanese girls with Class II division 1 malocclusion. J Orthod. 2001;28(3):211-5.

13. Ishii N, Deguchi T, Hunt NP. Morphological differences in the craniofacial structure between Japanese and Caucasian girls with Class II division 1 malocclusions. Eur J Orthod. 2002;24(1):61-7.

14. Jones BH, Meredith HV. Vertical change in osseous and odontic portions of human face height between the ages of 5 and 15 years. Am J Orthod. 1966;52(12):902-21.

15. Locks A. Análise das proporções verticais anteriores da face de indivíduos brasileiros, portadores de oclusão excelente e perfil agradável [mestrado]. Rio de Janeiro (RJ): Universidade Federal do Rio de Janeiro; 1981.

16. Locks A. Estudo cefalométrico das alturas faciais anterior e posterior, em crianças brasileiras, portadoras de má-oclusão Classe I de Angle, na fase de dentadura mista [tese]. Araraquara (SP): Universidade Estadual Paulista; 1996.

17. Merrifield LL. Analysis: concepts and values. Part II. J Charles H Tweed Int Found. 1989;17:49-64.

18. Miyajima K, McNamara JA Jr, Kimura T, Murata S, Iizuka T. Craniofacial structure of Japanese and European-American adults with normal occlusions and well-balanced faces. Am J Orthod Dentofacial Orthop. 1996;110(4):431-8.

19. Miyashita K. Contemporary cephalometric radiography. Tokyo: Quintessence; 1996.

20. Pinzan A. "Upgrade" nos conceitos da interpretação das medidas cefalométricas. In: Dominguez GC, organizador. Nova visão em ortodontia, ortopedia funcional dos maxilares. 1a ed. São Paulo: Ed. Santos; 2006. v. 1, p. 41-9.

21. Romani KL, Agahi F, Nanda R, Zernik JH. Evaluation of horizontal and vertical differences in facial profiles by orthodontists and lay people. Angle Orthod. 1993;63(3):175-82.

22. Schudy FF. Vertical versus anteroposterior growth as related to function and treatment. Angle Orthod. 1964;34(2):75-93.

23. Schudy FF. The rotation of the mandible resulting from growth: its implications in orthodontic treatment. Angle Orthod. 1965;35(1):36-50.

24. Siriwat PP, Jarabak JR. Malocclusion and facial morphology: is there a relationship? An epidemiologic study. Angle Orthod. 1985;55(2):127-38.

25. Steiner C. Cephalometrics in clinical practice. Angle Orthod. 1959;29(1):8-29.

26. Takahashi R. Determinação cefalométrica das alturas faciais anterior e posterior, em jovens brasileiros, descendentes de xandodermas e leucodermas, com oclusão normal [tese]. Bauru (SP): Universidade de São Paulo; 2002.

27. Ursi WJ, Trotman CA, McNamara JA Jr, Behrents RG. Sexual dimorphism in normal craniofacial growth. Angle Orthod. 1993;63(1):47-56.

28. Vion PE. Anatomia cefalométrica. São Paulo: Ed. Santos; 1994.

29. Wylie WL. The relationship between ramus height, dental height and overbite. Am J Orthod. 1946;32(2):57-67.

30. Wylie WL, Johnson EL. Rapid evaluation of facial dysplasia in the vertical plane. Angle Orthod. 1952;22(3):165-82.

17

A digital volumetric tomography (DVT) study in the mandibular molar region for miniscrew placement during mixed dentition

Mayur S. Bhattad[1], Sudhindra Baliga[2], Pavan Vibhute[3]

Objective: To assess bone thickness for miniscrew placement in the mandible during mixed dentition by using digital volumetric tomograph (DVT). **Material and methods:** A total of 15 healthy patients aged 8-10 years old, with early exfoliated mandibular second deciduous molar, were included. DVT images of one quadrant of the mandible were obtained using Kodak extraoral imaging systems and analyzed by Kodak dental imaging software. The error of the method (EM) was calculated using Dahlberg's formula. Mean and standard deviation were calculated at 6 and 8 mm from the cementoenamel junction (CEJ).Paired t-test was used to analyze the measurements. **Results:** Buccal cortical bone thickness, mesiodistal width and buccolingual bone depth at 6 mm were found to be 1.73 + 0.41, 2.15 + 0.49 and 13.18 + 1.22 mm, respectively; while at 8 mm measurements were 2.42 + 0.34, 2.48 + 0.33 and 13.65 + 1.25 mm, respectively. EM for buccal cortical bone thickness, mesiodistal width and buccolingual bone depth was 0.58, 0.40 and 0.48, respectively. The difference in measurement at 6 and 8 mm for buccal cortical plate thickness ($P < 0.05$) and buccolingual bone thickness ($P < 0.05$) was found to be significant, whereas for mesiodistal width it was insignificant ($P > 0.05$). **Conclusion:** Bone thickness measurement has shown promising evidence for safe placement of miniscrews in the mandible during mixed dentition. The use of miniscrew is the best alternative, even in younger patients.

Keywords: Miniscrews. Digital volumetric tomograph. Inter-radicular bone. Cortical bone.

» The authors report no commercial, proprietary or financial interest in the products or companies described in this article.

[1] Senior lecturer, Sharad Pawar Dental College and Hospital, Department of Pedodontics and Preventive Dentistry, Sawangi, Wardha, Maharashtra, India.
[2] Professor, Sharad Pawar Dental College and Hospital, Department of Pedodontics and Preventive Dentistry, Sawangi, Wardha, Maharashtra, India.
[3] Associate professor, Sharad Pawar Dental College and Hospital, Department of Orthodontics, Sawangi, Wardha, Maharashtra, India.

Mayur S Bhattad
Department of Pedodontics and Preventive Dentistry
HSRSSM Dental College and Hospital
Hingoli, Maharashtra, India - Ph. No. 09860273039
Email: mayur_b99@yahoo.co.in

INTRODUCTION

Maintenance of arch length during the primary, mixed and permanent dentition is of great significance for the normal development of future occlusion because premature loss of primary teeth due to caries, trauma, ectopic eruption, or other causes may lead to undesirable tooth movements of primary and/or permanent teeth including loss of arch length.[1] Space management is a key responsibility of dental practitioners who are concerned about monitoring the developing dentition, as the loss of arch length may lead to problems, such as crowding, dental impaction, crossbite formation, and dental midline discrepancies.[2] The use of space maintainers/retainers are advocated to maintain or regain lost arch length and may potentially obviate the need for later extractions and/or complex orthodontic treatment, hence space management continues to play a vital role in Dentistry.[3] However, these space maintaining devices in routine practice have shown appreciable adverse effects, such as plaque accumulation, dental caries, dislodged or broken appliances, interference with successor eruption, undesirable tooth movement and soft tissue impingement.[2,45]

In recent years, a new treatment method using miniscrews has been developed and applied to clinical orthodontic treatment. This technique enabled tooth movement that was impossible with conventional orthodontic treatment and served as an alternative method for absolute orthodontic anchorage.[6,7] Thus, miniscrews may have the potential to aid comprehensive space management and to overcome the disadvantages of conventional space maintaining devices.

Miniscrews offer the advantages of lower cost, smaller size, easy surgical placement/removal procedure, no additional laboratory work and minimum waiting period for osseointegration.[7,8] Numerous anatomic sites for miniscrew placement have been proven in adults; however, very few data are available for the mixed dentition age group.[6] The scope of miniscrews in Pediatric Dentistry for space maintenance and as an anchorage device in the late mixed dentition period may be possible and needs to be evaluated. Hence, this study aimed to assess the mesiodistal bone width, buccal cortical plate thickness and buccolingual bone thickness in the posterior region of the mandible for placement of miniscrews during mixed dentition.

MATERIAL AND METHODS

The study protocol was approved by DMIMS, Sawangi, Wardha, Mahrashtra state, India Institutional Review Board and an informed consent form was signed by parents/guardians accompanying the patients prior to the digital volumetric tomographic (DVT) scan. A total of 15 healthy patients, aged 8-10 years old, with early or recently exfoliated mandibular second deciduous molar and 2-4 mm bone covering erupting mandibular second premolar were included in the study. Patients with severe facial or dental asymmetries, systemic diseases or bone abnormalities, significant medical or dental history, vertical or horizontal periodontal bone loss were excluded.[6,9,10]

Digital volumetric tomographic images of one quadrant of the mandible in all 15 patients were obtained using Kodak 9000 extraoral imaging system. Either the right or left quadrant of the mandible was randomly chosen for measurement taking, as it was previously proven that there were no differences in cortical bone thickness between sides of the jaws.[11,12]

DATA ANALYSIS

The images obtained were analyzed by Kodak dental imaging software (3D module V 2.2). At the time of measurements, scanned images were oriented in all three planes: sagittal, axial and coronal. In the posterior inter-radicular areas of the mandible, the sagittal slice was used to locate the inter-radicular area of interest for measurements (Fig 1). The vertical reference plane was made parallel to the long axes of the roots, and the horizontal reference plane was marked along the cementoenamel junction (CEJ) of permanent mandibular first molar[10] (Fig 2). Measurements were carried out at 6 and 8 mm apical to the cementoenamel junction. Mesiodistal bone width in the mandibular first molar region was measured in sagittal slice (Fig 3) whereas the thickness of the buccal cortical plate (Fig 4) and buccolingual bone thickness or depth was measured in the areas between the second premolar and first molar in the coronal slice (Fig 5).

STATISTICAL ANALYSIS

Data obtained for measurements at 6 mm and 8 mm were statistically analyzed by means of paired t-test. The scanned images were measured by the same observer after a two week interval. The error of the method (EM) calculations were carried out by means of Dahlberg's formula.[6]

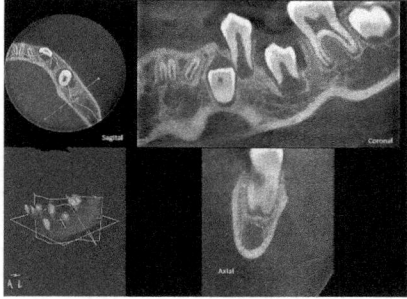

Figure 1 - Sagittal, coronal and axial slices.

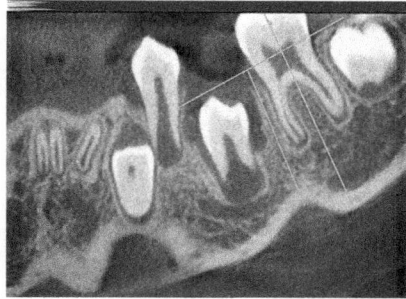

Figure 2 - Vertical and horizontal reference plane.

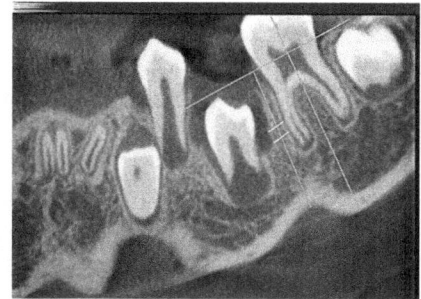

Figure 3 - Mesiodistal bone width at 6 and 8 mm.

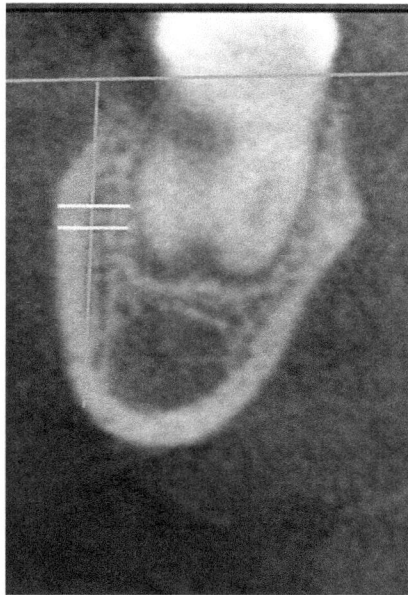

Figure 4 - Buccal cortical bone thickness at 6 mm and 8 mm.

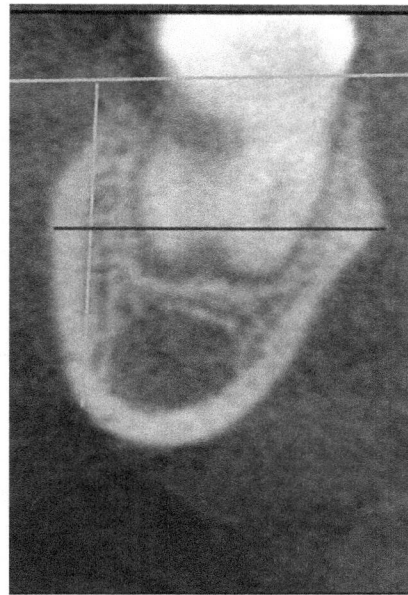

Figure 5 - Buccolingual bone depth at 6 mm and 8 mm.

RESULTS

Of the 15 images obtained, three were discarded due to poor image quality. Mean and standard deviation for each of the variables were calculated. Mesiodistal bone width measurements at 6 mm and 8 mm ranged from 1.3 to 2.9 mm. Results for buccal cortical plate thickness and buccolingual bone depth ranged between 1.5 - 2.9 mm and 11.9 - 15.4 mm, respectively. Mean values for mesiodistal bone width, buccal cortical plate thickness and buccolingual bone depth at 8 mm were found to be sufficient for miniscrews placement with a diameter of 1.2 - 1.4 mm and length of 10 - 14 mm (Table 1).

Differences in measurement at 6 and 8 mm for buccal cortical plate thickness ($P < 0.05$) and buccolingual bone thickness ($P < 0.05$) were found to be significant, whereas for mesiodistal width it was insignificant ($P > 0.05$) (Table 2). The error of the method (EM) for mesiodistal bone width, buccal and palatal cortical plate thickness and buccopalatal bone depth measurements were found to be 0.40, 0.58 and 0.48, respectively (Table 3).

DISCUSSION

Miniscrews[13-17] are now frequently used for establishing absolute anchorage for orthodontic tooth movement. They are easily inserted and removed without a mucoperiosteal flap, and can be loaded immediately after insertion.[18] Their potential applications include improving anchorage, increasing the horizontal component of force applied during space closure, posterior

Table 1 - Mean and standard deviation for mesiodistal bone width, buccal cortical plate thickness and buccolingual bone depth measurements.

Patient	Mesiodistal width		Buccal cortical plate		Buccolingual bone thickness	
	6 mm	8 mm	6 mm	8 mm	6 mm	8 mm
1	2.3 mm	2.6 mm	2.0 mm	2.9 mm	13.1 mm	13.7 mm
2	2.7 mm	2.6 mm	1.5 mm	2.6 mm	11.9 mm	12.1 mm
3	1.3 mm	2.2 mm	1.9 mm	1.9 mm	15.4 mm	15.4 mm
4	2.3 mm	2.8 mm	1.8 mm	2.4 mm	12.4 mm	12.8 mm
5	2.4 mm	2.9 mm	2.1 mm	2.5 mm	13.5 mm	14.8 mm
6	1.9 mm	2.6 mm	1.9 mm	2.2 mm	12.8 mm	13.1 mm
7	2.0 mm	2.8 mm	1.8 mm	2.6 mm	13.4 mm	15.1 mm
8	2.1 mm	2.7 mm	2.2 mm	2.7 mm	13.6 mm	14.3 mm
9	1.9 mm	2.4 mm	1.9 mm	2.5 mm	13.4 mm	13.7 mm
10	2.4 mm	2.8 mm	1.8 mm	2.3 mm	13.1 mm	13.5 mm
11	2.3 mm	2.5 mm	2.0 mm	2.0 mm	12.9 mm	12.5 mm
12	2.2 mm	2.5 mm	1.5 mm	2.4 mm	12.7 mm	12.8 mm
Mean ± SD	2.15 ± 0.49	2.48 ± 0.33	1.73 ± 0.41	2.42 ± 0.34	13.18 ± 1.22	13.65 ± 1.25

Table 2 - Paired t-test for mesiodistal bone width, buccal and palatal cortical plate thickness and buccolingual bone depth measurements.

	Mesiodistal width	Buccal cortical plate thickness	Buccolingual depth
T-test value	1.76	3.37	2.51
P value	0.13 (N.S., P > 0.05)	0.021 (Sig, P < 0.05)	0.044 (Sig, P < 0.05)

Table 3 - Error of the method for mesiodistal bone width, buccal and palatal cortical plate thickness and buccolingual bone depth measurements at 6 and 8 mm.

	Mesiodistal width	Buccal cortical plate thickness	Buccolingual depth
Error of the method	0.40	0.58	0.48

intrusion in open-bite cases, distalization of molars, extrusion of impacted teeth, molar uprighting and correction of midline diastema.[7,8,18]

The mandibular buccal region had the thickest cortical bone of all evaluated regions. Thicker cortical bone has been previously reported in the mandible than in the maxilla.[12,19] Increased cortical bone thickness and higher bone mineral density have been shown in the mandibular buccal region when compared to the maxillary buccal and lingual regions,[20-23] as the mandible is found to be always under torsional and bending strains or forces, whereas the maxilla is generally subjected to more compressive forces.[24] Also, in animal experiments, it has been demonstrated that regions which experience higher strain during function develop thicker cortical bones.[25]

Thus, in humans, cortical bone in the mandibular buccal region was found to be thicker posteriorly, and it becomes progressively thinner anteriorly.[12,26] This pattern might also be explained by the higher functional demands placed on posterior teeth. Van Eijden[24] reported an increase in the longitudinal elastic modulus (increase in stress per unit of strain) between the molar region and the symphysis. Stress and strain differences could give rise to the differences in cortical thickness in this region.

Age-related differences between younger, adolescent and older patients in cortical bone thickness might be explained by changes in functional capacity, because maximum bite forces, masticatory muscle size, and muscle activity have the tendency to increase with age. Changes in the functional capacity, which alter biomechanical stresses and strains, have shown to manipulate cortical bone thickness and bone density because increased strains and stresses within a certain limit increase cortical bone thickness and bone mineral density.[10]

In the mandible, the safest sites for miniscrew insertion have been found to be between the first and second molars, first and second premolars, first molar and first premolar and first premolar and canine. These sites provide moderate inter-radicular space and sufficient cortical plate thickness. However, due to root proximity, the area suitable for miniscrew insertion is over 8 mm from the alveolar crest.[6]

In this study, the CEJ was selected as the starting point for measurements, as compared to other studies in which alveolar crest was used, which could be affected by different periodontal problems.[27,28] The maximum level of measurement in this study was selected to be 6 and 8 mm from CEJ because miniscrew placement is most commonly advised in the area of attached gingiva.[29]

The selection of proper miniscrew diameter and length is important as it may hamper eruption or deflect erupting premolars during mixed dentition. Hence, selection will depend upon inter-radicular mesiodistal bone width, buccal cortical plate thickness and buccolingual bone depth.[28] Currently, most miniscrews have diameters ranging from 1.2 to 2 mm. Presently, there are no relative data available on the amount of bone that is to be present between miniscrews and dental roots for both periodontal health and miniscrew stability. Considering that the width of the periodontal ligament is approximately 0.25 mm, it is assumed that a minimum clearance of 1 mm of alveolar bone around the screw could be sufficient for periodontal health.[6,28] Combining this value with our data, the safe zone for a miniscrew 1.2 mm in diameter, placed in the inter-radicular spaces have been identified to be at 8 mm.

Radiographic analysis is a pre-requirement in determining anatomic sites for implant placement. Three-dimensional imaging techniques, such as CT or MRI imaging, have turned into important diagnostic imaging in the head and neck.[30] CT involves a considerably higher radiation dose[31] in comparison to conventional radiography, as well as high working costs and considerable investment in equipment.[32]

Digital volume tomograph (DVT) is a new imaging technique which produces three-dimensional images similar to CT, but at a low radiation dose which is comparable with panoramic radiograph, and at a lesser cost. DVT technology in clinical practice has numerous advantages, such as image accuracy, rapid scan time and display modes which are unique to maxillofacial imaging. Three-dimensional volumetric tomograph is also well suited for imaging the craniofacial area because it provides clear images of highly contrasted structures which are extremely useful for evaluating bone.[33,34] Hence, in this study, three-dimensional digital volumetric tomograph (DVT) was used to assess mesiodistal bone width, cortical bone thickness and buccolingual bone depth.

In the mandibular molar region, mini-implants placement between premolars is not recommended due to the presence of mental foramen.[29] Hence, the proximity of the mental foramina and bone density in the posterior region needs to be assessed in mixed dentition in order to provide a three-dimensional analysis for miniscrew placement. However, the results of the present study need to be correlated with clinical assessment so as to maintain optimum periodontal health and miniscrew stability.

CONCLUSION

After evaluating the amount of bone thickness in the inter-radicular spaces of the mandibular posterior region, the results of the present study show promising evidence for safe miniscrews placement in the mixed dentition period. This results need to be reevaluated in a larger scale.

Miniscrew has proved to be the best alternative to routinely use clinical appliances for space management, uprighting and distalization of molars, and intrusion and extrusion of teeth. It can also be used as a temporary prosthesis abutment in younger patients.

REFERENCES

1. Guidelines on the use of space maintainers following premature loss of primary teeth. J Can Dent Assoc. 1997;63(10):753-66.

2. Laing E, Ashley P, Naini FB, Gill DS. Space maintenance. Int J Paediatr Dent. 2009;19(3):155-62.

3. Ngan P, Randy GA, Fields JRH. Management of space problems in the primary and mixed dentitions. J Am Dent Assoc. 1999;130:1330-9.

4. Dincer M, Haydar S, Unsal B, Turk TS. Space maintainer effects on intercanine arch width and length. J Clin Pediatr Dent. 1996;21(1):47-50.

5. Cuoghi OA, Bertoz FA, de Mendonca MR, Santos EC. Loss of space and dental arch length after the loss of the lower first primary molar: A longitudinal study. J Clin Pediatr Dent 1998;22(2):117-20.

6. Paola MP, Cristina I, Sefano V, Aldo C. Safe Zones: a guide for miniscrew positioning in the maxillary and mandibular arch. Angle Orthod. 2006;76(2):191-7.

7. Carano A, Velo S, Leone P, Siciliani G. Clinical applications of the Miniscrew Anchorage System. J Clin Orthod. 2005;39(1):9-24.

8. Mark R, Yanosky, Holmes JD. Mini-implant temporary anchorage devices: orthodontic applications. Compend. 2008;29(1):12-20.

9. Kim SH, Yoon HG. Evaluation of interdental space of the maxillary posterior area for orthodontic mini-implants with cone-beam computed tomography. Am J Orthod Dentofacial Orthop. 2009;135(5):635-41.

10. Farnsworth D, Rossouw PE, Ceen RF, Buschangd PH. Cortical bone thickness at common miniscrew implant placement sites. Am J Orthod Dentofacial Orthop. 2011;139(4):495-503.

11. Kang S, Lee SJ, Ahn SJ, Heo MS, Kim TW. Bone thickness of the palate for orthodontic mini-implant anchorage in adults. Am J Orthod Dentofacial Orthop. 2007;131(4 Suppl):S74-81.

12. Schwartz CL, Dechow PC. Variations in cortical material properties throughout the human dentate mandible. Am J Phys Anthropol. 2003;120(3):252-77.

13. Costa A, Raffainl M, Melsen B. Miniscrews as orthodontic anchorage: a preliminary report. Int J Adult Orthodon Orthognath Surg. 1998;13(3):201-9.

14. Kanomi R. Mini-implant for orthodontic anchorage. J Clin Orthod. 1997;31:763-7.

15. Park HS, Bae SM, Kyung HM, Sung JH. Micro-implant anchorage for treatment of skeletal Class I bialveolar protrusion. J Clin Orthod. 2001;35(7):417-22.

16. Paik CH, Woo YJ, Boyd R. Treatment of an adult patient with vertical maxillary excess using miniscrew fixation. J Clin Orthod. 2003;37(8):423-8.

17. Xun CL, Zeng XL, Wang X. Clinical application of miniscrew implant for maximum anchorage treatment. Chin J Stomatol. 2004;39:505-8.

18. Fortini A, Cacciafesta V, Sfondrini MF, Cambi S, Lupoli M. Clinical applications and efficiency of miniscrews for extradental anchorage. Orthodontics. 2004;1(2):1-12.

19. Peterson J, Wang Q, Dechow PC. Material properties of the dentate maxilla. Anat Rec A Discov Mol Cell Evol Biol. 2006;288(9):962-72.

20. Ono A, Motoyoshi M, Shimizu N. Cortical bone thickness in the buccal posterior region for orthodontic mini-implants. Int J Oral Maxillofac Surg. 2008;37(4):334-40

21. Deguchi T, Nasu M, Murakami K, Yabuuchi T, Kamioka H, Takano-Yamamoto T. Quantitative evaluation of cortical bone thickness with computed tomographic scanning for orthodontic implants. Am J Orthod Dentofacial Orthop. 2006;129(6):721.e7-12.

22. Park HS, Lee YJ, Jeong SH, Kwon TG. Density of the alveolar and basal bones of the maxilla and the mandible. Am J Orthod Dentofacial Orthop. 2008;133(1):30-7.

23. Mitsuru M. Clinical indices for orthodontic mini-implants. J Oral Sci. 2011;3(4):407-12.

24. Van Eijden TM. Biomechanics of the mandible. Crit Rev Oral Biol Med. 2000;11(1):123-36.

25. Daegling DJ, Hylander WL. Experimental observation, theoretical models, and biomechanical inference in the study of mandibular form. Am J Phys Anthropol. 2000;112(4):541-51.

26. Katranji A, Misch K, Wang HL. Cortical bone thickness in dentate and edentulous human cadavers. J Periodontol. 2007;78(5):874-8.

27. Fayed MM, Pazera P, Katsaros C. Optimal sites for orthodontic mini-implant placement assessed by cone beam computed tomography. Angle Orthod. 2010;80(5):939-51.

28. Monnerat C, Restle L, Mucha JN. Tomographic mapping of mandibular interradicular spaces for placement of orthodontic mini-implants. Am J Orthod Dentofacial Orthop. 2009;135(4):428.e1-9; discussion 428-9

29. Melsen B. Mini-implants: where are we? J Clin Orthod 2005;39:539-47.

30. Fuhrmann R, Klein HM, Wehrbein H, Guènther RW, Dietrich P. Hochaufö sende computertomographie fazialer und oraler knochendehiszenzen. Dtsch ZahnaÈrztl Z. 1993;48:242-6.

31. Hassfeld S, Streib S, Stahl H, Stratmann U, Fehrentz D, ZoÈller J. Low-dose-computertomographie des kieferknochens in derpraÈ implantologischen Diagnostik. Mund Kiefer Gesichts Chir. 1998;2:188-93.

32. Arai Y, Tammisalo E, Iwai K, Hashimoto K, Shinoda K. Development of a compact computed tomographic apparatus for dental use. Dentomaxillofac Radiol. 1999;28(4):245-8.

33. Ziegler CM, Woertche R, Brief J, Hassfeld S. Clinical indications for digital volume tomography in oral and maxillofacial surgery. Dentomaxillofac Radiol. 2002;31(2):126-30.

34. Scarfe WC, Farman AG, Sukovic P. Clinical applications of cone-beam computed tomography in dental practice. J Can Dent Assoc. 2006;72(1):75-80.

18

Comparison of clinical bracket point registration with 3D laser scanner and coordinate measuring machine

Mahtab Nouri[1], Arash Farzan[2], Ali Reza Akbarzadeh Baghban[3], Reza Massudi[4]

Objective: The aim of the present study was to assess the diagnostic value of a laser scanner developed to determine the coordinates of clinical bracket points and to compare with the results of a coordinate measuring machine (CMM). **Methods:** This diagnostic experimental study was conducted on maxillary and mandibular orthodontic study casts of 18 adults with normal Class I occlusion. First, the coordinates of the bracket points were measured on all casts by a CMM. Then, the three-dimensional coordinates (X, Y, Z) of the bracket points were measured on the same casts by a 3D laser scanner designed at Shahid Beheshti University, Tehran, Iran. The validity and reliability of each system were assessed by means of intraclass correlation coefficient (ICC) and Dahlberg's formula. **Results:** The difference between the mean dimension and the actual value for the CMM was 0.0066 mm. (95% CI: 69.98340, 69.99140). The mean difference for the laser scanner was 0.107 ± 0.133 mm (95% CI: -0.002, 0.24). In each method, differences were not significant. The ICC comparing the two methods was 0.998 for the X coordinate, and 0.996 for the Y coordinate; the mean difference for coordinates recorded in the entire arch and for each tooth was 0.616 mm. **Conclusion:** The accuracy of clinical bracket point coordinates measured by the laser scanner was equal to that of CMM. The mean difference in measurements was within the range of operator errors.

Keywords: Laser. Orthodontics. Computer-assisted image processing.

» The authors report no commercial, proprietary or financial interest in the products or companies described in this article.

[1] Associate professor, Dentofacial Deformities Research Center of Shahid Beheshti University of Medical Sciences, Iran.

[2] Postgraduate student of Orthodontics, Research Center of Shahid Beheshti University of Medical Sciences, Iran.

[3] Assistant professor of Biostatistics, Faculty of Paramedicine, Shahid Beheshti, University of Medical Sciences, Iran.

[4] Professor, Laser and Plasma Research Institute, Shahid Beheshti University, Iran.

Arash Farzan - Orthodontics Dep., Shahid Beheshti University of Medical Sciences, Evin, 11, Tehran, 1998777339 — Iran.
E-mail: dr.arash.farzan@gmail.com

INTRODUCTION

In order to prevent relapse during the retention period, it is paramount that the arch form be maintained. Therefore, before orthodontic treatment onset, patient's initial arch form should be determined and wires with the same arch form should be used throughout treatment so as to ensure stability of treatment results.

Various landmarks and tools have been used to assess patient's arch form. In previous studies, the midpoint of incisal edges and buccal cusp tips have been used as landmarks.[1,2] However, with the technological advances in three-dimensional devices, buccal landmarks at bracket attachment points became available to be used for this purpose.[3-6] This new technique helps in generating a more precise arch form, especially at force application points.

Various imaging techniques, such as radiography, photocopy, two-dimensional scanning,[5] three-dimensional scanning[5] and coordinate measuring machine (CMM),[7] have been used to determine patient's dental arch form.

CMM is found to be the most accurate device for this purpose. Due to its mechanical nature and the presence of a touch probe, this technique has a high precision of approximately 10 μm and can be considered as the gold standard.[7] Stereophotogrammetry and CBCT have also been introduced for 3D imaging with the use of laser or regular light. Of the mentioned techniques, laser scanner is found to be an accurate method. OraScanner, for instance, was reported to have an accuracy of approximately 30-50 μm.[8] The voxel size in CBCT is of approximately 0.125 mm.[9]

After determining the landmarks with an accurate imaging technique, a mathematical model is adopted to these points, following a straight curve to be used in straight wire techniques. Currently, second and third order bends can be performed by the use of robotics; however, these methods have not gained much popularity due to the complexity and high costs of the technique. Although different mathematical models, such as the fourth-degree polynomial equation, beta-function and cubic spline, have been used in different studies, mostly, the use of polynomial equation has been suggested.[10-18]

In Iran, as in other Middle Eastern countries, the use of these technologies is not feasible, since the majority of companies do not operate in this area. Therefore, we developed a laser scanner as well as its associated software to generate arch form using a fourth-degree polynomial equation. The scanner was developed at the Orthodontics and Dentofacial Orthopedics Department of Shahid Beheshti Medical University.

The aim of the present study is to assess the diagnostic value of this laser scanner designed to determine the coordinates of clinical bracket points, and to compare the results with the results yielded by CMM.

MATERIAL AND METHODS

This diagnostic experimental study was conducted on maxillary and mandibular orthodontic study casts of 18 adults with normal Class I occlusion and fully erupted permanent teeth including second molars. Patients did not have crowding or midline shift and teeth had no abrasion, fracture, or ectopic eruption.

In order to create maximum contrast for visual detection, all casts were colored black, using water-soluble dye (Pars Co., Tehran, Iran) and a brush. Afterwards, clinical bracket points were marked on each tooth according to the bracket placement guide for prefabricated appliances.[19] An orthodontic gauge (Unitek, USA) and a fine tip white nail polish measuring 2 mm in diameter (Nail Design Polish, Victoria, Taiwan, Taiwan) were used (Figs 1A-C).

In the first part of the study, the coordinates of bracket points were measured on all casts by a coordinate measuring machine (CMM) (Mora, Aschaffenburg, Germany) with 10 ± 0.01 micrometer precision. Files were digitally saved in .txt format (Figs 2 A, B). This device has a touch probe with a diameter of 2 mm. When the operator touched the respective point with the probe, the machine read the input from the probe and recorded the X, Y and Z coordinates of the point. In the second part of the study, the three-dimensional coordinates (X, Y, Z) of bracket points were measured on the same casts by a 3D laser scanner designed at Shahid Beheshti University, Tehran, Iran.[20] Files were also saved in .txt format. The scanner consisted of two class 2 laser diodes and two charge-coupled devices (CCD) used to capture and transfer images into a computer.

Scanner

Scanning was carried out with a 3D surface laser scanner. Our scanner[20] consisted of two class 2 laser diodes operating at 685 nm with output power of

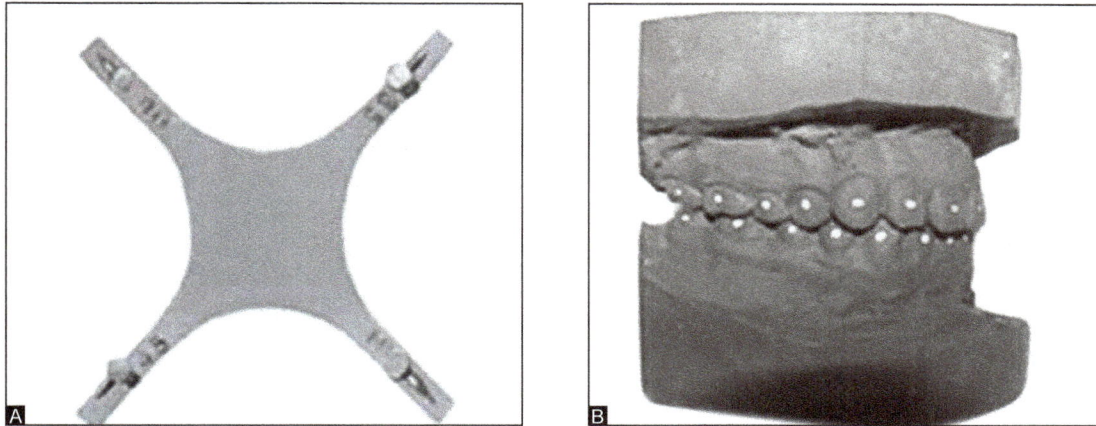

Figure 1 - Preparation of dental cast for digitiza-tion by CMM and laser scanner. **A)** Orthodontic measuring gauge used to determine CBPs. **B)** Fi-nal dental casts after being painted and marked for CBPs.

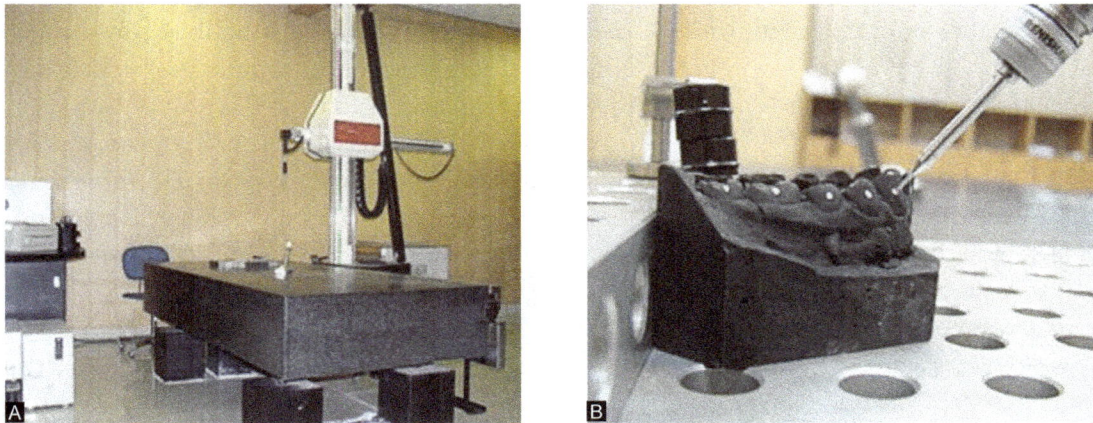

Figure 2 - Coordinate measuring machine (CMM). **A)** Device setting general view. **B)** Dental casts are placed to have CBPs digitized by the touch probe of the CMM.

1 mW. Each laser produced a line 100-mm thick at a distance of 180 mm from the laser. Two CCDs (768 x 493 pixels, Hitachi KPM1, Japan) captured and transferred the image of the cast into a computer. The distance between the cameras and the object varied from 12 to 26 cm. The maximum area of test scanning was 6 x 6 cm². The cast was secured to the horizontal surface of a rotating table controlled by a step motor which rotated the table with an accuracy of 0.009 degrees (Figs 3 A, B). To calibrate the scanner system, we attached two metal backing plates separating the rectangular grids (16 x 16 cm) with circles printed on paper. The diameter of each circle was 6 mm and the distance

between them was 12 mm. The grid had an angle of 30 degrees relative to the side of the rectangle. The vertical distance between the two plates was 20 mm. For calibration, the grids were placed on the rotating table and the CCDs were adjusted so that the whole grid pattern could be imaged. Each CCD captured an image and the software merged both images into a final image. A program written in Visual Basic 6 environment was used to calculate the relative position of different points on the cast. To acquire such position, we first determined the location of the CCD and the laser relative to a specified point on the rotating table. Next, the cast, marked with a point painted on

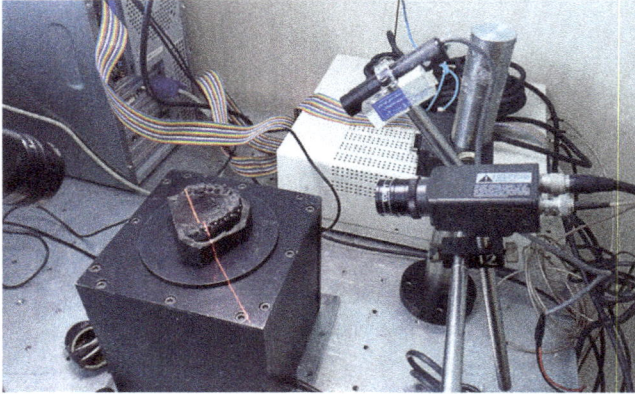

Figure 3 - Dental casts are placed on the rotor for CBP digitization. Laser beam is irradiated onto the cast while it is rotated by the rotor.

its surface, was adjusted on the rotating table. Having the resolution of the stepper motor and considering different reflections of the laser from the white color points on the cast, one can determine the position of those points in relation to the center of the coordinate.

DATA ANALYSIS
Reproducibility and Validity

Normally, the validity of CMM is annually controlled by the manufacturer. Additionally, a certificate of validity is issued. However, in this study, validity and reproducibility of the device were ensured by measuring the diameter of a reference metal master disc (Gauge disc, Mitutoyo, Osaka, Japan) with a known diameter of 69.994 mm at 20 °C. Measurements were taken by the operator for 10 times with at least one-day interval between each measurement. To assess reproducibility of the 3D laser scanner, a Teflon cube with dimensions of 31.90 x 31.90 mm was scanned. The values obtained were compared with actual dimensions of the cube. The dimensional measurements were exactly the same as the actual dimensions of the cube.

To assess the laser scanner validity in measuring clinical bracket point coordinates, the Y and X coordinates recorded on each cast were compared using the Y and X coordinates obtained from CMM readings as reference. Since the Z coordinate is not required for drawing dental arch curve, this coordinate was considered as zero for each point. To assess reproducibility of CMM, CMM measurements of the reference master gauge disc were compared with the actual measurements of the disc at 20 °C. To assess reproducibility of the laser scanner, CMM

measurements of the Teflon cube were compared with 3D scanner measurements of the cube. The magnitudes of errors were determined by means, standard deviation and 95% confidence intervals. To assess the laser scanner validity in measuring the coordinates of clinical bracket points, the coordinates recorded by the laser scanner were compared with CMM reading using ICC. The numerical value of this error was calculated for each group of maxillary and mandibular teeth and compared with CMM measurements using Dahlberg's[21] formula as the reference.

RESULTS

The results of CMM reproducibility testing that included measurements of the diameter of a reference master gauge disc (Mitutoyo, Osaka, Japan) with a known diameter of 69.994 mm at 20 °C measured 10 times by the same operator showed that the mean recorded value was 69.98740 mm, with a range of 0.004 mm and standard deviation of 0.016 mm. The difference between the measured mean dimension and the actual value was 0.0066 mm. At 95% CI, this difference was not statistically significant.

Comparisons of the 10 measurements of the cube are presented in Table 1. The mean difference is 0.107 ± 0.133 mm (95% CI: -0.002, 0.24). Since zero falls within the confidence interval, there was no statistically significant difference between the two methods used to calculate the dimensions of the cube.

ICC was 0.998 for the X coordinate and 0.996 for the Y coordinate; which were indicative of a very high similarity between measurements yielded by both methods: CMM and laser scanner. The numerical differences for the X and Y coordinates, according to Dahlberg's formula applied to various areas of the dental arch, are demonstrated in Table 2. It was the least for central incisors and the greatest for molars. The numerical differences in the X and Y coordinates of incisors were 0.345 and 0.426, respectively. The numerical differences in the X and Y coordinates of canines were 0.661 and 0.606, respectively. Also, the numerical differences in the X and Y coordinates of posterior teeth were 0.860 and 0.817, respectively. The greater the convexity of the tooth surface, the greater the difference between measurements. Thus, the maximum error value is usually observed in molars and first premolars. There was no difference between maxillary and mandibular measurements.

The mean difference in the coordinates recorded in the entire arch and for each tooth was 0.616 mm. These differences do not cause clinically significant changes when drawing patient's arch form (Figs 4A, B).

DISCUSSION

In this study, a newly developed 3D laser scanner was compared with a CMM with regards to measuring the dimensions of a Teflon cube and recording the coordinates of clinical bracket points. The coordinates of clinical bracket points are helpful in drawing a polynomial curve of the dental arch. No significant differences were detected in the dimensions of the Teflon cube measured by the two devices. However, according to Dahlberg's formula, the difference

Table 1 - Ten measurements of the Teflon cube.

Scanner measurements	31.92	32.15	32.07	32.11	32.01	31.79	32.17	32.05	31.80	32.01
Difference*	C.02	0.25	0.17	0.21	0.11	-0.11	0.27	0.15	-0.10	0.11

*Scanner value - reference value (31.90 mm).

Table 2 - Numerical differences for the X and Y coordinates according to Dahlberg's formula.

X centrals	Y centrals	X laterals	Y laterals	X canines	Y canines	X premolars	Y premolars	X molars	Y molars	
0.252	0.365	0.439	0.487	0.661	0.606	0.776	0.695	0.945	0.939	Total
0.285	0.368	0.36	0.400	0.655	0.466	0.749	0.580	0.953	0.924	Upper arch
0.218	0.355	0.498	0.556	0.667	0.704	0.801	0.796	0.937	0.939	Lower arch

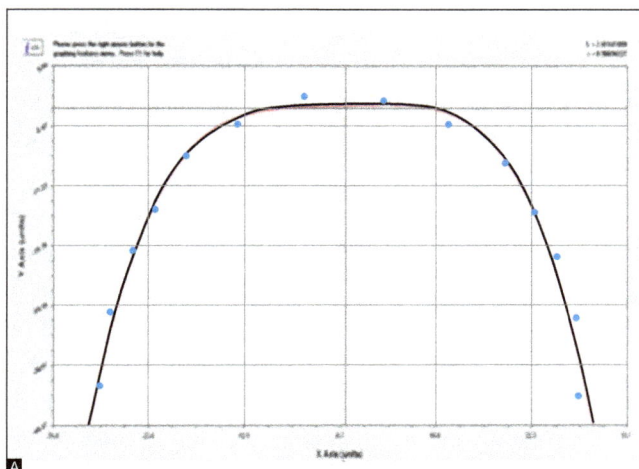

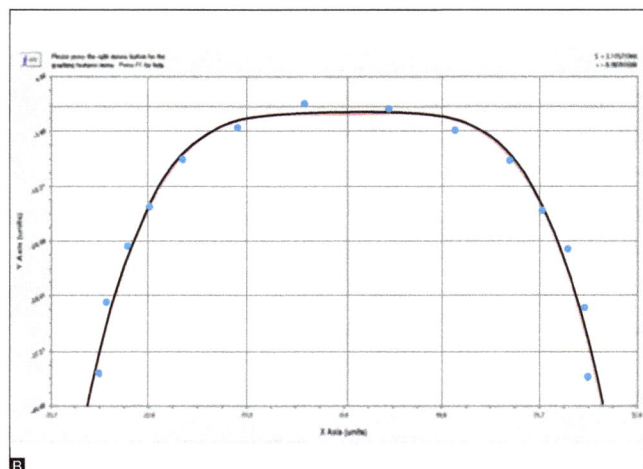

Figure 4 - **A)** A sample of dental arch drawn by 4ᵗʰ degree polynomial, using coordinates obtained by CMM. **B)** A sample of maxillary arch drawn by 4ᵗʰ degree polynomial, using coordinates obtained by the laser scanner.

between the mean values of the coordinates of clinical bracket points was found to be 0.616 mm in the X and Y coordinates when the readings of the 3D laser scanner and the reference device (CMM) were compared. This difference between the two devices may be due to the different linear measurements and due to recording only one point. For example, the linear distance between two distinct points may be nearly the same, although the exact coordinates may differ. There is also another fact that should be taken into account when digitizing CBPs by a 3D laser scanner: the difference between CBP's width (1 mm, on average) and irradiated laser beam width (100 μm or 0.1 mm, on average). Even though the software used to perform landmark digitization calculated the geometric center of each point, a difference between the center point determined by two devices may have contributed to potential differences in measurements.

This difference may also be attributed to the different spatial location of these points (due to the position of clinical bracket points in different spatial planes). The variability of this difference in different tooth series is another important issue that needs to be considered. An increasing gradient exists in the amount of this difference as moving from anterior towards posterior teeth, since the least difference was observed at central incisors and the maximum difference at molar teeth. Considering the fact that convexity of teeth increases in the dental arch from anterior towards posterior teeth (labial surface of incisors is more flat than the buccal surface of posterior teeth), it can be suggested that the difference between the two devices is due to the different placement of the CMM probe compared to the point captured by the 3D scanner on more convex surfaces in comparison to straighter surfaces. The amount of this difference was calculated separately for the maxilla and mandible. It seems that no difference exists in recording coordinates at different areas of the the mandible and the maxilla. In general, the amount of difference between the X and Y coordinates of different tooth series was slightly different and less than the clinically perceptible level, since this difference was less than 1 mm which is the human eye accuracy.

To date, several studies have assessed the accuracy of 3D methods. Nearly all of them were based on assessment and comparison between linear dimensions (such as tooth size,[20,22-26] intercanine distance, interpremolar distance, intermolar distance,[24,24,27,28] tooth crown height,[29] and arch length[23,24,28,30,31]) and a reference method (for instance, manual measurement on dental casts). In the present study, we compared Descartes' coordinates of specific points. To this end, we compared the coordinates recorded by our newly designed 3D laser scanner with readings yielded by an accurate reference device (CMM). Once the spatial coordinates of specific points required by the clinician are recorded with an acceptable accuracy, linear (related to two points) and angular (related to three points) measurements will have an acceptable accuracy as well.

According to a systematic review,[32] the mean difference between 3D techniques and reference methods in measurement of mesiodistal width of teeth was 0.01 to 0.3 mm. Also, the mean difference between 3D techniques and reference methods was 0.04 to 0.4 mm when measuring intercanine, interpremolar and intermolar distances, as well as 0.1 mm when measuring tooth crown height, and 0.19 to 0.8 mm when measuring arch length. With our laser scanner, the differences in Descartes' coordinates of clinical bracket points varied from 0.2 to 0.9 mm at various areas of the dental arch with a mean difference of 0.616 mm.

Furthermore, the reproducibility (reliability coefficient) of measurements performed by our 3D laser scanner ranged from fair to good.[33]

Accuracy of our laser scanner, especially at the anterior arch, was acceptable for clinical purposes (the overall mean difference of 0.468 mm with the area between central incisors and canine teeth used as reference). The lower accuracy of the device in recording the coordinates of points at the posterior arch is less critical considering the U-shaped form of the dental arch and the main goal of measuring these coordinates, which is to determine the clinical bracket points or drawing the arch form. A slight difference between the coordinates of these points and their actual coordinates was within the error range of our device and does not cause significant changes when drawing the arch form (Figs 4A, B).

It is suggested that the accuracy of measurements be increased in future studies by improving the rotational mechanics of the device, enhancing the accuracy of CCD imaging and using a thinner probe in the CMM.

Within the limitations of this study, the following conclusions were drawn:

The accuracy of clinical bracket point coordinates measured by our laser scanner was equal to that of CMM. The mean difference in measurements was within the range of operator errors (mean of 0.616 mm). One error in recording point coordinates by CMM is due to the operator and the width of the probe. However, this error has no clinical significance. In the laser scanner technique, error is attributed to the width of the marked point which is much wider than the width of the irradiated laser.

REFERENCES

1. Bonwill WGA. Geometrical and mechanical laws of articulation. Tr Ortod Soc. 1985;119-33.

2. Broomell IN. Anatomy and histology of the mouth and teeth. 2nd ed. Philadelphia: Blackiston's Son; 1902.

3. Stanton FL. Arch predetermination and a method of relating predetermind arch to the malocclusion to show the minimum tooth movement. Int J Orthod Oral Surg Radiogr. 1922;8(12):757-78.

4. Brader AC. Dental arch form related with intraoral forces: PR=C. Am J Orthod. 1972;61(6):541-61.

5. Beagle EA. Application of the cubic spline function in the description of dental arch form. J Dent Res. 1980;59:1549-56.

6. Sampson PD. Dental arch shape: a statistical analysis using conic sections. Am J Orthod. 1981;79(5):535-48.

7. Lili M, Xu T, Lin J. Validation of a three-dimensional facial scanning system based on structured light techniques. Comput Methods Programs Biomed. 2009;94(3):290-8.

8. Graber LW, Vanarsdall RL, Vig KWL. Orthodontics: current principles and techniques. 5th ed. Philadelphia: Mosby. 2012.

9. Hajeer MY, Millett DT, Ayoub AF, Siebert JP. Applications of 3D imaging in orthodontics: part II. J Orthod. 2004;31(2):154-62.

10. Triviño T, Vilella OV. Forms and dimensions of the lower dental arch. Rev Soc Bras Ortodon 2005;5:19-28.

11. Kageyama T, Domínguez-Rodríguez GC, Vigorito JW, Deguchi T. A morphological study of the relationship between arch dimensions and craniofacial structures in adolescents with Class II Division 1 malocclusions and various facial types. Am J Orthod Dentofacial Orthop. 2006;129(3):368-75.

12. Lu KH. An orthogonal analysis of the form, symmetry, and asymmetry of the dental arch. Arch Oral Biol. 1966;11:1057-69.

13. Sanin C, Savara BS, Thomas DR, Clarkson QD. Arc length of the dental arch estimated by multiple regression. J Dent Res. 1970;49(4):885.

14. Pepe SH. Polynomial and catenary curve fits to human dental arches. J Dent Res. 1975;54(6):1124-32.

15. Hechter FJ. Symmetric and dental arch form of orthodontically treated patients. Dent J. 1978;44(4):173-84.

16. Ferrario VF, Sforza C, Miani AJ, Tartaglia G. Mathematical definition of the shape of dental arches in human permanent healthy dentitions. Eur J Orthod. 1994;16(4):287-94.

17. Wakabayashi K, Sohmura T, Takahashi J, Kojima T, Akao T, Nakamura T, et al. Development of the computerized dental cast form analyzing system: three dimensional diagnosis of dental arch form and the investigation of measuring condition. Dent Mater J 1997;16(2):180-90.

18. Ferrario VF, Sforza C, Dellavia C, Colombo A, Ferrari RP. Three-dimensional hard tissue palatal size and shape: a 10-year longitudinal evaluation in healthy adults. Int J Adult Orthod Orthognath Surg. 2002;17(1):51-8.

19. BeGole EA. A computer program for the analysis of dental arch form using the catenary curve. Comput Programs Biomed. 1981;13(1-2):93-9.

20. Nouri M, Massudi R, Bagheban AA, Azimi S, Fereidooni F. The accuracy of a 3D laser scanner for crown width measurements. Aust Orthod J. 2009;25(1):41-7.

21. Dahlberg G. Statistical methods for medical and biological students. London: George Allen & Unwin; 1940.

22. Santoro M, Galkin S, Teredesai M, Nicolay OF, Cangialosi TJ. Comparison of measurements made on digital and plaster models. Am J Orthod Dentofacial Orthop. 2003;124(1):101-5.

23. Redlich M, Weinstock T, Abed Y, Schneor R, Holdstein Y, Fischer A. A new system for scanning, measuring and analyzing dental casts based on a 3D holographic sensor. Orthod Craniofac Res. 2008;11(2):90-5.

24. Goonewardene RW, Goonewardene MS, Razza JM, Murray K. Accuracy and validity of space analysis and irregularity index measurements using digital models. Aust Orthod J. 2008;24(2):83-90.

25. Watanabe-Kanno GA, Abrao J, Miasiro Junior H, Sanchez-Ayala A, Lagravere MO. Reproducibility, reliability and validity of measurements obtained from Cecile3 digital models. Braz Oral Res. 2009;23(3):288-95.

26. Horton HM, Miller JR, Gaillard PR, Larson BE. Technique comparison for efficient orthodontic tooth measurements using digital models. Angle Orthod. 2010;80(2):254-61.

27. Bell A, Ayoub AF, Siebert P. Assessment of the accuracy of a three-dimensional imaging system for archiving dental study models. J Orthod. 2003;30(3):219-23.

28. Quimby ML, Vig KW, Rashid RG, Firestone AR. The accuracy and reliability of measurements made on computer-based digital models. Angle Orthod. 2004;74(3):298-303.

29. Keating AP, Knox J, Bibb R, Zhurov AI. A comparison of plaster, digital and reconstructed study model accuracy. J Orthod. 2008;35(3):191-201.

30. Stevens DR, Flores-Mir C, Nebbe B, Raboud DW, Heo G, Major PW. Validity, reliability, and reproducibility of plaster vs digital study models: comparison of peer assessment rating and Bolton analysis and their constituent measurements. Am J Orthod Dentofacial Orthop. 2006;129(6):794-803.

31. Leifert MF, Leifert MM, Efstratiadis SS, Cangialosi TJ. Comparison of space analysis evaluations with digital models and plaster dental casts. Am J Orthod Dentofacial Orthop. 2009;136(1):16 e1-4.

32. Fleming PS, Marinho V, Johal A. Orthodontic measurements on digital study models compared with plaster models: a systematic review. Orthod Craniofac Res. 2011;14(1):1-16.

33. Roberts CT, Richmond S. The design and analysis of reliability studies for the use of epidemiological and audit indices in orthodontics. Br J Orthod. 1997;24:139-47.

19

Prevalence of dental anomalies of number in different subphenotypes of isolated cleft palate

João Paulo Schwartz[1], Daniele Salazar Somensi[1], Priscila Yoshizaki[1], Luciana Laís Savero Reis[1], Rita de Cássia Moura Carvalho Lauris[2], Omar Gabriel da Silva Filho[2], Gisele Dalbén[3], Daniela Gamba Garib[4]

Objective: This study aimed at carrying out a radiographic analysis on the prevalence of dental anomalies of number (agenesis and supernumerary teeth) in permanent dentition, in different subphenotypes of isolated cleft palate pre-adolescent patients. **Methods:** Panoramic radiographs of 300 patients aged between 9 and 12 years, with cleft palate and enrolled in a single treatment center, were retrospectively analyzed. The sample was divided into two groups according to the extension/severity of the cleft palate: complete and incomplete . The chi-square test was used for intergroup comparison regarding the prevalence of the investigated dental anomalies (P < 0.05). **Results:** Agenesis was found in 34.14% of patients with complete cleft palate and in 30.27% of patients with incomplete cleft palate. Supernumerary teeth were found in 2.43% of patients with complete cleft palate and in 0.91% of patients with incomplete cleft palate. No statistically significant difference was found between groups with regard to the prevalence of agenesis and supernumerary teeth. There was no difference in cleft prevalence between genders within each study group. **Conclusion:** The prevalence of dental anomalies of number in pre-adolescents with cleft palate was higher than that reported for the general population. The severity of cleft palate did not seem to be associated with the prevalence of dental anomalies of number.

Keywords: Cleft palate. Tooth abnormalities. Panoramic radiograph.

[1] Specialist in Orthodontics, Hospital for Rehabilitation of Craniofacial Anomalies – São Paulo University (HRAC-USP).
[2] MSc in Orthodontics, HRAC-USP.
[3] PhD in Pediatric Dentistry, HRAC-USP.
[4] Full professor and assistant professor of Orthodontics, School of Dentistry — University of São Paulo/Bauru.

» The authors report no commercial, proprietary or financial interest in the products or companies described in this article.

Daniela Gamba Garib
Rua Rio Branco, 19-18 – Bauru/SP – Brazil — CEP: 17.040-480
E-mail: dgarib@uol.com.br

INTRODUCTION

The embryonic explanation for isolated cleft palate is the lack of fusion of the palatal shelves that form the secondary palate. In this type of cleft, the palatine processes do not fuse neither in the midline nor with the nasal septum, keeping the communication between oral and nasal cavities, while the formation of lips and alveolar ridge is processed normally.[1]

Isolated cleft palate may be complete or incomplete.[1] It is considered complete when it affects the hard and soft palate, extending to the incisive foramen (Fig 1A). On the other hand, it is considered incomplete when it partially affects the soft and/or hard palate, not reaching the incisive foramen (Figs 1B, 1C and 1D).

The prevalence of cleft lip and palate is approximately 1:1000 births.[1] In general, individuals of Asian descent have higher prevalence while those of African descent have lower prevalence when compared to Caucasian individuals.[2] The etiology of cleft lip and palate is complex, with multifactorial causality, in which case both genetic and environmental factors play a major role in determining the malformation.[3] From an embryological standpoint, cleft palate is a disorder that differs from cleft lip and palate. Differences in epidemiology and etiologic factors have also been reported in the literature.[3]

Similarly to the general population, odontogenic disorders are also found in patients with clefts. It is assumed that cleft and dental anomalies present a common or inter-related genetic origin, considering the high prevalence of dental anomalies in cleft patients.[4] In other words, patients with clefts present more incidence of dental anomalies than individuals without clefts.[5] Moreover, the prevalence of dental anomalies seems to be related to the extension/severity of cleft lip and palate.[6]

The diagnosis of dental anomalies of number is essential to define the treatment plan in the rehabilitation process of patients with cleft palate, either orthodontic, with prosthesis or implants. The purpose of this study was to radiographically assess the prevalence of dental anomalies of number in different subphenotypes of isolated cleft palate.

MATERIAL AND METHODS

This study was conducted in the department of Orthodontics at the Hospital for Rehabilitation of Craniofacial Anomalies, University of São Paulo (HRAC-USP), after approval by the respective Institutional Review Board. The study analyzed the radiographs of 300 patients from the HRAC-USP files. The sample comprised 117 (39%) males and 183 (61%) females who were in late mixed dentition (second transitional period of mixed dentition according to the Van der Linden classification) and early permanent dentition. The patients aged between 9 and 12 years old (chronological age). At this age, the third molars were excluded from the evaluation.

The total sample was divided into two study groups, according to the extension of cleft palate indicated in the medical records of patients: Group 1 - complete cleft palate; and Group 2 - incomplete cleft palate.

The occurrence of permanent teeth agenesis and supernumerary permanent teeth was evaluated in panoramic radiographs by a calibrated observer with the aid of a film viewer in a room with appropriate lightening. The study included only radiographs with good technical quality that allowed good visualization of teeth, erupted or not, and their surrounding structures.

After the prevalence of dental anomalies was calculated in each study group, the chi-square test was used for comparison. It was also used to verify intragroup differences in the prevalence of anomalies between sexes. The results were considered at a significance level of 5%.

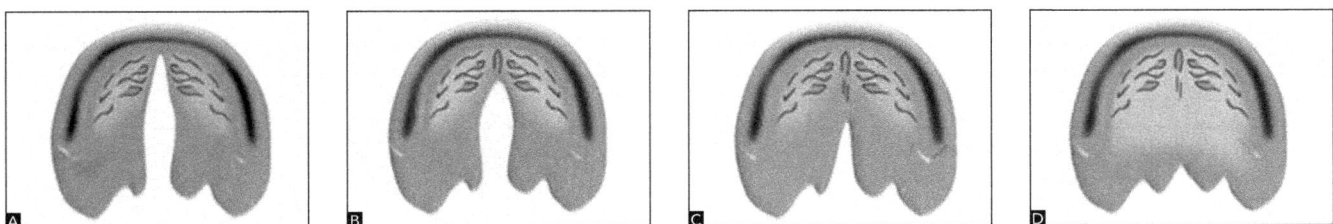

Figure 1 - Complete cleft palate invariably extends from the incisive foramen to the uvula (A). Incomplete cleft palate involves the posterior region of the palate without reaching the incisive foramen (B); affects the soft palate and part of the hard palate (C); or may affect only the soft palate (D).

RESULTS

Out of the 300 patients analyzed, 82 (27.33%) had complete cleft palate, whereas 218 (72.66%) had incomplete cleft palate. Among individuals with complete cleft palate, 31 (37.8%) were males and 51 (62.19%) females. As for patients with incomplete cleft palate, 86 (39.44%) were males and 132 (60.55%) females. In both groups, the proportion between male and female was approximately 1:2.

The prevalence of dental anomalies in Group 1 (complete cleft palate) and Group 2 (incomplete cleft palate) is expressed in percentage and presented in Table 1. In Group 1, tooth agenesis of permanent teeth excluding the third molars was observed in 28 (34.14%) patients, while supernumerary teeth were found in 2 (2.43%). In Group 2, tooth agenesis was observed in 66 (30.27%) patients, while supernumerary teeth was found in 2 (0.91%). No significant difference in the prevalence of hypodontia

and supernumerary teeth was found between Groups 1 and 2 (Table 1). Additionally, there was no difference between groups in the prevalence of agenesis for the most commonly affected teeth: second premolars and maxillary lateral incisors (Table 1).

Figures 2 and 3 show the prevalence of agenesis of each permanent tooth in Groups 1 and 2, respectively. With regard to supernumerary teeth, in Group 1 they were found in the region of the maxillary left lateral incisor and the maxillary left second premolar, while in Group 2 supernumerary teeth were observed in the region of the maxillary right lateral incisor and between the central incisors (mesiodens).

The distribution of dental anomalies according to sex is shown in Table 2. In both groups, there was no statistically significant difference between males and females for the prevalence of tooth agenesis and supernumerary teeth (Table 2).

Table 1 - Prevalence of dental anomalies in groups 1 and 2, and intergroup comparison results (chi-square test).

	G1 + G2	G1	G2	χ^2	p
Hypodontia	31.33%	34.14%	30.27%	0.0064	0.9359
Supernumerary	1.33%	2.43%	0.91%	0.0000	1.0000
Hypodontia MxLI	8.50%	7.92%	8.71%	1.9340	0.1644
Hypodontia Mx2P	7.50%	9.14%	6.88%	0.0000	1.0000
Hypodontia Md2P	8.66%	6.70%	9.40%	0.2545	0.6139

* MxLI = maxillary lateral incisor, Mx2P = maxillary second premolar, Md2P = mandibular second premolar.

Table 2 - Prevalence of dental anomalies according to sex and intragroup comparison results (chi-square test).

	Complete cleft palate				Incomplete cleft palate			
	Female	Male	χ^2	p	Female	Male	χ^2	p
Hypodontia	35.29%	32.25%	0.0390	0.8434	32.57%	26.74%	0.2798	0.5968
Supernumerary	0%	6.45%	1.0960	0.2952	0%	2.32%	1.0300	0.3101

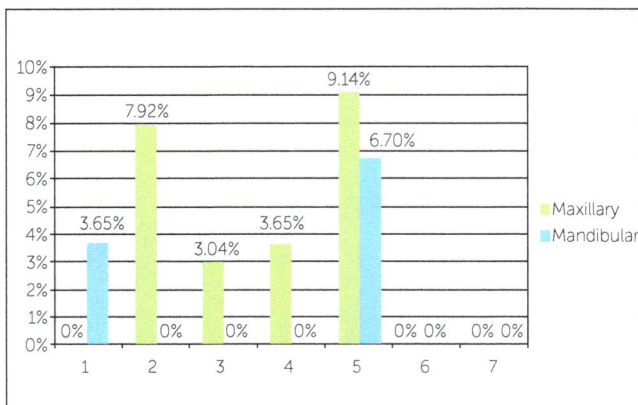

Figure 2 - Prevalence of agenesis of each permanent tooth (excluding third molars) in the complete cleft palate group (group 1).

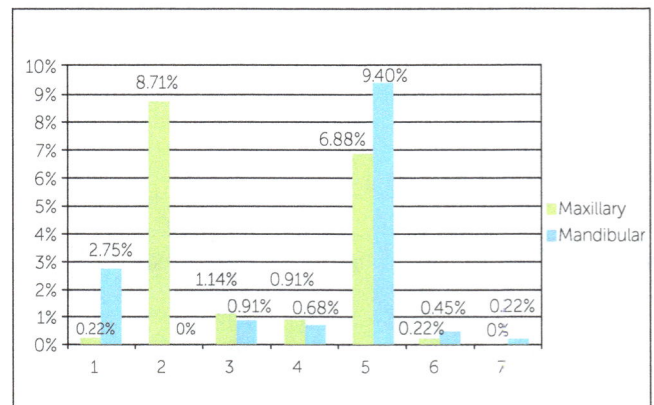

Figure 3 - Prevalence of agenesis of each permanent tooth (excluding third molars) in the incomplete cleft palate group (group 2).

DISCUSSION

Cleft palate is more common among female patients.[1,7] In this study, both complete and incomplete cleft palate prevailed in females. In individuals without clefts, excluding the third molars, the prevalence of tooth agenesis in the population varies from 4.3% to 7.8%, primarily affecting the mandibular second premolar, followed by the maxillary lateral incisor and maxillary second premolar.[8] The present results show that the prevalence of tooth agenesis is much higher in individuals with cleft palate than in the general population.

According to this study, the prevalence of hypodontia of permanent teeth, excluding the third molars, in patients with cleft palate was 31.33% and was similar to that reported in the literature for patients with these malformations. Previous studies reported a prevalence of permanent tooth agenesis in patients with cleft lip and palate of 25.5% to 33% in Czech patients,[9] 30% in Swedish patients,[10] 25% to 40%[11] and 33% in Finnish patients[12] and 28.5% in Norwegian patients.[13] Another previous study reported that tooth agenesis was observed more frequently in patients with complete cleft palate than in patients with incomplete cleft palate.[11] However, our study did not find any difference in the occurrence of hypodontia according to the subphenotypes (Table 1).

As for the subphenotypes, in both complete and incomplete cleft palate the teeth most affected by hypodontia were the maxillary and mandibular second premolars as well as maxillary lateral incisors, particularly the maxillary second premolars in complete cleft palate and the mandibular second premolars in incomplete cleft palate (Figs 2 and 3). These data are in accordance with other reports in the literature,[9,10,14] and are similar to those found for the general population.[4]

The prevalence of supernumerary teeth in patients with cleft palate found in our study is similar to the prevalence found for the general population, with no significant difference between complete and incomplete cleft subphenotypes. Supernumerary teeth were prevalent in 2.43% of group 1 and 0.91% of group 2 (Table 1). In patients with complete palatine cleft, supernumerary teeth were found in the region of maxillary left lateral incisors and maxillary left second premolars. In patients with incomplete cleft palate, they were found in the region of maxillary right lateral incisors and between the central incisors (mesiodens). The prevalence of supernumerary teeth in adolescents without clefts is 1% to 2%.[15] A previous investigation found no supernumerary teeth in patients with isolated cleft palate.[10]

A recent study found that the presence of dental anomalies may represent an additional clinical marker for oral clefts, suggesting a common genetic origin for these anomalies.[16] The development of tooth germs and the occurrence of cleft palate are closely related during embryological development, both anatomically and chronologically, and many studies have reported the manifestation of dental anomalies associated with various forms of cleft lip, cleft palate or both.[16] It has been proposed that individuals with cleft have higher prevalence of dental anomalies than the general population, and that the severity of the malformations seems to be directly related to the extension of the cleft.[16] In this study, the prevalence of tooth agenesis and the total prevalence of dental anomalies, except for supernumerary teeth, was slightly higher in female patients, although no statistically significant difference was found. The same was observed for the occurrence of complete and incomplete isolated cleft palate.

CONCLUSION

The prevalence of dental anomalies of number seems not to be related to the subphenotypes of cleft palate. Individuals with complete and incomplete cleft palate showed a similar prevalence of permanent tooth agenesis and supernumerary teeth. Further studies are necessary to determine the exact inter-relation between cleft palate and the prevalence of other dental anomalies.

REFERENCES

1. Silva Filho OG, Freitas JAS. Caracterização morfológica e origem embriológica In: Trindade IEK, Silva Filho OG. Fissuras Labiopalatinas: uma abordagem interdisciplinar. São Paulo: Ed. Santos; 2007. cap. 2, p.17-49.

2. Murray JC. Gene/environment causes of cleft lip and/or palate. Clin Genet. 2002;61(4):248-56.

3. Garib DG. Etiologia das más oclusões: implicações clínicas em ortodontia. In: Lubiana NF, Garib DG, Silva Filho OG. Pro-Odonto Ortodontia: programa de atualização em Ortodontia. Porto Alegre: ABO, Artmed, Panamericana; 2009. cap. 3.1, p. 1-37.

4. Garib DG. Padrão de anomalias dentárias associadas. In: Lubiana NF, Garib DG, Silva Filho OG. Pro-Odonto Ortodontia: programa de atualização em Ortodontia. Porto Alegre: ABO, Artmed, Panamericana; 2009. cap. 5, p. 59-102.

5. Da Silva AP, Costa B, Carvalho Carrara, CF. Dental anomalies of number in the permanent dentition of patients with bilateral cleft lip: radiographic study. Cleft Palate Craniofac J. 2008;45(5):473-6.

6. Eerens k, Vlietinck R, Heindbünchel K, Van Olmen A, Derom C, Willems G, et al. Hypodontia and tooth formation in groups of children with cleft and, nonrelated controls. Cleft Palate Craniof J. 2001;38(4):374-8.

7. Derijcke A, Eerens A, Carels C. The incidence of oral clefts: a review. Br J Oral Maxillofac Surg. 1996;34(6):488-94.

8. Garib DG, Peck S, Gomes SC. Increased occurrence of dental anomalies associated with second-premolar agenesis. Angle Orthod. 2009;79(3):436-41.

9. Jiroutová O. Hypodontia in patients with isolated cleft palate, its relationship to etiopathogenesis. Acta Chir Plast. 1991;33(1):57-63.

10. Larson M, Hellquist R, Jakobsson OP. Dental abnormalities and ectopic eruption in patients with isolated cleft palate. Scand J Plast Reconstr Surg Hand Surg. 1998;32(2):203-12.

11. Ranta R, Stegars T, Rintala A. Correlations of hypodontia in children with isolated cleft palate. Cleft Palated J. 1983;20(2):163-5.

12. Ranta R. A review of tooth formation in children with cleft lip/palate. Am J Orthod Dentofacial Orthop. 1986;90(1):11-8.

13. Andersson EM, Sandvik L, Abyholm F, Semb G. Clefts of the secondary palate referred to the Oslo cleft team: epidemiology and cleft severity in 994 individuals. Cleft Palate Craniofac J. 2010;47(4):335-42.

14. Haataja J, Haavikko K, Ranta R. Hypodontia and supernumerary teeth in Finnish children affected with facial clefts. An orthopantomographic and clinical study. Suom Hammaslaak Toim. 1971;67(6):303-11.

15. Bergström K. An orthopantomographic study of hypodontia, supernumeraries and other anomalies in schoolchildren between ages of 8-9 years. Swed Dent J. 1977;1(1):45-57.

16. Letra A, Menezes R, Granjeiro JM, Vieira AR. Defining subphenotypes for oral clefts based on dental development. J Dent Res. 2007;86(10):986-91.

20

Mandibular asymmetry: A proposal of radiographic analysis with public domain software

Alexandre Durval Lemos[1], Cintia Regina Tornisiello Katz[2], Mônica Vilela Heimer[2], Aronita Rosenblatt[3]

Objective: This preliminary study aimed to propose a new analysis of digital panoramic radiographs for a differential diagnosis between functional and morphological mandibular asymmetry in children with and without unilateral posterior crossbite. **Methods:** Analysis is based on linear and angular measurements taken from nine anatomic points, demarcated in sequence directly on digital images. A specific plug-in was developed as part of a larger public domain image processing software (ImageJ) to automate and facilitate measurements. Since panoramic radiographs are typically subject to magnification differences between the right and left sides, horizontal linear measurements were adjusted for greater accuracy in both sides by means of a Distortion Factor (DF). In order to provide a preliminary assessment of proposed analysis and the developed plug-in, radiographs of ten patients (5 with unilateral posterior crossbite and 5 with normal occlusion) were analyzed. **Results:** Considerable divergence was found between the right and left sides in the measurements of mandibular length and position of condyles in patients with unilateral posterior crossbite in comparison to individuals with normal occlusion. **Conclusion:** Although there are more effective and accurate diagnostic methods, panoramic radiography is still widespread, especially in emerging countries. This study presented initial evidence that the proposed analysis can be an important resource for planning early orthodontic intervention and, thus, avoid progression of asymmetries and their consequences.

Keywords: Panoramic radiography. Imaging diagnosis. Mandible.

[1] Professor, Department of Dentistry, State University of Paraíba, UEPB.

[2] Assistant professor, Department of Social Dentistry, Federal University of Pernambuco, UFPE.

[3] Full professor, Department of Social Dentistry, University of Pernambuco, UPE.

» The authors report no commercial, proprietary or financial interest in the products or companies described in this article.

Alexandre Durval Lemos
Rua Afonso Campos, 48 – Sl.216 – Centro – Campina Grande/PB — Brazil
CEP: 58400-235 – E-mail: adurval@ibest.com.br

INTRODUCTION

Advances in medical and biological sciences in recent years and the growing importance of determining the relationship between structure and function have made imaging analysis an increasingly important discipline.[1] Healthcare professionals, especially dentists, depend on analyses from radiology centers; however, the software programs designed for this purpose are expensive and restricted to the services of these centers. Thus, the use and disclosure of an easy-to-use public domain program for analysis of digital images is of paramount importance.

ImageJ occupies a unique position as a public domain software (www.rsb.info.nih.gov/ij/) that can run on any operating system (Macintosh, Windows, Linux and even a PDA operating system). This software is easy to use, can perform a full set of imaging manipulations and has a huge and knowledgeable user community.[1] Wayne Rasband is the core author of ImageJ. Its first release (version 0.50) was on September 23rd, 1997 and its most recent version (1.47h) was released on December 23rd, 2012. After developing the Macintosh-based image bank for the National Institutes of Health (NIH) during 10 years, Rasband made the brave decision to start afresh with ImageJ using the Java programming language (the letter J in the name stands for Java), which freed the software from an individual operating system.[2] According to the NIH, the software has been downloaded from its web site tens of thousands of times, with a current rate of about 24,000 downloads per month.

ImageJ incorporates a number of useful tools for digital image processing, including determination of linear and angular measurements, calculation of areas, particle analysis, cell counts, etc. This tool has been employed in Medicine (with more than 200 published researches) as well as in other fields of knowledge, such as Engineering, Physics, Astronomy, Computer Science and Chemistry. However, few studies involving the use of ImageJ in the field of Dentistry have been published.[2,3,4] A search of Pubmed, EBSCO and Scopus databases using the keywords Dentistry and ImageJ revealed 39 studies, only three of which were in the field of Orthodontics.

Studies suggest that patients with unilateral posterior crossbite often exhibit mandibular asymmetry stemming from a functional deviation of the mandible.[5-8] Routine screening procedures for dental and craniofacial disorders and bilateral examinations of the stomatognathic system are needed. Since panoramic radiographs provide this information, such images could be used as a routine tool for diagnosis and treatment planning. Panoramic radiographs have been used to assess right and left height differences in the condyle, ramus and total mandible height for the definition of asymmetries.[9-12]

Radiographic analyses found in the literature are restricted to the diagnosis of morphological asymmetry in the mandible.[7,8,13,14,15] Thus, the aim of the present study was to propose a new analysis of panoramic radiographs for a differential diagnosis between functional and morphological asymmetry in children with and without unilateral posterior crossbite using the ImageJ software.

MATERIAL AND METHODS

The aim of the present preliminary study on differential diagnosis between morphological and functional mandibular asymmetry was to propose a new analysis method involving the use of a public domain software. To this end, digital radiographs from ten patients were analyzed – five with unilateral posterior crossbite and five with normal occlusion. Patients' average age was nine years old. The present study was performed in the city of Campina Grande, in the state of Paraíba, in the northeast of Brazil. It was approved by Paraíba State University Institutional Review board (CAAE: 3201.0.000.133-10).

The criteria for patients with normal occlusion were as follows: Class I canine and molar relationships with minor or no crowding, normal growth and development and well-aligned maxillary and mandibular dental arches; presence of all teeth except for third molars; good facial symmetry (clinically determined); no significant medical history; no functional deviation of the mandible; and no history of trauma or previous orthodontic treatment.

The criteria for patients with posterior crossbite were as follows: unilateral posterior crossbite with at least two posterior teeth in crossbite; mandibular dental midline deviation of at least 1 mm to the crossbite side; functional deviation of the mandible; no systemic disease and no developmental or acquired craniofacial or neuromuscular deformities;

no remarkable facial or occlusal asymmetry; no history of orthodontic treatment; no missing teeth (excluding third molars); and no extensive carious lesions or pathologic periodontal condition.

Images were taken with a digital Orthophos DS panoramic radiograph machine (Sirona Dental Systems, Germany) previously standardized (62 Kv, 8 mA and 14.1s exposure time). All radiographs were standardized and taken by the same operator. Patients were positioned with the lips in resting position and the head oriented to Frankfurt horizontal plane.[16]

Anatomical points were marked directly on the digital images using ImageJ software. Based on the objectives of the study, the following landmarks were used: 1- right pterygomaxillary fossa (RPF); 2- anterior nasal spine (ANS); 3- left pterygomaxillary fossa (LPF); 4- most cranial point of left condyle (LHC);[14] 5- left gonion (LGo); 6- most cranial point of right condyle (RHC);[14] 7- right gonion (RGo); 8- Pogonion (Pg – midpoint of mandible often seen in panoramic radiographs as a white spot on the midline);[14] 9- inter-incisive point (IP).

A plug-in was created to automate and facilitate measurement-taking (download and instructions - http://rsbweb.nih.gov/ij/plug-ins/lemos-asymmetry-analysis/index.html).

The following linear (mm) and angular (degree) measurements were taken on both sides of each digital panoramic radiograph:

Linear measurements
Morphological variables:
- Ramus height (RH): distance between the most cranial point of the condyle (points 4 and 6, as described by Deleurant et al[14]) and the gonion (points 5 and 7).
- Corpus length (CL): distance between gonion (Go) and pogonion (Pg); the gonion was defined as a random midpoint on the posterior curvature of the mandible (intersection points between corpus and ramus).

Functional variables:
- Pg-MSP: distance between pogonion and median sagittal plane, represented by a horizontal link connecting the Pg to the plane.
- IP-MSP: distance between IP and MSP, represented by a horizontal line connecting the IP to the plane.

- CHD: difference between the heights of the right and left condyle (beginning with most superior to the most inferior position; represented by a horizontal line automatically drawn from the CH point of the taller condyle, proceeding to the contralateral side for better visualization in relation to the opposing condyle.

Pg-MSP, IP-MSP and CHD variables were considered as functional, once the panoramic images were taken with subjects in protrusion position; in other words, in functional movement.

Angular measurement
- Gonial Angle (GA): formed between RH and CL on both sides; results expressed in degrees.

After marking the points and determining lines and planes, angular and linear measurements were analyzed (Figs 1 and 2).

Assessment of mandibular asymmetry was performed using the criteria described by Ramirez-Yanes et al,[15] and categorized as follows: non-significant asymmetry (difference of 0 to 2 mm between the sides of the mandible); light asymmetry (difference of 2 to 3 mm); moderate asymmetry (difference of 3 to 5 mm); and severe asymmetry (difference > 5 mm).

RESULTS
Tables 1, 2 and 3 display patients' measurements assessed by means of the proposed analysis method. Figures 1 and 2 show the radiographs with the analyses preformed. Considerable divergence was found between the sides in the crossbite group in relation to the corpus length measurement (CL), and positioning of the condyles (CHD) in patients with posterior crossbite in comparison to patients with normal occlusion (Tables 1, 2, 3).

DISCUSSION
Although it is not considered a public health problem, posterior crossbite stands out as one of the most frequently studied malocclusions in the primary dentition and onset of mixed dentition. Once occurring in the early stages of dental development, self-correction does not generally occur.[18,19] Early diagnosis and orthodontic intervention allow adequate guidance of

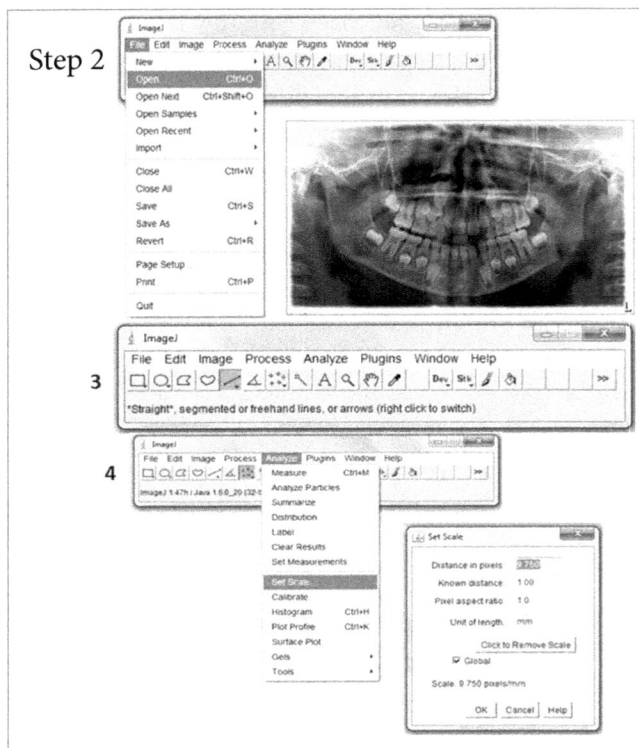

Figure 1 - Lemos asymmetry analysis performed on patient with normal occlusion.

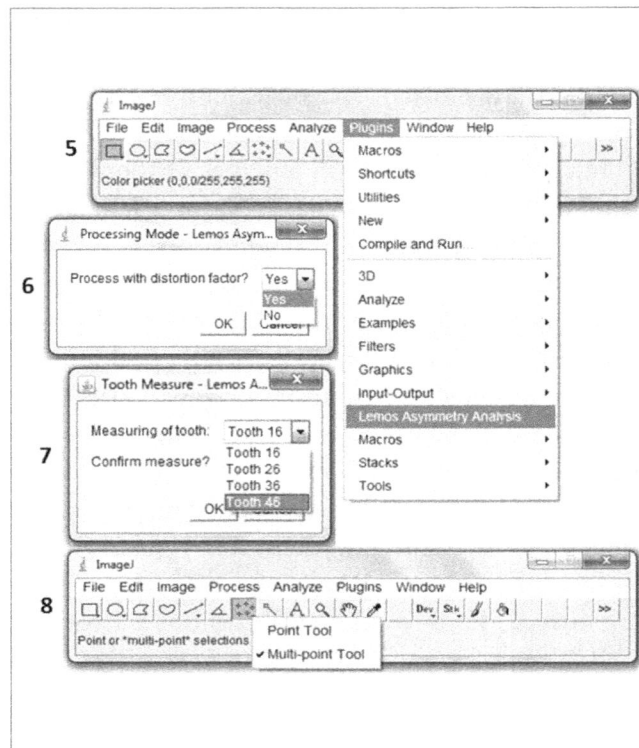

Figure 2 - Lemos asymmetry analysis performed on patient with unilateral (right side) posterior crossbite.

maxillary and mandibular growth as well as establishment of an adequate, stable functional pattern in the entire associated musculature, in addition to harmonious development of occlusion.[6,20] If treatment is not instituted early enough, skeletal remodeling of the temporomandibular joint can occur, thereby leading to permanent deviation from the lower midline and facial asymmetry.[21] Thus, late treatment is normally more complex, expensive and time-consuming and may involve auxiliary surgical procedures.[22,23]

The present study sought to demonstrate the viability of using ImageJ software as a tool to diagnose mandibular asymmetry in patients with posterior crossbite. Moreover, a plug-in was created to facilitate analysis. This plug-in is a diagnostic tool that can be extended and improved at any time.

Habets et al[9] proposed one of the first analyses for assessment of mandibular asymmetry developed on a sample of patients with temporomandibular joint problems. Other authors adopted this analysis to measure mandibular asymmetry in patients with posterior crossbite.[7,8] Although widely employed due to its ease

of use, this analysis is restricted to the assessment of vertical measurements (height of corpus and condyle of the mandible) and does not consider horizontal and angular measurements.

Ramirez-Yanes et al[15] carried out a study to determine the prevalence of mandibular asymmetry, proposing the analysis of digitized panoramic radiographs of 327 children. They found that half of the sample had moderate to severe mandibular asymmetry. The authors used the inter-incisive point as reference to determine the corpus of the mandible. However, prevalence may be overestimated, as a patient may exhibit a dental deviation that alters the point of reference and consequently affects measurement of mandible length.

One difference in the present analysis is the use of points on the maxilla (ANS, RPF and LPF), which is a stable bone and serves as reference for tracing the median sagittal plane. The advantage of this plane is that it corresponds to the true midline, thereby facilitating diagnosis of skeletal (Pg-MSP) and dental (IP-MSP) deviation. With regard to the length of the

Table 1 - Statistics for the following variables: ramus height + condyle, corpus length and gonial angle according to side and differences in the crossbite group.

Variable	Side	
	Crossed	Non-crossed
	Mean ± SD	Mean ± SD
Ramus height + condyle	51.9 ± 6.6	51.7 ± 5.2
Corpus length	68.4 ± 6.2	69.9 ± 7.3
Gonial angle	112.6 ± 6.4	112.8 ± 6.3

Table 2 - Statistics for the following variables: ramus height + condyle, corpus length and gonial angle according to side and differences in the normal occlusion group.

Variable	Side	
	Right	Left
	Mean ± SD	Mean ± SD
Ramus height + condyle	50.9 ± 1.9	51.3 ± 1.9
Corpus length	75.5 ± 4.7	75.3 ± 4.1
Gonial angle	109.4 ± 3.1	110.0 ± 2.8

Table 3 - Statistics for the following variables: Pog-MSP, IP-MSP, CHD according to groups.

Variable	Group	
	Experimental	Control
	Mean ± SD	Mean ± SD
Pog-MSP	2.8 ± 2.2	0.8 ± 1.3
IP-MSP	2.0 ± 1.9	0.9 ± 0.9
CHD	3.2 ± 1.7	1.2 ± 0.7

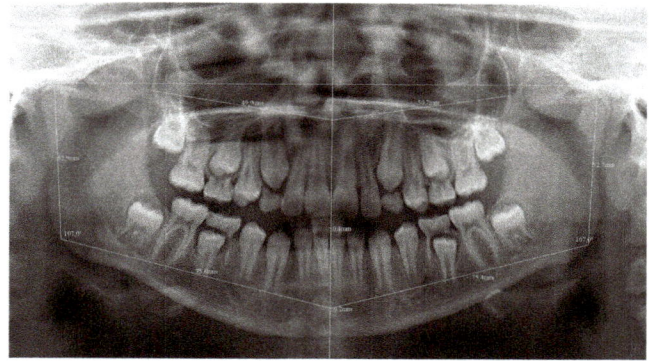

Figure 3 - Lemos asymmetry analysis performed on patient with normal occlusion.

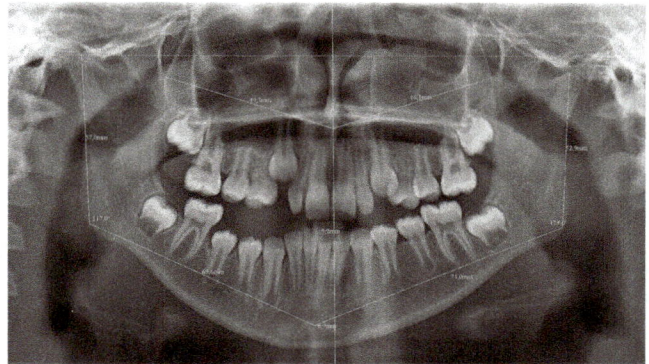

Figure 4 - Lemos asymmetry analysis performed on patient with unilateral (right side) posterior crossbite.

corpus of the mandible on both sides (LCL, RCL), the reference in the present study was an anatomic point on the mandible (Pg), which is the midpoint of the mandible often seen in orthopantomograms as an white spot on the midline.[14] Thus, this analysis can also be applied to patients with missing incisors, regardless of the type of malocclusion.

Comparison of measurements revealed considerable discrepancy in the length of mandibular corpus as well as the positioning of the condyles in the patient with posterior crossbite. According to the criteria proposed by Ramirez-Yanes et al,[15] this suggests significant asymmetry. Analysis of measurements demonstrates that patients (crossbite group) had both skeletal (CL) and positional (CHD) asymmetry. At times, even in cases of obvious mandibular asymmetry, it is

not self-evident whether one side has overgrown or the other has undergrown,[24,25] which underscores the applicability of the analysis proposed herein.

Unlike other analyses available in the literature,[7,8,9,14,15] this analysis is also based on the visualization of positional asymmetry of condyles through CHD measurement as well as skeletal asymmetry through measurements of the ramus (LRH and RRH), providing a differential diagnosis and assisting in the choice of adequate treatment. It is worth noting that the mandible adapts to mandibular deviations by modeling the condyle and glenoid fossae,[26] suggesting that asymmetry may be an adaptive response to functional demands.[27] Animal studies as well as studies involving humans with crossbite have shown that functional shift can produce asymmetric mandibular growth.[7,22] Children in deciduous and mixed dentition with unilateral posterior crossbite have asymmetrically positioned condyles and asymmetric muscle function. The condyles on the crossbite side are positioned relatively more upwardly and backwardly in the glenoid fossae than the condyles on the non-crossbite side.[29] Therefore, the prevalence of mandibular asymmetries in young growing patients must be further studied, along with the impact these asymmetries may have on facial growth.[15]

The use of panoramic radiographs to diagnose mandibular asymmetries is subject to distortions, especially in horizontal and oblique measurements;[12,13,17] thus, a Distortion Factor (DF) is recommended.[15] It should be calculated for each hemimandible so as to ensure greater accuracy in horizontal measurements (more subject to distortion),

and, as a consequence, in diagnosis. This tool (DF) is available in the plug-in. Although there are more effective and accurate diagnostic methods, for instance cone-beam computed tomography (CBCT), panoramic radiography is still widespread,[29] especially in emerging countries.

CONCLUSIONS

The analysis proposed herein has the advantage of simultaneously assessing horizontal, vertical and angular mandibular measurements in patients with and without posterior crossbite, thereby allowing differential diagnosis between functional and morphological asymmetry. This easy-to-use public domain tool proves to be an important resource for planning of early orthodontic intervention, in addition to avoiding the progression of asymmetries and their consequences.

REFERENCES

1. Abramoff MD, Magalhães PJ, Ram SJ. Image processing with Image. J Biophotonics Int. 2004;11(7):36-42.
2. Yasar F, Yesilova E, Akgünlü F. Alveolar bone changes under overhanging restorations. Clin Oral Investig. 2010;14(5):543-9.
3. Araki M, Kawashima S, Matsumoto N, Nishimura S, Ishii T, Komiyama K, et al. Tree-dimensional reconstruction of a fibro-osseous lesion using binary images transformed from histopathological images. Dentomaxillofac Radiol. 2010;39(4):246-51.
4. Özer SY. Comparison of root canal transportation induced by three rotary systems with noncutting tips using computed tomography. Oral Surg Oral Med Oral Pathol Oral Radiol Endod. 2011;111(2):244-50.
5. Lam PH, Sadowsky C, Omerza F. Mandibular asymmetry and condylar position in children with unilateral posterior crossbite. Am J Orthod Dentofacial Orthop. 1999;115(5):569-75.
6. Pinto AS, Buschang PH, Throckmorton GS, Chen P. Morphological and positional asymmetries of young children with functional unilateral posterior crossbite. Am J Orthod Dentofacial Orthop. 2001;120(5):513-20.
7. Kilic N, Kiki A, Oktay H. Condylar asymmetry in unilateral posterior crossbite patients. Am J Orthod Dentofacial Orthop. 2008;133(3):382-7.
8. Uysal T, Sisman Y, Kurt G, Ramoglu SI. Condylar and ramal vertical asymmetry in unilateral and bilateral posterior crossbite patients and a normal occlusion sample. Am J Orthod Dentofacial Orthop. 2009;136(1):37-43.
9. Habets LL, Bezuur JN, Naeiji M, Hansson TL. The orthopantomogram, an aid in diagnosis of temporomandibular joint problems. II. The vertical symmetry. J Oral Rehabil. 1988;15(5):465-71.
10. Kiki A, Kilic N, Oktay H. Condylar asymmetry in bilateral posterior crossbite patients. Angle Orthod. 2007;77(1):77-81.
11. Kurt G, Uysal T, Sisman Y, Ramoglu SI. Mandibular asymmetry in Class II subdivision malocclusion. Angle Orthod. 2008;78(1):32-7.
12. Van Elslande DC, Russett SJ, Major PW, Flores-Mir C. Mandibular asymmetry diagnosis with panoramic imaging. Am J Orthod Dentofacial Orthop. 2008;134(2):183-92.
13. Habets LL, Bezuur JN, VanOoij CP, Hansson TL. The orthopantomogram, an aid in diagnosis of temporomandibular joint problems. I. The factor of vertical magnification. J Oral Rehabil. 1987;14(5):475-80.
14. Deleurant Y, Zimmermann A, Peltomäki T. Hemimandibular elongation: treatment and long-term follow-up. Orthod Craniofac Res. 2008;11(3):172-9.
15. Ramirez-Yañes GO, Stewart A, Franken E, Campos K. Prevalence of mandibular asymmetry in growing patients. Eur J Orthod. 2011;33(3):236-42.
16. Azevedo AR, Janson G, Henriques JF, Freitas MR. Evaluation of asymmetries between subjects with Class II subdivision and apparent facial asymmetry and those with normal occlusion. Am J Orthod Dentofacial Orthop. 2006;129(3):376-83.
17. Laster WS, Ludlow JB, Bailey LJ, Hershey HG. Accuracy of measurements of mandibular anatomy and prediction of asymmetry in panoramic radiographic images. Dentomaxillofac Radiol. 2005;34(6):343-9.
18. Heimer MV, Katz CR, Rosenblatt A. Non-nutitive sucking habits, dental malocclusions, and facial morphology in Brazilian children: a longitudinal study. Eur J Orthod. 2008;30(6):580-85.
19. Godoy F, Godouy-Bezerra J, Rosenblatt A. Treatment of posterior crossbite comparing 2 appliances: a community-based trial. Am J Orthod Dentofacial Orthop. 2011;139(1):e45-52.
20. Kecik D, Kocadereli I, Saatci I. Avaliation of the treatment changes of functional posterior crossbite in the mixed dentition. Am J Orthod Dentofacial Orthop. 2007;131(2):202-15.
21. Bishara SE, Burkey PS, Kharouf JG. Dental and facial asymmetries: a review. Angle Orthod. 1994;64(2):89-98.
22. Thilander B, Lennartsson B. A study of children with unilateral posterior crossbite treated and untreated, in the deciduous dentition-occlusal and skeletal characteristics of significance in predicting the long-term outcome. J Orofac Orthop. 2002;63(5):371-83.
23. Pêtren S, Bondemark L, Söderfeldt B. A systematic review concerning early orthodontic treatment of unilateral posterior crossbite. Angle Orthod. 2003;73(5):588-96.
24. Liukkonen M, Sillanmäki L, Peltomäki T. Mandibular asymmetry in healthy children. Acta Odontol Scand. 2005;63(3):168-72.
25. Melnik AK. A cephalometric study of mandibular asymmetry in a longitudinally followed sample of growing children. Am J Orthod Dentofacial Orthop. 1992;101(4):355-66.
26. Liu C, Kaneko S, Soma K. Glenoid fossa responses to mandibular lateral shift in growing rats. Angle Orthod. 2007;77(4):660-7.

27. Duthie J, Bharwani D, Tallents R H, Bellohusen R, Fishman L. A longitudinal study of normal asymmetric mandibular growth and its relationship to skeletal maturation. Am J Orthod Dentofacial Orthop. 2007;132(2):179-84.

28. Hesse KL, Årtun J, Joondeph DR, Kennedy DB. Changes in condylar position and occlusion associated with maxillary expansion for correction of functional unilateral posterior crossbite. Am J Orthod Dentofacial Orthop. 1997;111(4):410-8.

29. Hazan-Molina H, Molina-Hazan V, Schendel SA, Aizenbud D. Reliability of panoramic radiographs for the assessment of mandibular elongation after distraction osteogenesis producers. Orthod Craniofac Res. 2011;14(1):25-32.

21

Enamel surface evaluation after bracket debonding and different resin removal methods

Michele Machado Vidor[1], Rafael Perdomo Felix[2], Ernani Menezes Marchioro[3], Luciane Hahn[4]

Objective: To assess enamel surface under scanning electron microscopy (SEM) after resin removal and enamel polishing procedures following brackets debonding, as well as compare the time required for these procedures. **Methods:** A total of 180 deciduous bovine incisors were used. The enamel surface of each tooth was prepared and brackets were bonded with light cured Transbond XT composite resin. Brackets were removed in a testing machine. The samples were randomized and equally distributed into nine groups according to the resin removal and polishing technique: Group 1, 30-blade tungsten carbide bur in high speed; Group 2, 30-blade tungsten carbide bur in high speed followed by a sequence of 4 Sof-lex polishing discs (3M); Group 3, 30-blade tungsten carbide bur in high speed followed by Enhance tips (Dentsply). All groups were subdivided into (a) unpolished; (b) polished with aluminum oxide paste; and (c) polished with water slurry of fine pumice. Subsequently, the enamel surface was assessed and statistical analysis was carried out. **Results:** There were statistically significant differences in enamel roughness and removal time among all groups. Groups 3a, 3b and 3c appeared to be the most efficient methods of removing resin with low damages to enamel. Groups 2a, 2b and 2c were the most time consuming procedures, and Group 2a caused more damages to enamel. **Conclusion:** The suggested protocol for resin removal is the 30-blade tungsten carbide bur in high speed followed by Enhance tips and polishing with aluminum oxide paste. This procedure seems to produce less damages and is less time consuming.

Keywords: Dental enamel. Dental debonding. Dental polishing.

[1] Masters student in Clinical Dentistry, Radiology, Universidade Federal do Rio Grande do Sul (UFRGS), Santa Cecília, Rio Grande do Sul, Brazil.
[2] Masters student in Dental Prosthesis, Pontifícia Universidade Católica do Rio Grande do Sul (PUCRS), Porto Alegre, Rio Grande do Sul, Brazil.
[3] Adjunct professor, Pontifícia Universidade Católica do Rio Grande do Sul (PUCRS), Department of Dentistry, Porto Alegre, Rio Grande do Sul, Brazil.
[4] Professor, São Leopoldo Mandic, School of Dentistry, Postgraduate program in Orthodontics, Porto Alegre, Rio Grande do Sul, Brazil.

Acknowledgements: We thank to Centro de Microscopia Eletrônica e Microanálise (CEMM) from PUCRS.

» The authors report no commercial, proprietary or financial interest in the products or companies described in this article.

Michele Machado Vidor
Rua 24 de outubro, 650 – Cj 208 – Porto Alegre/RS — Brazil
CEP: 90.510-000 – E-mail: michele.vidor@ufrgs.br

INTRODUCTION

In Orthodontics, as in other dental specialties, there is an ongoing urge to simplify technical procedures in order to achieve the goals with quality and minimal discomfort.[1] Acid etching of tooth surface, introduced by Buonocore[2] in 1955, is an example and represents a major breakthrough in Dentistry. The adhesive technique allowed bracket direct bonding with significant reduction of bands placement around teeth, resulting in faster, easier and more accurate accessories positioning, also making the procedure more comfortable to patients.[1] Advances in the technology of bonding material allowed this procedure to become safe and efficient due to its good mechanical and physical properties. However, bracket removal and enamel surface polishing after debonding have become a concern. The search for a safe and efficient method attracted the attention of many researchers, which resulted in the introduction of numerous tools and techniques.[2-21] Nevertheless, the techniques that provide efficient enamel surface polishing present a wide clinical sequence. Thus, many clinicians create their own methods of resin removal and enamel polishing based on trial and error without knowing the actual damage they may be causing to patient's enamel.[3] Therefore, no consensus has been reached regarding the best resin removal technique promoting less damage to enamel surface.[4,5]

Thus, the main purpose of this study is to assess the enamel surface after different resin removal and enamel polishing techniques after bracket debonding. Assessment was carried out by means of scanning electron microscopy (SEM). Moreover, the present study also aimed to compare the time required for these procedures, and present a simplified and efficient protocol aiming at lower loss and damage to the enamel.

MATERIAL AND METHODS

A total of 180 bovine deciduous incisors were used in this study. In selecting the sample, the following inclusion criteria were applied: integrity of tooth enamel, no caries, fractures or cracks visible to the naked eye. For preparation of specimens, the teeth were sectioned at the tooth cervix, and only the dental crowns were used. The remaining dental pulp in the crown was removed using a dental probe.

Subsequently, the crowns were placed on wax, with the buccal surface against a glass plate so as to allow most part of the flat surface of enamel to stay parallel to the ground and perpendicular to the sidewalls of the PVC ring. In this position, the crowns were fixed by heating the wax around the teeth with a heated wax scraper. Afterwards, standard PVC rings, with 20 mm of internal diameter and height, were positioned in such a way so as to involve the entire crown. Self-curing acrylic resin was then poured on them. Once the setting time of acrylic resin had passed, the samples were washed with water vapor pressure in order to remove all the wax. Samples were then stored under immersion in distilled water, at room temperature, in a sealed plastic container until bracket bonding.

The bracket bonding area was determined clinically and by inspection on the flat portion of the buccal surface of the dental crown and closest to its center. Enamel surfaces were prepared for bonding as described below:

1) Prophylaxis with rubber cup in low rotation, using pumice and water for 10 seconds.
2) Washing with distilled water for 10 seconds.
3) Drying with compressed air, free from oil and water, for 10 seconds at a distance of 5 cm.
4) Acid etching with 37% phosphoric acid for 15 seconds, subsequently washed with distilled water for 10 seconds and dried with compressed air for 10 seconds.
5) Adhesive application on etched enamel (Transbond XT).
6) Application of composite resin (Transbond XT) on the bracket basis and positioning on the tooth with a bracket placing forceps with enough manual pressure for the disposal of excess material removed with a dental probe.
7) Light curing of adhesive and composite resin.

A stainless steel lower incisor bracket was bonded by one single operator on each one of the 180 teeth used in the sample. Bracket base surface was 10.47 mm², as measured by a digital caliper. After the bonding procedure, the samples were immersed in distilled water and stored in a closed container, in an incubator, set at 37° C for 24 hours. Accessories removal was accomplished through a mechanical testing machine, operated at 0,5 mm/min, in which a round section stainless steel wire (0.018-in) was positioned holding the bracket wings while keeping it parallel to the direction of the force. After debonding, the samples were assessed using a stereoscopic microscope (10x magnification) operated by a single calibrated investigator so as to evaluate adhesive remnant index (ARI) according to the classification criteria established by Årtun and Bergland[6] (Table 1). Excess resin surrounding the bracket base was not considered.

The samples were randomly divided into nine groups (n = 20) according to the resin removal technique and the polishing procedure executed or not at the enamel surface (Table 2).

Resin removal in Groups 1a, 1b and 1c was carried out only with tungsten carbide drill (30 blades, 9714FFJET) in high speed, without irrigation and light force application moving in one direction. In Groups 2a, 2b and 2c, the same technique was used with the tungsten carbide drill for removal of the largest volume of resin, followed by the sequence of four Sof-lex (3M) discs in low rotation. In Groups 3a, 3b and 3c, after the use of a tungsten carbide drill, resin removal was performed with Enhance finishing tips (Dentsply). Tungsten carbide burs, Sof-lex (3M) discs and Enhance finishing tips were replaced every five samples. Resin removal was deemed complete when the surface seemed to be smooth and without resin by the naked eye under illumination of the light reflector. The time for complete removal was registered in seconds. After the removal procedure, enamel surface polishing of Groups 1b, 2b and 3b was carried out with aluminum oxide paste (Enamelize Cosmedent) and felt disc (Flexibuff Cosmedent); while in Groups 1c, 2c and 3c polishing was performed with pumice and a rubber cup. In Groups 1a, 2a and 3a, no surface polishing was performed.

Specimens were examined by scanning electron microscopy (Philips XL 30), under magnification of 500 and 1500 x. Images were printed for evaluation of enamel surface by a single, previously calibrated investigator. Assessment was based on the surface roughness index (SRI) according to the classification criteria shown in Table 3.

The non-parametric Kruskal-Wallis test was employed to assess adhesive remnant index (ARI) and surface roughness index (SRI). In order to compare resin removal time, factorial analysis of variance test

was carried out. This test compares a study variable (time) considering two factors (polishing and group) in order to verify whether the polishing-group interaction is significant. In other words, whether or not these two factors combined interfere in the variable. The groups were compared by means of analysis of variance (ANOVA) and Tukey's multiple comparison tests.

Table 1 - Adhesive remnant index idealized by Årtun and Bergland.[6]

Score 0	No adhesive left on the tooth enamel
Score 1	Less than half adhesive left on the tooth enamel
Score 2	More then half adhesive left on the tooth enamel
Score 3	All adhesive left on the tooth enamel with a distinct impression of the bracket mesh

Table 2 - Division of groups regarding resin removal and polishing techniques.

	Unpolished	Polished with aluminium oxide	Polished with pumice
Tungsten drill – 30 blades	Group 1a	Group 1b	Group 1c
Tungsten drill – 30 blades + sequence of four Sof-lex disc–discs	Group 2a	Group 2b	Group 2c
Tungsten drill – 30 blades + Enhance finishing tips	Group 3a	Group 3b	Group 3c

Table 3 - Surface roughness index.

Score 1	Acceptable surface with thin and scattered grooves
Score 2	Slightly rough surface, with some thin and other thicker grooves
Score 3	Rough surface, several thick grooves over the entire tooth surface
Score 4	Very rough surface, deep and thick grooves over the entire surface

Source: Closs, Reston and Falster.[7]

RESULTS AND DISCUSSION

The present study aimed to assess the enamel surface resulting from different resin removal techniques after bracket debonding, followed or not by polishing. Assessment was conducted to determine which technique causes less damage to enamel surface and provides better clinical time for execution. Despite the more frequent use of human premolars in adhesion tests in Orthodontics,[3] the use of bovine teeth became a viable alternative due to difficulty obtaining human teeth for *in vitro* studies.[9] Even though bovine deciduous teeth offer lower bond strength, researches have concluded that they can be used as substitutes in laboratory studies, since they present a fairly regular surface and similarities in composition and mechanical properties to human teeth.[10] In view of difficulties obtaining human teeth and scientific support concerning the use of bovine teeth, we opted to use the latter for the present study.

After bracket removal, the teeth surface were assessed as to the amount of remaining resin, according to the classification criteria of Årtun and Bergland[6] for ARI. The non-parametric Kruskal-Wallis test revealed that there was no significant difference for the adhesive remnant index (ARI) among the nine groups compared (P = 0.395) (Table 4), with predominance of scores 2 and 3. These results indicate that more than half of resin was left on the tooth (score 2) or all resin was left on the tooth with the bracket mash impression (score 3). Since there were no statistically significant differences regarding the amount of resin remaining after bracket debonding, it was possible to compare resin removal time and enamel polishing.

The results obtained with regard to resin removal and enamel surface polishing time by means of factorial analysis of variance showed that the effect of group / type of polishing procedure interaction was not significant; however, the factors polishing and group, when analyzed separately, revealed a statistically significance difference (Table 5).

By means of this test, comparisons were made between groups and between the types of polishing procedures in relation to the variable time. Analysis of variance (ANOVA) and Tukey's multiple comparison test results revealed a statistically significant difference between the types of polishing procedure for all groups,

Table 4 - Comparison among adhesive remnant index scores among the nine groups.

Group	Score 0		Score 1		Score 2		Score 3	
	n	%	n	%	n	%	n	%
1a	-	-	-	-	5	25.0	15	75.0
1b	-	-	-	-	2	10.0	18	90.0
1c	-	-	-	-	4	20.0	16	80.0
2a	-	-	-	-	2	10.0	18	90.0
2b	-	-	-	-	1	5.0	19	95.0
2c	-	-	-	-	1	5.0	19	95.0
3a	-	-	-	-	5	25.0	15	75.0
3b	-	-	-	-	2	10.0	18	90.0
3c	-	-	-	-	4	20.0	16	80.0
Total	-	-	-	-	26	14.4	154	85.6

Table 5 - Results of the factorial analysis of variance when comparing time considering two factors: group and type of polishing procedure.

Sources of variation	Sum of squares	DF	Medium square	F	P
Group	73166.8	2	36583.4	115.75	0.000
Type of polishing procedure	14595.2	2	7297.6	23.09	0.000
Group x type of polishing procedure	470.3	4	117.5	0.37	0.828
Error	54045.2	171	316.1		
Total	898364	180			

Table 6 - Comparison of time (seconds) between the types of polishing procedure for each group.

Polishing procedure	Number of cases	Mean ± SD	F	P
Tungsten drill				
Unpolished	20	46.95^A ± 17.58	6.35	0. 003
Polished with aluminium oxide	20	67.85^B ± 20.41		
Polished with pumice	20	60.00^B ± 18.11		
Tungsten drill + Sof-lex disc				
Unpolished	20	79.30^A ± 19.32	8.56	0. 001
Polished with aluminium oxide	20	105.95^B ± 20.98		
Polished with pumice	20	91.10^{AB} ± 20.89		
Tungsten drill + Enhance finishing tips				
Unpolished	20	34.25^A ± 14.07	9.64	0. 000
Polished with aluminium oxide	20	52.80^B ± 12.03		
Polished with pumice	20	45.10^B ± 14.07		

* SD = Standard deviation.
** Means followed by the same letter do not differ.

also showing that the time spent in the unpolished samples is significantly lower than that spent in the samples polished with aluminum oxide and pumice, which did not differ among each other (Table 6).

There were significant differences between all groups in terms of resin removal time. The tungsten drill + Sof-lex discs groups featured significantly superior time in comparison to the other groups, associated or not with enamel polishing. The tungsten drill + Enhance finishing tips groups presented the smallest resin removal time among the polished groups. The time for tungsten drill + Enhance finishing tips unpolished group did not significantly differ from procedures involving tungsten drill, only (Table 7). Our findings regarding the longer resin removal time associated with the use of Sof-lex disc corroborate those found in the literature.[9]

Scanning electron microscopy (SEM) allows better visualization of the enamel surface after different methods of resin removal and enamel polishing are carried out.[1,11,13,16,17,18,23] In order to enable a comparative analysis of the different techniques employed, the enamel surface was assessed according to the surface roughness index (SRI).[19] A healthy deciduous bovine tooth was used as control (Fig 1).

All methods effectively removed all adhesive remnant after debonding, and also produced grooves on the enamel surface that varied in depth, thereby corroborating several studies which have obtained the same results.[7,12,14,22,24]

The results of the Kruskal-Wallis non-parametric test for the surface roughness index demonstrated statistically significant differences among the nine groups compared (Table 8). In which it is observed:

» Group 2a presented the highest scores (Fig 2);
» Groups 1a, 1b, 1c, 2b and 2c featured intermediate scores (Figs 3 to 7);
» Groups 3a, 3b and 3c featured the lowest scores (Figs 8, 9, 10).

Table 7 - Comparison of time (seconds) among groups for each type of polishing procedure.

Group	Number of cases	Mean ± SD	F	P
Unpolished				
Tungsten drill	20	46.95^A ± 17.58		
Tungsten drill + Sof-lex disc	20	79.30^B ± 19.32	36.78	0.000
Tungsten drill + Enhance finishing tips	20	34.2^A ± 14.07		
Polished with aluminium oxide				
Tungsten drill	20	67.85^A ± 20.41		
Tungsten drill + Sof-lex disc	20	105.95^B ± 20.98	44.96	0.000
Tungsten drill + Enhance finishing tips	20	52.80^C ± 12.03		
Polished with pumice				
Tungsten drill	20	60.00^A ± 18.11		
Tungsten drill + Sof-lex disc	20	91.10^B ± 20.89	34.33	0.000
Tungsten drill + Enhance finishing tips	20	45.10^C ± 14.07		

* SD = Standard deviation.
** Means followed by the same letter do not differ.

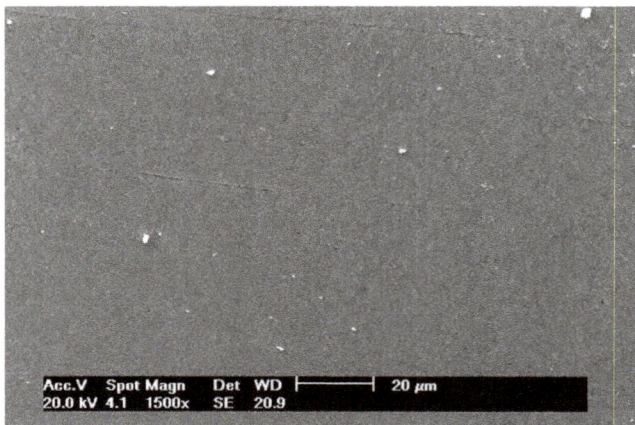

Figure 1 - Micrography of healthy bovine tooth enamel surface–(control).

Table 8 - Scores of surface roughness index comparison among the nine groups.

Group	Surface roughness index							
	Score 1		Score 2		Score 3		Score 4	
	n	%	n	%	n	%	n	%
1a	3	15.0	12	60.0	5	25.0	-	-
1b	7	35.0	8	40.0	3	15.0	2	10.0
1c	4	20.0	11	55.0	5	25.0	-	-
2a	-	-	6	30.0	10	50.0	4	20.0
2b	2	10.0	9	45.0	9	45.0	-	-
2c	3	15.0	10	50.0	6	30.0	1	5.0
3a	10	50.0	8	40.0	2	10.0	-	-
3b	13	65.0	6	30.0	1	5.0	-	-
3c	10	50.0	7	35.0	2	10.0	1	5.0
Total	52	28.9	77	42.8	43	23.9	8	4.4

Results showed that the group causing more damage to enamel surface was Group 2a (tungsten drill + Sof-lex discs without enamel polishing), and that the methods that provided an enamel surface with fewer grooves were those in which resin removal was performed with tungsten drill + Enhance finishing tips, followed or not by enamel surface polishing. According to Tüfekçi et al,[11] remnant resin removal with Sof-lex discs produces deeper wear, beyond maximum average depth, causing more damage to the enamel. Opposed to these findings, Zarrinnia, Eid and Kehoe[18] found best results when polishing the enamel surface with Sof-lex discs. Nevertheless, some researchers[18] observed greater roughness when resin was removed with Enhance finishing tips; however, previous studies[17] have suggested the use of these abrasive tips on resin removal protocol with a view to minimizing the grooves produced by drills and discs. These findings corroborate the results obtained in the present study in which finishing tips produced the lowest roughness scores, thereby microscopically showing better surface smoothness, similarly to healthy enamel.

Several authors emphasize the importance of enamel polishing after bracket debonding and resin removal based on improvements of enamel surface after this procedure.[1,12,13,17,19,20,22,24,26]

In addition, Fonseca et al[25] reported that polishing not only increases surface smoothness, but also provides a

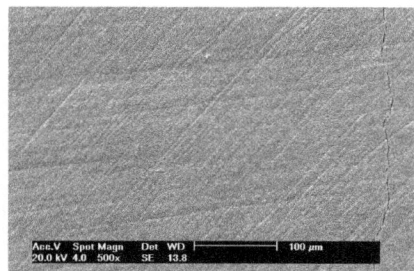

Figure 2 - Micrography of enamel surface after resin removal with Tungsten drill + Sof-lex® discs without polishing (Group 2a).

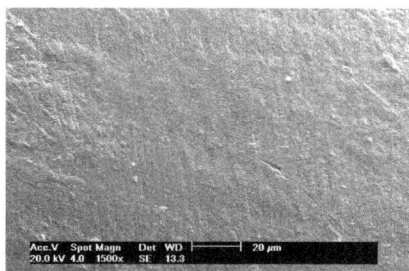

Figure 3 - Micrography of enamel surface after resin removal with tungsten drill without polishing (Group 1a).

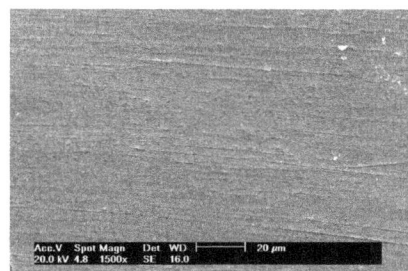

Figure 4 - Micrography of enamel surface after resin removal with tungsten drill and polishing with aluminum oxide (Group 1b).

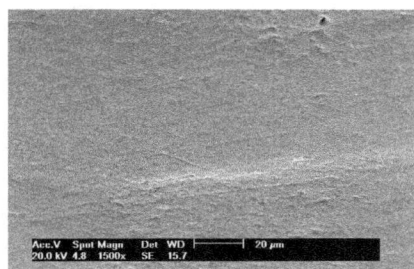

Figure 5 - Micrography of enamel surface after resin removal with tungsten drill and polishing with pumice (Group 1c).

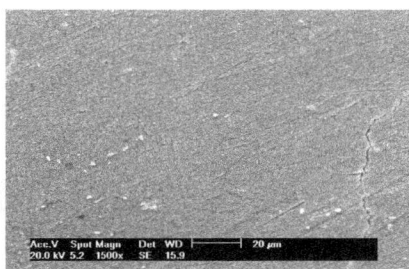

Figure 6 - Micrography of enamel surface after resin removal with tungsten drill + Sof-lex discs and polishing with aluminium oxide (Group 2b).

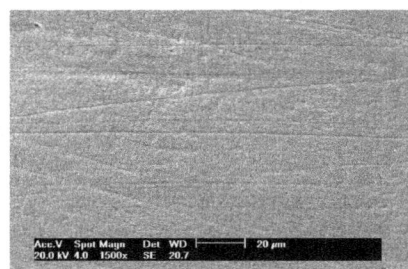

Figure 7 - Micrography of enamel surface after resin removal with tungsten drill + Sof-lex discs and polishing with pumice (Group 2c).

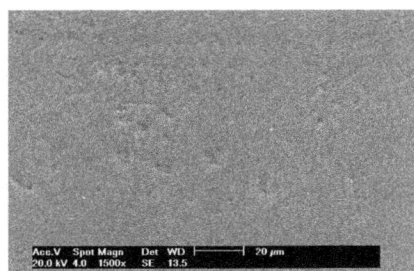

Figure 8 - Micrography of enamel surface after resin removal with tungsten drill + Enhance finishing tips without polishing (Group 3a).

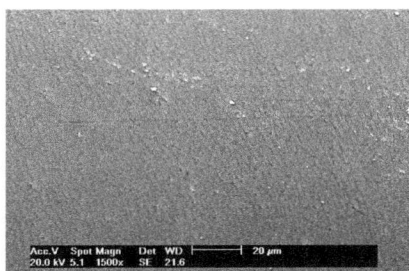

Figure 9 - Micrography of enamel surface after resin removal with tungsten drill + Enhance finishing tips and polishing with aluminium oxide (Group 3b).

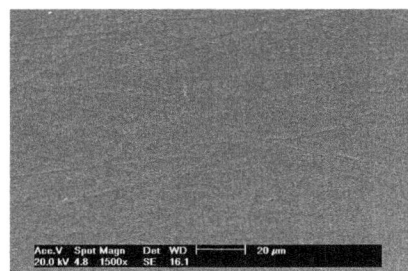

Figure 10 - Micrography of enamel surface after resin removal with tungsten drill + Enhance finishing tips and polishing with pumice (Group 3c).

special shine and prevents plaque retention. Although we have not found statistically significant differences among groups, the literature shows the importance of final polishing. Additionally, even though there is no statistical difference regarding the best polishing technique, electron microscopy suggests smoother enamel surfaces when polishing is carried out with aluminum oxide paste in comparison to pumice stone. Visually, it also presented a glossy surface.

CONCLUSION

Based on the results of this study it is reasonable to conclude that all techniques employed to remove remnant resin from enamel surface promoted grooves and, although no statistically significant difference was found with regard to polishing in the present study, we fully agree with the literature about the importance of enamel polishing. Additionally, even though there were no statistical differences concerning the best polishing technique, electron microscopy suggests smoother enamel surfaces when polishing is performed with aluminum oxide paste in comparison to pumice stone. Visually, it also presented a glossy surface.

Among the aspects analyzed herein, the use of tungsten drill (30 blades), in unidirectional movements, is recommended to remove large volumes of resin remnant, followed by Enhance finishing tips with gentle pressure and polishing with aluminum oxide paste. This protocol promotes better enamel surface smoothness in addition to a reduced procedure time.

REFERENCES

1. Retief DH, Denys FR. Finishing of enamel surface after debonding of orthodontics attachments. Angle Orthod. 1979;49(1):1-10.

2. Buonocore MG. A simple method of increasing the adhesion of acrylic filling materials to enamel surfaces. J Dent Res. 1955;34(6):849-53.

3. Hong YH, Lew KK. Quantitative and qualitative assessment of enamel surface following five composite removal methods after bracket debonding. Eur J Orthod. 1995;17(2):121-8.

4. Ozer T, Basaran A, Kama JD. Surface roughness of the restored enamel after orthodontic treatment. Am J Orthod Dentofacial Orthop. 2010;137(3):368-74.

5. Eliades T, Gioka C, Eliades G, Makou M. Enamel surface roughness following debonding using two resin grinding methods. Eur J Orthod. 2004;26(3):333-8.

6. Årtun J, Bergland S. Clinical trials with crystal growth conditioning as an alternative to acid – etch enamel pretreatment. Am J Orthod. 1984;85(4):333-40.

7. Closs LQ, Reston EG, Falster CA. Rugosidade da superfície do esmalte x descolagem de bráquetes: avaliação de técnicas de polimento. J Bras Ortodon Ortop Facial. 2006;11(62):158-64.

8. Fox NA, McCabe JF, Buckley JG. A critique of bond strength testing in orthodontics. Br J Orthod. 1994;21(1):33-43.

9. Retief H, Mandras RS, Russel CM, Denys FR. Extracted human versus bovine teeth in laboratory studies. Am J Dent. 1990;3(6):253-8.

10. Osterle LJ, Shellhart WC, Belanger GK. The use of bovine enamel in bonding studies. Am J Orthod Dentofacial Orthop. 1998;114(5):514-9.

11. Tüfekçi E, Merrill TE, Pintado MR, Beyer JP, Brantley WA. Enamel loss associated with orthodontic adhesive removal on teeth with white spot lesion: an in vitro study. Am J Orthod Dentofacial Orthop. 2004;125(6):733-9.

12. Gwinnet AJ, Gorelick L. Microscopic evaluation of enamel after debonding: clinical application. Am J Orthod. 1977;71(6):651-65.

13. Burapavong V, Marshall GW, Apfel DA, Perry HT. Enamel surface characteristics on removal of bonded orthodontic brackets. Am J Orthod. 1978;74(2):176-87.

14. Zachrisson BU, Årtun J. Enamel surface appearance after various debonding techniques. Am J Orthod. 1979;75(2):121-7.

15. Rouleau BD, Grayson WM, Cooley RO. Enamel surface evaluation after clinical treatment and removal of orthodontics brackets. Am J Orthod. 1982;81(5):423-6

16. Krell KV, Courey JM, Bishara SE. Orthodontic bracket removal using conventional and ultrasonic debonding techniques, enamel loss and time requirements. Am J Orthod Dentofacial Orthop. 1993;103(3):258-66.

17. Campbell PM. Enamel surfaces after orthodontics bracket debonding. Angle Orthod. 1995;65(2):103-10.

18. Zarrinnia, K. et al. The effect different debonding techniques on the enamel surface: an in vitro qualitative study. Am J Orthod Dentofacial Orthop. 1995;108(3):284-93.

19. Tonial AP, Bizetto MP. Aspectos técnicos e conservadores na remoção de bráquetes de resina remanescente do esmalte dentário. Ortodon Gaúch. 2000;6(1):59-66.

20. Naccarato SRF, Nauff F, Azambuja Jr N, Jaeger RG, Tortamano A. Avaliação de diferentes métodos de remoção de resina após a descolagem de bráquetes e seus efeitos sobre o esmalte. Anais da Revista de Pesquisas Brasileiras; 2003. p. 265.

21. Tavares SW. Análise in vitro de diferentes métodos de remoção da resina residual no esmalte dentário [tese]. Piracicaba (SP); UNICAMP; 2006.

22. Pignatta LMB. Avaliação da superfície do esmalte dentário por Microscopia Eletrônica de Varredura após a remoção do bráquete e polimento [dissertação]. Araçatuba (SP): Universidade Estadual Paulista "Júlio de Mesquita Filho"; 2006.

23. Eminkahyagil N, Arman A, Çetinahin A, Karabulut E. Effect of resinremoval methods on enamel and shear bond strength of rebonded brackets. Angle Orthod. 2006;76(2):314-21.

24. Arhun N, Arman A. Effects of orthodontic mechanics to tooth enamel: a review. Semin Orthod. 2007;13(4):281-91.

25. Fonseca DM, Pinheiro FHSL, Medeiros SF. Sugestão de um protocolo simples e eficiente para remoção de bráquetes ortodônticos. Rev Dental Press Estét. 2004;1(1):112-9.

26. Macieski K, Rocha R, Locks A, Ribeiro GU. Effects evaluation of remaining resin removal (three modes) on enamel surface after bracket debonding. Dental Press J Orthod. 2011;16(5):146-54.

22

Cephalometric analysis for the diagnosis of sleep apnea: A comparative study between reference values and measurements obtained for Brazilian subjects

Patrícia Superbi Lemos Maschtakow[1], Jefferson Luis Oshiro Tanaka[2], João Carlos da Rocha[3], Lílian Chrystiane Giannasi[4], Mari Eli Leonelli de Moraes[5], Carolina Bacci Costa[6], Julio Cezar de Melo Castilho[7], Luiz Cesar de Moraes[8]

Objective: To verify if the reference values of Sleep Apnea cephalometric analysis of North American individuals are similar to the ones of Brazilian individuals presenting no craniofacial anomalies. The study also aimed to identify craniofacial alterations in Obstructive Sleep Apnea-Hypopnea Syndrome (OSAHS) patients in relation to individuals without clinical characteristics of the disease through this cephalometric analysis. **Method:** It were used 55 lateral cephalograms consisting of 29 for the control group of adult individuals without clinical characteristics of OSAHS and 26 apneic adults. All radiographs were submitted to Sleep Apnea cephalometric analysis through Radiocef Studio 2.0. The standard values of this analysis were compared, by means of z test, to the ones obtained from the control group and these were compared to values from apneic group through Student's *t* test. **Results:** There were no significant differences between values obtained from control group and standard values. On the group of OSAHS patients it was observed a decrease on the dimensions of upper airways and an increase on the soft palate length. **Conclusions:** The standard values of Sleep Apnea analysis can be used as reference in Brazilian individuals. Besides, through lateral cephalograms it was possible to identify craniofacial alterations in OSAHS patients.
Keywords: Obstructive sleep apnea. Comparative study. Cephalometry

[1] Doctorate Student of the Program of Oral Biopathology at FOSJC-UNESP.
[2] Professor of the Specialization Course in Orthodontics APCD.
[3] Assistant Professor of Pediatric Dentistry at FOSJC-UNESP
[4] Adjunct Professor, UNINOVE.
[5] Assistant Professor of Dental Radiology at FOSJC-UNESP.
[6] Doctorate Student of the Program of Oral Biopathology at FOSJC-UNESP.
[7] Assistant Professor, Dental Radiology at FOSJC-UNESP.
[8] Full Professor, Dental Radiology at FOSJC-UNESP.

» The authors report no commercial, proprietary or financial interest in the products or companies described in this article.

Patrícia Superbi Lemos Maschtakow
pat.lems@yahoo.com.br / rocha@fosjc.unesp.br

INTRODUCTION

The radiographic cephalometry is an important element for investigation of alterations that occur during craniofacial growth and development. This technique transcended the boundaries of odontology and, today, presents significative importance in other areas, such as Otorhinolaryngology, as an important tool for the evaluation of upper airways (UA) and diagnosis of the obstructive sleep apnea-hypopnea syndrome (OSAHS).[25]

The OSAHS consists in repeated apneic events, resultant from total or partial collapse of the pharynx during sleep. It was identified, predisposing factors such as obesity, alterations on the neuromuscular pattern and skeletal or soft tissue anatomical alterations.[24] Many authors[1,4,7,9,21] discussed and validated the lateral cephalometric radiograph for evaluation of the UA. Although it consists in method of diagnosis through two-dimensional image, the lateral cephalometric radiograph provides linear and angular measurements that are essential to locate the spots of obstruction of the pharynx.[17,18]

Simões[24] evaluated through lateral cephalometric radiographs, the pharyngeal space in north American individuals with normal occlusions belonging to Ann Arbor's sample. This work generated a table with standard values that is widely used as reference in Brazilian radiological and orthodontic clinics. However, studies that validated this analysis were not found for the use in the Brazilian population.

In this context, the objective of this study was to verify if reference values of Sleep Apnea cephalometric analysis relative to North American individuals are similar to the ones of Brazilian individuals with no craniofacial anomalies. The study also aimed to identify craniofacial alterations in OSAHS patients in relation to individuals without clinical characteristics of the disease.

MATERIAL AND METHODS

The present study was approved by the Ethics Committee in Research of the State University of São Paulo, São José dos Campos, School of Dentistry, under the protocol number 103/2007/2006-PH/CEP.

Sample selection

In the present study, 55 lateral cephalometric radiographs were used. Twenty-six from individuals with diagnosis of OSAHS confirmed by polysomnographic exam, consisted of 18 males ranging from 20 to 70 years of age, and 8 females from 30 to 57 years of age. The radiographs were obtained at the same center of dental radiology. Polysomnographic exams were also performed in a single clinic specialized in sleep disorders.

Twenty nine radiographs of individuals presenting no symptoms relative to OSAHS were also used, comprising 11 males from 18 to 29 years of age and 18 females from 19 to 35 years of age.

The criteria for inclusion of the cephalometric radiographs of OSAHS patients were: Polysomnographic examination report that corroborated the diagnosis of OSAHS available and performed in specialized clinic according to protocol recommended by the Brazilian Society of Sleep on the I Consensus in Snore and Sleep Apnea,[27] including the AHI values, body mass index (BMI), total period of sleep and period of sleep in each stage, average heart rate and baseline oxyhemoglobin saturation (SO_2).

Regarding the control group, the criteria were: Existence of medical report with full information about the systemic conditions of the individuals: Not syndromic, did not snore, did not use medicines to induce sleep (hypnotic or neuroleptic), had not been subjected to orthognathic surgical treatment, upper airways treatment or previous orthodontic treatment, did not have respiratory or neurological problems, were not obese and with harmonious facial profile and Class I skeletal pattern.

It were excluded the radiographs that presented the image of the soft palate in format of inverted V, which, according to McNamara Jr.,[19] indicates that the individual swallowed at the moment of obtaining the image, which can interfere on measurements related to this structure.

Cephalometric analysis

The cephalometric radiographs were digitized with resolution of 300 dpi through flatbed scanner EPSON Perfection 4990 (Epson America Inc., Long Beach, California,USA) with transparency reader attached and its respective software SilverFast® SE 6. The images were saved in TIFF format (Tagged Image File Format) without compression. The cephalometric analysis were performed by a single evaluator and digitized through the software Radiocef Studio 2.0 (Radiomemory, Belo Horizonte/MG).

In the present study, for the classification of individuals on the control group regarding the sagittal skeletal pattern, it was used the ANB angle. Only individuals with ANB between 0° and 4° were selected.

For evaluation of the UA and related structures, it was used the Sleep Apnea analysis which is in the list of analysis of the software and is based on works by Simões[24] and Pinto.[21] This cephalometric analysis is constituted of 28 points forming 14 factors (linear measures), shown in Figure 1.

Statistical analysis

For evaluation of method error, the measures were obtained twice with 30 days interval. The results of both readings were compared through simple Linear Regression Analysis and Student's *t* test with level of significance at 5% ($\alpha = 0.05$).

The mean for every factor obtained on the control group was compared to the standard value of the Sleep Apnea analysis through the test. Posteriorly, to verify differences between the group of OSAHS patients and the control group, it was used the Student's *t* test with $\alpha = 0.05$.

RESULTS

The mean between the first and the second reading of each measure was used to calculate the analyzed factors. The results of z test, used for comparison of means of the control group and of standard values of Sleep Apnea analysis,[24] are represented on Table 1 and Figure 2 for females and on Table 2 and Figure 3 for males.

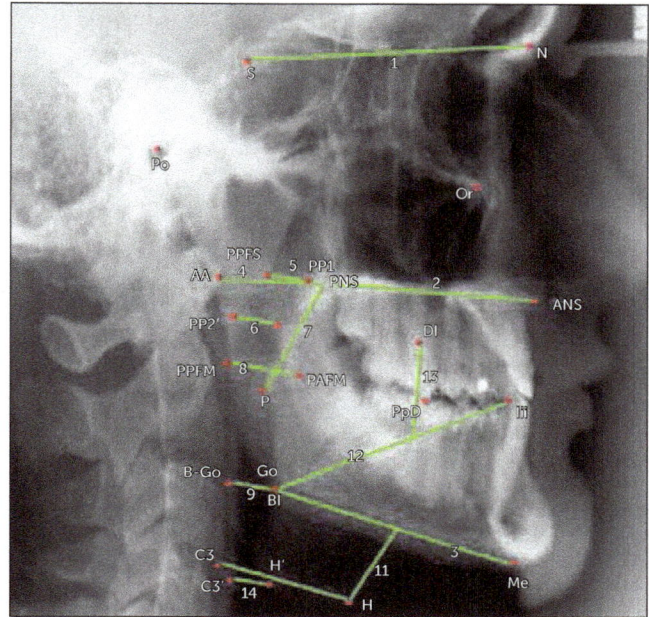

Figure 1 - Representation of points and factors evaluated on Sleep Apnea cephalometric analysis.

Table 1 - Mean, standard deviation (SD) and p value of the 14 linear measures (mm) on control group and standard for females, after application of z test.

Factor	Group control Mean ± SD	Standard Value Mean ± SD	p value
1) S-N	69.70 ± 3.11	73 ± 3.0	0.2858
2) ANS-PNS	53.20 ± 2.82	54 ± 3.0	0.7964
3) Goc-Me	73.92 ± 6.37	74 ± 5.0	0.9883
4) AA-PNS	39.88 ± 5.42	36 ± 3.0	0.2335
5) PPFS-PP1	20.09 ± 3.50	24 ± 3.5	0.2780
6) PP2-PP2'	13.90 ± 2.48	14 ± 2.0	0.9618
7) PNS-P	33.02 ± 4.83	35 ± 4.5	0.6703
8) PPFM-PAFM	17.77 ± 3.36	21 ± 3.5	0.3683
9) B-Go/BI	11.87 ± 2.93	13 ± 2.5	0.6643
10) C3-H	34.27 ± 3.70	36 ± 3.0	0.5808
11) PM-H	20.51 ± 15.32	15 ± 3.0	0.2398
12) BI-PI	69.87 ± 6.14	72.5 ± 3.0	0.4308
13) DI-PI/BI	22.38 ± 3.76	24 ± 3.0	0.6049
14) C3'-H'	11.74 ± 2.85	13.5 ± 2.0	0.4049

* Significant level: 5%.

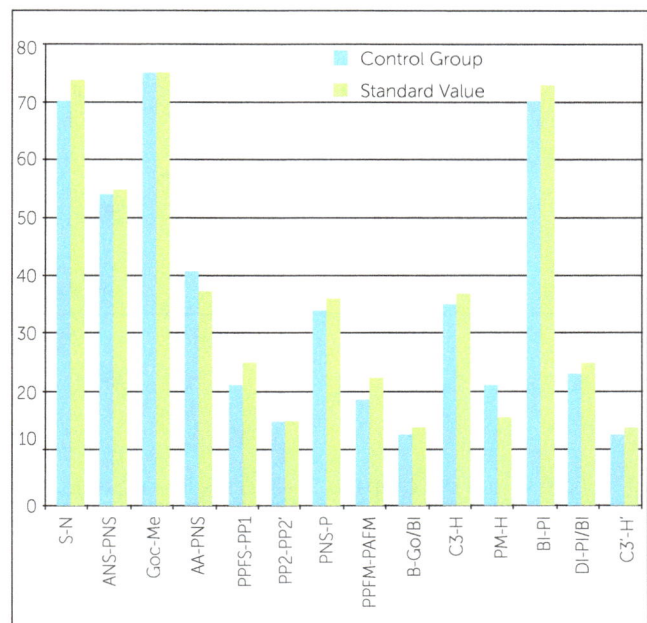

Figure 2 - Graphic of comparison between the factors values, in millimeters, of the control group and standard values in female individuals.

Table 2 - Mean, standard deviation and p value of the 14 linear measures (mm) on the control group and standard values for male individuals after application of z test.

Factor	Control Group Mean ± S.D.	Standard values Mean ± S.D.	p value
1) S-N	76.10 ± 4.34	80 ± 2.00	0.1031
2) ANS-PNS	60.02 ± 4.97	62.5 ± 4.00	0.5625
3) Goc-Me	79.26 ± 4.12	84.5 ± 5.00	0.3099
4) AA-PNS	40.83 ± 2.32	36 ± 3.50	0.1758
5) PPFS-PP1	19.91 ± 2.84	26 ± 4.00	0.1367
6) PP2-PP2'	14.11 ± 2.04	12 ± 3.00	0.4894
7) PNS-P	34.68 ± 3.75	34 ± 5.00	0.8944
8) PPFM-PAFM	19.45 ± 2.41	22 ± 4.50	0.5761
9) B-Go/BI	14.45 ± 3.57	15.5 ± 3.50	0.7749
10) C3-H	40.81 ± 4.29	41 ± 3.50	0.9614
11) PM-H	19.79 ± 4.80	19 ± 6.00	0.8969
12) BI-PI	73.39 ± 4.88	79 ± 5.00	0.2819
13) DI-PI/BI	24.38 ± 3.56	29.5 ± 3.00	0.1084
14) C3'-H'	16.77 ± 5.37	17.5 ± 4.00	0.8617

* Significance level: 5%.

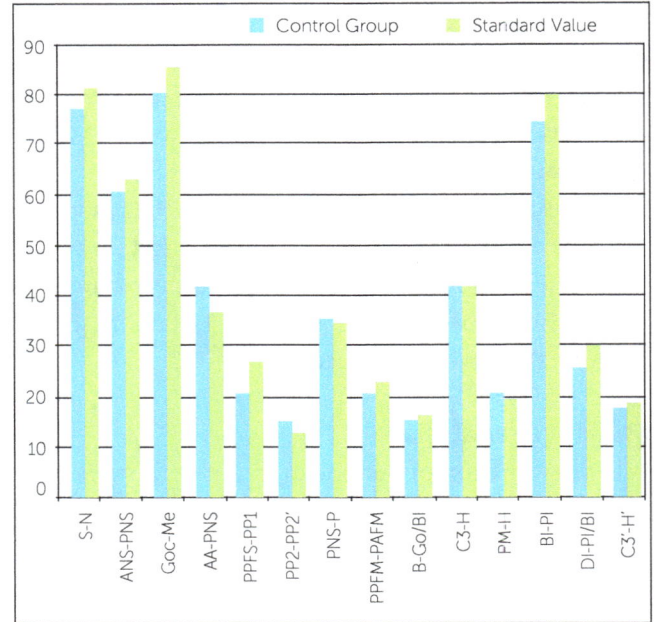

Figure 3 - Graphic of comparison between the factors values, in millimeters, of the control group and standard values in male individuals.

Table 3 - Mean, standard deviation and p value of linear measures in males on the control group and on the OSAHS group after application of Student's t test.

Factor	OSAHS (n = 18) Mean ± S.D.	Control (n = 11) Mean ± S.D.	p value
1) S-N	74.8 ± 3.3	76.1 ± 4.3	0.3734
2) ANS-PNS	56.9 ± 5.1	60 ± 5	0.3734
3) Goc-Me	71.1 ± 3.2	79.3 ± 4.1	0.3734
4) AA-PNS	37.3 ± 4.1	40.8 ± 2.3	0.0431
5) PPFS-PP1	14.4 ± 3.5	19.9 ± 2.9	0.0000*
6) PP2-PP2'	7.5 ± 2.5	14.1 ± 2.1	0.0000*
7) PNS-P	43.3 ± 4.5	34.7 ± 3.8	0.0000*
8) PPFM-PAFM	15.1 ± 2.8	19.5 ± 2.4	0.0000*
9) B-Go/BI	12.1 ± 3.2	14.5 ± 3.6	0.0796
10) C3-H	43.4 ± 5.1	40.8 ± 4.3	0.1545
11) PM-H	26 ± 6.5	19.8 ± 4.8	0.0223
12) BI-PI	73.9 ± 4.9	73.4 ± 4.9	0.8921
13) DI-PI/BI	24 ± 2.7	24.4 ± 4.2	0.9500
14) C3'-H'	6.1 ± 2	16.8 ± 5.4	0.0000*

* Significance level: 5%.

Table 4 - Graphic of comparison between the factors values, in millimeters, of the control group and of the standard values in female individuals.

Factor	OSAHS (n = 8) Mean ± S.D.	Control (n = 18) Mean ± S.D.	p value
1) S-N	68.4 ± 3.93	69.7 ± 3.12	0.0021*
2) ANS-PNS	48.8 ± 4.64	53.21 ± 2.83	0.0021*
3) Goc-Me	68.68 ± 6.96	73.92 ± 6.38	0.1869
4) AA-PNS	37.25 ± 6.9	39.89 ± 4.41	0.5570
5) PPFS-PP1	16.75 ± 3.78	20.1 ± 3.51	0.1222
6) PP2-PP2'	6.67 ± 2.51	13.9 ± 2.48	0.0000*
7) PNS-P	41.14 ± 3.14	33.02 ± 4.84	0.0003*
8) PPFM-PAFM	12.01 ± 2.74	17.77 ± 3.36	0.0005*
9) B-Go/BI	7.12 ± 1.57	11.87 ± 2.94	0.0003*
10) C3-H	41.68 ± 7.09	34.27 ± 3.71	0.0005*
11) PM-H	23.88 ± 7.26	20.52 ± 15.32	0.6133
12) BI-PI	67.76 ± 6.21	69.88 ± 6.15	0.5514
13) DI-PI/BI	19.98 ± 3.03	22.38 ± 3.76	0.0000*
14) C3'-H'	6.08 ± 2.35	11.74 ± 2.86	0.0000*

* Significance level: 5%.

The p values of comparisons and results of Student's t test for studied groups are represented on Tables 3 and 4.

DISCUSSION

Through the results of the present study it was observed that, despite the evident physical differences between Brazilian and north American individuals, there was no significative difference on the cephalometric dimensions relative to UA among the individuals of these two nationalities, indicating that there is possibility of using the table of standard values for OSAHS on the evaluation of Brazilian individuals.

Today, the diagnosis and treatment of OSAHS depend on a multidisciplinary team of health professionals. The dentist, specially the orthodontist, maxillary functional orthopedist and oral and maxillofacial surgeon have fundamental role on the diagnosis of obstruction of UA through radiographs that are part of their work routine. Besides, they participate actively on the treatment of apneic individuals through intraoral appliances[11,12,22] or orthognathic surgeries.

Several methods of diagnosis by image can be used in order to evaluate the dimensions of UA, however in this study, it was chosen the lateral cephalometric radiograph because this exam is considered the most accessible and widely requested method according to other authors.[1,4,17,18]

The choice for the cephalometric analysis used in this study was due to its large use in radiological and orthodontic clinics and for it embraces measures in all regions susceptible to obstruction.

It was considered important to verify if reference values for the craniofacial measures based in studies with American individuals can be used for Brazilian individuals since in a study comparing OSAHS patients from two distinct ethnicities, Cakirer et al[6] found significant differences on the craniofacial characteristics associated to UA between these groups.

The narrowing of the nasopharynx observed in OSAHS male patients (Table 3) was a finding similar to presented by other authors.[1,4,17,21,23] According to some studies,[5,19,21] the upper pharyngeal space is one of the regions most susceptible to collapse due to frequent hypertrophy of the pharyngeal tonsils. In the present study, the tonsils were not separately evaluated, however, it was considered the dimensions of the soft tissue on the nasopharynx by marking the posterior point where there was greater obstruction of the airway according to McNamara Jr.[19]

King[15] mentioned that the forward and downward growth of the face is affected by the anterior growth of the cranial base and posterior growth of the occipital bone or by the association of both, and this growth will contribute to the increase of the pharynx's diameter. In female OSAHS patients was observed a reduction on the cranial base and on the dimensions in all regions of the pharynx. Some authors[3,2,8,26] mentioned the decrease of the cranial base as one of the cephalometric findings characteristics of OSAHS.

The hyoid bone was more anteriorly positioned in females on the group of OSAHS subjects and did not present significant difference in males on the present research, similar to the findings by Tsai et al,[26] who found that this factor is associated to greater severity of OSAHS in females.

It is known that the hyoid bone has no bone articulation and is suspended by a grid of muscles and ligaments. Therefore, its position is largely dependent of muscle ligaments, such as tongue, and it is also influenced by the individual's posture.[8] This fact explains the importance of evaluating this structure in apneic individuals.

Battagel and L'Estrange[4] asserted that the greater alterations on dimensions of UA in OSAHS patients occur in the oropharynx, agreeing with Lowe et al,[16] and were related to the reduction of the median posterior palatal space that, in the present work, was also reduced on the group of OSAHS subjects. This space has close relation to the dimensions of the soft palate which increased length was related to presence of OSAHS in several researches[3,4,10,20,25,26] and the present study.

The lower airspace is significantly reduced on the group of OSAHS patients agreeing with Lyberg et al.[17] This obstruction of the hypopharynx is related to the epiglottic region that corresponds to the area of great interest for orthognathic surgeries.[13]

On Figure 4, it can be compared lateral cephalometric radiographs correspondent to group of OSAHS subjects and the control group, in which is observed the most common alterations of UA and related structures found on the group of OSAHS patients in relation to the control group.

The hypothesis that anatomic factors, are involved on the etiology of OSAHS has great support in literature. Therefore, it is important to know the anatomic alterations predominant in apneic individuals so that professionals that work directly with lateral cephalometric radiograph can identify risk factors and refer the patient to specialists and specific exams such as polysomnography, considered the gold standard exam for diagnosis of OSAHS. This will contribute to the early diagnosis of the disease, avoiding the severe sequelae related to it.

CONCLUSIONS

» Craniofacial measures used as reference on the diagnosis of OSAHS, can be applied to Brazilian individuals.

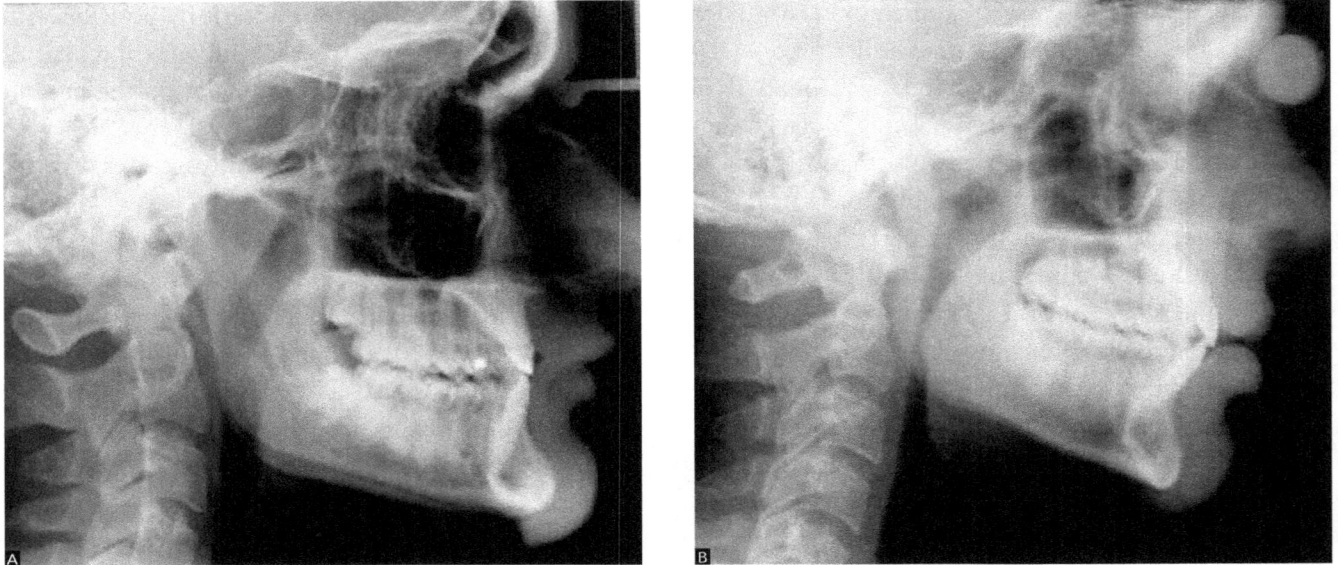

Figure 4 - A) Example of radiographs of control group's individual **B)** example of radiographs of OSAHS individuals.

» There were significative craniofacial alterations in OSAHS patients when compared to individuals without clinical characteristics of this disease.

» In male apneics it were observed reductions of the upper, mean, inferior and retropalatal air spaces and increase of the soft palate length.

» In female apneics, reduction of the dimensions in all evaluated pharyngeal regions, of anterior cranial base and maxilla length.

REFERENCES

1. Andersson L, Brattström V. Cephalometric analysis of permanently snoring patients with and without obstructive sleep apnea syndrome. Int J Oral Maxillofac Surg. 1991;20(3):159-62.

2. Bacon WH, Turlot JC, Krieger J, Stierle JL. Cephalometric evaluation of pharyngeal obstructive factors in patients with sleep apneas syndrome. Angle Orthod. 1990;60(2):115-22.

3. Bacon WH, Krieger J, Turlot JC, Stierle JL. Craniofacial characteristics in patients with obstructive sleep apneas syndrome. Cleft Palate J. 1988;25(4):374-8.

4. Battagel JM, L'Estrange PR. The cephalometric morphology of patients with obstructive sleep apnoea (OSA). Eur J Orthod. 1996;18(6):557-69.

5. Bell WH. Modern practice in orthognathic and reconstructive surgery. Philadelphia: WB Saunders; 1992.

6. Cakirer B, Hans MG, Graham G, Aylor J, Tishler PV, Redline S. The relationship between craniofacial morphology and obstructive sleep apnea in Whites and in African-Americans. Am J Respir Crit Care Med. 2001;163(4):947-50.

7. Castellucci E, Barbosa M, Knop LAH, Lessa MM, Araujo TM. Avaliação da radiografia cefalométrica lateral como meio de diagnóstico da hipertrofia de adenóide. Rev Dental Press Ortod Ortop Facial. 2009;14(4):83-91.

8. Chaves Júnior CM. Indivíduos com síndrome da apnéia e hipopnéia do sono obstrutiva avaliados pela análise cefalométrica das contra partes de Enlow [tese]. Piracicaba (SP): Universidade Estadual de Campinas; 2000.

9. David FA, Castilho CM. Estudo comparativo entre os traçados manual e computadorizado da análise do espaço aéreo faríngeo em radiografias cefalométricas laterais. Ortodontia. 1999;3(2):288-93.

10. Faria AC, Ramos MC, Fonseca RG, Paschoal JR. Estudo cefalométrico em indivíduos com distúrbios ventilatórios obstrutivos do sono. J Bras Ortodon Ortop Facial. 2006;63(11):281-8.

11. Giannasi LC, Magini M, Oliveira CS, Oliveira LVF. Treatment of obstructive sleep apnea using an adjustable mandibular repositioning appliance fitted to a total prosthesis in a maxillary edentulous patient. Sleep Breath. 2008;12(1):91-5.

12. Giannasi LC, Mattos LC, Magini M, Costa MS, Oliveira CS, Oliveira LVF. The impact of the Adjustable PM Positioner appliance in the treatment of obstructive sleep apnoea. Arch Med Sci. 2008;4(3):336-41.

13. Gonçales ES. Estudo cefalométrico computadorizado do espaço aéreo faríngeo de indivíduos submetidos à cirurgia ortognática para correção de prognatismo mandibular [tese]. Bauru (SP): Universidade de São Paulo; 2006.

14. Houston WJB. The analysis of errors in orthodontic measurements. Am J Orthod. 1971;83(5):382-90.

15. King EW. A roentgenographic study of pharyngeal growth. Angle Orthod. 1952;22(1):23-6.

16. Lowe AA, Santamaria JD, Fleetham JA, Price C. Facial morphology and obstructive sleep apnea. Am J Orthod Dentofacial Orthop. 1986;90(6):484-91.

17. Lyberg T, Krogstad O, Djupesland G. Cephalometric analysis in patients with obstructive sleep apnoea syndrome. I. Skeletal morphology J Laryngol Otol. 1989;103(3):287-92.

18. Lyberg T, Krogstad O, Djupesland G. Cephalometric analysis in patients with obstructive sleep apnoea syndrome. II. Soft tissue morphology. J Laryngol Otol. 1989;103(3):293-7.

19. McNamara Jr JA. A method of cephalometric evaluation. Am J Orthod Dentofacial Orthop. 1984;86(6):449-69.

20. Partinen M, Guilleminault C, Quera-Salva MA, Jamieson A. Obstructive Sleep Apnea cephalometric roentgenograms the role of anatomic upper airway abnormalities in the definition of abnormal breathing during sleep. Chest. 1988;93(6):1199-205.

21. Pinto AJ. Ronco e apnéia do sono. Rio de Janeiro: Revinter; 2000.

22. Rodrigues AAAAS, Rodrigues RND. Aparelho intrabucal para o tratamento dos transtornos respiratórios do sono: qual a sua influência nos parâmetros cardiológicos do paciente? Rev Dental Press Ortod Ortop Facial. 2008;13(3):20-2.

23. Silva ELC, Campos PSF, Fontes FHO, Macedo Sobrinho JB, Panella J. Accuracy of cephalometric pharyngeal analysis for diagnosis of obstructive sleep apnea syndrome (OSA). Rev Ci Med Biol. 2005;4(2):118-24.

24. Simões DO. Cefalometria em apnéia do sono. In: Colombini NEP. Cirurgia da face: Interpretação funcional e estética. Síndrome da apnéia obstrutiva do sono: enfoque maxilofacial e otorrinolaringológico. Rio de Janeiro: Revinter; 2002. p. 572-96.

25. Strauss RA, Burgoyne CC. Diagnostic imaging and sleep medicine. Dent Clin North Am. 2008;52(4):891-915.

26. Tangugsorn V, Krogstad O, Espeland L, Lyberg T. Obstructive sleep apnoea: multiple comparisons of cephalometric variables of obese and non-obese patients. J Craniomaxillofac Surg. 2000;28(4):204-12.

27. Tsai HH, Ho CY, Lee PL, Tan CT. Sex differences in anthropometric and cephalometric characteristics in the severity of obstructive sleep apnea syndrome. Am J Orthod Dentofacial Orthop. 2009;135(2):155-64.

28. Tufik S, Sampaio PL, Weckx LLM, et al. Consenso em ronco e apnéia do sono. São Paulo: Sociedade Brasileira de Sono; Rinologia e Otorrinolaringologia; 2000.

23

Analysis of correlation between initial alveolar bone density and apical root resorption after 12 months of orthodontic treatment without extraction

Paula Cabrini Scheibel[1], Adilson Luiz Ramos[2], Lilian Cristina Vessoni Iwaki[3], Kelly Regina Micheletti[4]

Objective: The aim of the present study was to investigate the correlation between initial alveolar bone density of upper central incisors (ABD-UI) and external apical root resorption (EARR) after 12 months of orthodontic movement in cases without extraction. **Methods:** A total of 47 orthodontic patients 11 years old or older were submitted to periapical radiography of upper incisors prior to treatment (T_1) and after 12 months of treatment (T_2). ABD-UI and EARR were measured by means of densitometry. **Results:** No statistically significant correlation was found between initial ABD-UI and EARR at T_2 (r = 0.149; p = 0.157). **Conclusion:** Based on the present findings, alveolar density assessed through periapical radiography is not predictive of root resorption after 12 months of orthodontic treatment in cases without extraction.

Keywords: Root resorption. Tooth movement. Dental radiography. Bone density.

» The authors report no commercial, proprietary or financial interest in the products or companies described in this article.

[1] MSc in Integrated Dentistry, State University of Maringá, UEM.
[2] Adjunct professor, Department of Dentistry, State University of Maringá, UEM.
[3] Associate professor of Dental radiology and Stomatology, Department of Dentistry, State University of Maringá, UEM.
[4] PhD resident in Orthodontics, State University of São Paulo, UNESP.

Paula Cabrini Scheibel
Av Luiz Teixeira Mandes, 2266. Centro de Otorrino / Sala 06 CEP 87105-001
Maringá - PR — Brazil — E-Mail: pscheibel13@gmail.com

INTRODUCTION

Orthodontic movement often results in external apical root resorption (EARR).[1-6] While this event does not significantly affect teeth support in most patients, severe root resorption occurs in 5% to 14.5% of cases.[1-5]

As the risk factors identified for EARR stemming from orthodontic treatment have limited effectiveness, studies involving multivariate analyses have suggested that individual factors may contribute to the etiology of this condition.[1,3,4,7,8,9] This belief has led researchers to investigate the influence of maxillary bone density. Kaley and Phillips[10] as well as Horiuchi et al[11] found that dental movement in areas of greater bone density, such as cortical bone, is associated with greater root resorption. Goldie and King[12] found that low bone mineral density (BMD) in rats induced by lactation and calcium deficiency (increased secretion of parathyroid hormone) led to less root resorption during orthodontic movement in comparison to the control group. However, Otis et al[13] found no significant effect of alveolar bone density around roots over the amount of root resorption.

Considering the divergent results of previous studies, the aim of the present investigation was to test the hypothesis that increased alveolar bone density is an individual predisposing factor for EARR during orthodontic treatment, especially in cases without extraction.

MATERIAL AND METHODS

A prospective study was carried out with a sample of 91 upper incisors in 47 patients, 11 years old or older who had participated in a previous study.[6] All patients had a complete fixed appliance installed with straight-wire orthodontics at the clinics of the Orthodontic Postgraduate Program of the State University of Maringá and at Maringá Dental Association (Brazil) between July 2008 and April 2009. In selecting the sample, the following inclusion criteria were applied: Signed informed consent form; patients who were 11 years old or older; fully intact crown of upper incisors or only with proximal restorations; and scheduled orthodontic treatment without extractions and/or incisor intrusion. The exclusion criteria were: Previous history of fixed orthodontic treatment; previous root resorption; history of dentoalveolar trauma to upper incisors; history of osteoporosis or rickets and hyperparathyroidism.

All procedures were approved by the State University of Maringá Institutional Review Board, Brazil (190/2008). Each volunteer was submitted to periapical radiography of the upper incisor region either immediately prior to or immediately after bracket bonding (T_1), as well as 12 months after orthodontic treatment (T_2). Radiographs were taken using the RX Timex 70 C (Gnatus, Ribeirão Preto, SP, Brazil) and Pro 70-Intra (Prodental, Ribeirão Preto, São Paulo, Brazil) x-ray equipment operating with 70 kVp, 7 mA and a 0.25-second exposure time.[6] A five-step 2 x 20 x 3.5 mm aluminum wedge (Al step-wedge) was attached to the apical region perpendicular to the film (Agfa Dentus M2 "Comfort"). Kodak developing and fixing solutions (Kodak do Brazil, Comércio e Indústria Ltda, São José dos Campos, SP, Brazil) were used to develop the radiographs. The radiographic film was processed manually using the time-temperature method.[14] Development time was determined after verifying the liquid temperature (2 minutes in developer with temperature between 20 and 26°C). Intermediate washing was standardized at 30 seconds and fixing time was standardized at 10 minutes.[15] Radiographic images were digitized using a scanner under 400 ppi resolution (ArtixScan 18000F, Microtek, São Paulo, SP, Brazil).

Measure of alveolar bone density

By means of the histogram tool provided by Photoshop CS3 software (Adobe System, California, USA), a trapezoidal region of interest was outlined in the alveolar bone process of the apical region of upper central incisors to estimate optical density expressed in grey level values ranging from 0 (black) to 255 (white).[14] Each trapezoidal region of interest consisted of approximately 2000 pixels and was selected in such a way so as to avoid roots, lamina dura and nasal spine. The digital reading of each step was performed by selecting a rectangular trapezoidal region of interest of approximately 2500 pixels (Fig 1). Using the optical densities of aluminum step wedge, mean optical density of bone between both central incisors was converted into milimeters aluminum equivalent (mmAl/Eq).

Measure of external apical root resorption

Tooth length (TL) and crown length (CL) of upper incisors (#11 and #21) at both evaluation times (TLT_1 and TLT_2; CLT_1 and CLT_2) were measured at

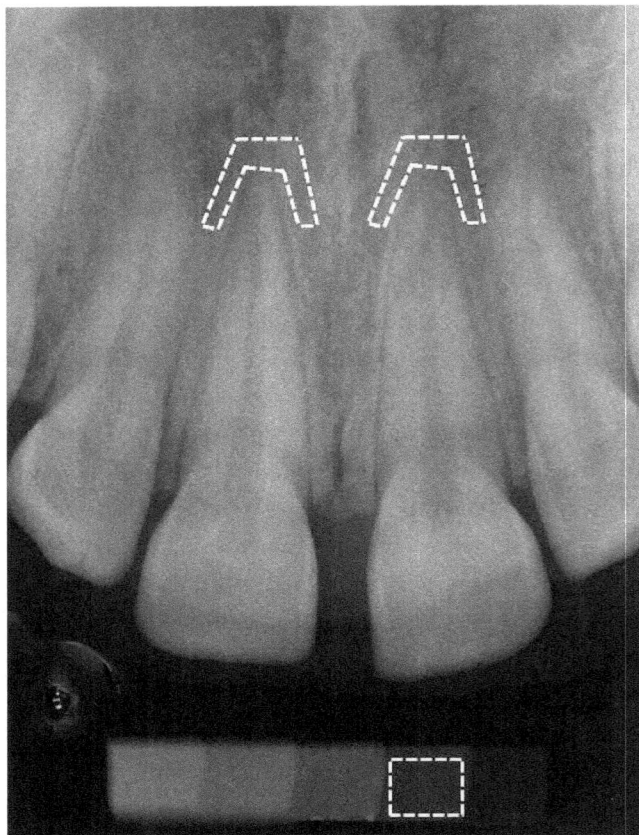

Figure 1 - Scanned periapical radiograph; region of interest selected in the apical region of upper central incisors and second step of aluminum step-wedge (evaluated by histogram tool of Adobe Photoshop CS2 program).

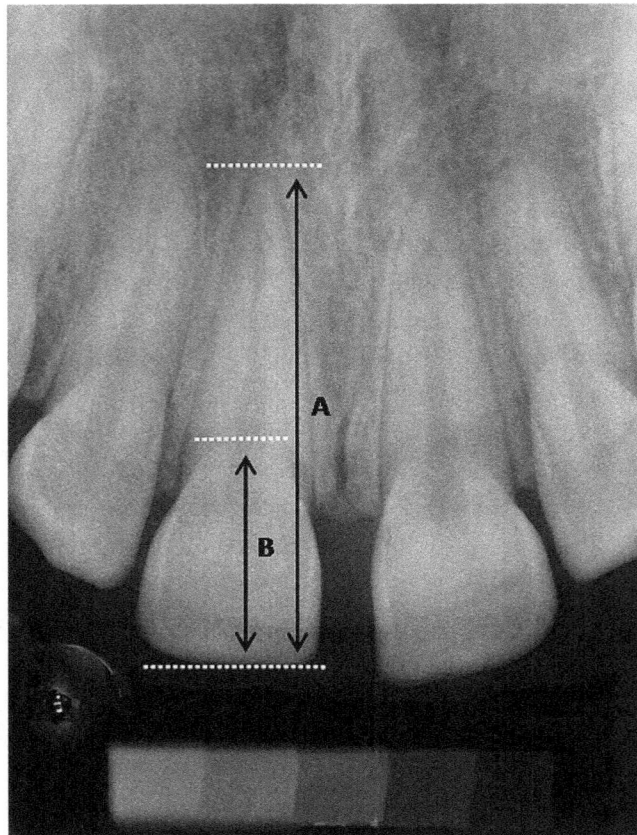

Figure 2 - Radiograph illustrating measures: (**A**) incisal-apical distance (tooth length) used to calculate root resorption; (**B**) distance from incisal edge to cementum-enamel junction (crown length) used for correction of radiograph inclination.

a precision of 0.1 mm with the aid of CorelDRAW X4 software.[6,16,17,18] These measures corresponded to the distance from the incisal edge to the root apex and the greatest distance between the incisal edge and the cementum-enamel junction. The long axis of the tooth was used as reference (Fig 2). To compensate for possible variations in inclination during radiograph taking at different times (presuming that the crown measure remains unaltered during treatment),[17,19,20] expected tooth length at T_2 was calculated using the following equation:[6,18,21]

$$\text{TLT}_2 \text{ expected} = \text{CLT}_2 \cdot \text{TLT}_1/\text{CLT}_1$$

The amount of EARR was determined by subtracting expected tooth length at T_2 by tooth length at T_2:

$$\text{EARR } T_2 = \text{TLT}_2 \text{ expected} - \text{TLT}_2$$

The amount of EARR was expressed in percentage in relation to initial tooth length. 0% resorption was classified as absent; 1 to 4% was classified as rounding of roots; 4 to 8% was classified as mild; and 8 to 12% was classified as moderate.[6] Intra-examiner reliability was statistically assessed by analyzing the differences between duplicate measures on the radiographic images of 25 randomly selected patients (tooth and crown length, optical densities of the alveolar bone and second step of the aluminum wedge) with a 15-day interval between measures at both T_1 and T_2. The error of the method was calculated using Dahlberg's formula:

$$Se = \sqrt{\frac{\sum d^2}{2n}}$$

In which 'd' is the difference between pairs of measurements and 'n' is the number of pairs of measurements.

Spearman's correlation coefficient (r) was also employed. Although no statistically significant differences were found between the first and second measures, the mean of each variable was used in the subsequent statistical tests to minimize random error.

Statistical analysis

Neither EARR nor ABD-UI had normal distribution (Lilliefors test). Thus, nonparametric Spearman correlation test was used to determine potential correlations between initial ABD-UI and EARR at T_2. Significance level was set at 5% ($P < 0.05$) for all statistical tests.

RESULTS

No significant differences were found between teeth #11 and #21 regarding EARR and ABD-UI. After 12 months of treatment, mean EARR was 3.5% (standard deviation: 3.03%; range: 0 to 12.1%) (Table 1). Three patients (6%) had no root resorption; 18 patients (38%) had resorption between 1 and 4%; 18 patients (38%) had resorption between 4 and 8%; and eight patients (17%) had resorption between 8 and 12% (Table 2). No statistically significant correlation was found between initial ABD-UI and EARR after 12 months ($r = 0.149$; $p = 0.157$).

DISCUSSION

Apical root resorption can occur in the early stages of orthodontic treatment, especially in upper incisors which generally undergo greater movement in comparison to other teeth.[3,8,9,17,20] The degree of compression of periodontal ligament is believed to influence the extent of EARR, as greater compression is accompanied by an increase in the area of hyalinization and, theoretically, an increase in EARR severity. However, the force produced by an orthodontic appliance is not necessarily the same force distributed along the periodontal ligament. A number of aspects influence the degree of final root compression and consequent tissue damage, such as mechanical factors (direction of movement; duration and intensity of force applied) and biological factors (crown to root ratio, root anatomy and density of trabecular bone).[21]

Periapical radiography is the method of choice to assess apical root resorption stemming from orthodontic treatment, mainly due to the cost-benefit

Table 1 - Descriptive characterization of sample (n = 47) according to age, mean percentage of EARR after 12 months of treatment and initial ABD-UI in mmEq/Al of 91 upper incisors.

	Minimum	Maximum	Mean ± SD
Age (years)	11	51	20 ± 10.52
EARR (%)	0	12.1	3.5 ± 3.03
ABD-UI (mmEq/Al)	1.24	4.97	2.55 ± 0.89

Table 2 - Descriptive characterization of sample (n = 47) according to percentage of EARR in more resorbed upper central incisors.

EARR (%)	Patients n (%)
0%	3 (6%)
≥ 1 and ≤ 4%	18 (38%)
> 4 and ≤ 8%	18 (38%)
> 8 and ≤ 12%	8 (17%)
	47 (100%)

ratio of this method. Periapical radiographs are known to have greater reliability in comparison to lateral and panoramic radiographs.[22] However, periapical radiographs have less sensitivity and specificity in comparison to volumetric tomography. The three-dimensional visualization of teeth is the major advantage of computed tomography over conventional radiographic exams,[23,24] but the disadvantages of this method are greater cost and greater exposure to x-rays in comparison to periapical radiography.

In previous studies employing dual-energy x-ray absorptiometry (DXA), systemic BMD (lumbar spine and femur) was not correlated with maxillo-mandibular alveolar BMD.[14,25] However, Scheibel and Ramos[25] found a correlation between alveolar bone density in the region of upper incisors and neck of the femur using periapical radiography. Other studies have also found a correlation between systemic BMD and alveolar bone mass assessed by periapical radiography and expressed in mmEqAl.[26-29] Thus, the choice of periapical radiography is based on the possibility of selecting trabecular alveolar bone and avoiding the lamina dura, roots and other structures in comparison to DXA.

A study investigating alveolar density of anterior and posterior regions of the maxilla and mandible found that only the densities of the anterior maxilla and posterior mandible were correlated.[25] This study and other investigations therefore suggest the specific densitometric evaluation of the region of interest.[30,31] Anterior alveolar regions of the maxilla and mandible have greater densitometric values in comparison to posterior regions,[14,31,32] which may be related to the greater occurrence of root resorption in upper incisors together with other factors such as root anatomy and orthodontic mechanics.

The dentoalveolar complex of each patient is unique in terms of size, orientation and density, and associations between EARR and alveolar density and morphology have not yet been established.[13] In the literature, only Otis et al[13] performed a direct investigation on these associations. Using digital techniques on cephalometric radiographs, the authors measured the dimensions of lower incisors and surrounding bone structures (quantitative aspect) as well as density of trabecular bone (qualitative aspect). The present study also investigated the correlation between alveolar bone mass and EARR; however, the methodologies differed with regard to the region examined, type of radiographic exam and methods employed to determine bone density. In the present study, no significant correlation was found between ABD-UI and EARR 12 months after orthodontic treatment. Similarly, setting aside methodological differences, Otis et al[13] found that the amount of alveolar bone adjacent to the root, cortical bone thickness, trabecular bone density and fractal dimension were not significantly correlated with the extent of EARR.

As cortical bone is denser than trabecular bone, a number of studies have investigated associations between bone density and root resorption in an indirect manner by analyzing the proximity of roots and cortical bone during orthodontic movement.[1,10,11,33] In a histological study involving monkeys, Wainwright[33] found no differences in the amount of root resorption between movement against cortical bone and trabecular bone. A clinical study also found no greater root resorption in patients with roots and apices subjectively judged to be in close proximity with palatal cortical bone.[1]

Kaley and Philips[10] studied a case series of 200 patients submitted to orthodontic treatment with the edgewise technique. The authors reported findings that contrast those of the studies cited above.

Six patients (3%) had severe resorption (greater than one quarter of the length of the root) in both upper central incisors. For other teeth, this extent of resorption occurred in less than 1% of patients. Using a case-control model, the characteristics of 21 patients with severe resorption were compared to randomly selected controls from the same case series. Risk factors of root resorption related to orthodontic treatment included increased proximity of maxillary incisors roots to palatal cortical bone (odds ratio: 20), maxillary surgery (odds ratio: 8) and root torque (odds ratio: 4.5). According to the authors, proximity of roots to palatal cortical bone may be directly related to other statistically significant measures observed in the study, such as torque of upper incisors, changes in angle, duration of use of rectangular arch wires and extractions in the upper arch.

Horiuchi et al[11] suggest that proximity of upper central incisors roots to palatal cortical bone during orthodontic treatment may explain approximately 12% of variation in root resorption, whereas alveolar bone thickness explains about 2%. The authors also state that tooth extrusion and lingualization of the crown also contribute to root resorption. In another study, the amount of incisor movement was significantly correlated to the amount of EARR, with even greater movement in cases in which prior extraction of premolars was performed ($r = 0.61$; $P < 0.05$).[34]

It makes sense to measure the total displacement of a tooth by the root apex which is where pathological resorption occurs.[35] In a number of studies, apical displacement, especially in the anteroposterior direction and against cortical bone, was found to be significantly correlated with apical root resorption.[1,10,11] In a meta-analysis,[35] mean apical resorption was correlated with apical displacement ($r = 0.822$) and total treatment duration ($r = 0.852$). However, prolonged treatment alone did not appear to be related to greater root resorption. Although certain procedures, such as torque of upper incisors, changes in angle, duration of rectangular arch wires and extractions in the upper arch, are not found to be direct factors, they seem to be correlated with greater EARR.[10] The findings suggest the need for further investigations of this possible association with larger samples and cases involving greater movement, such as cases with extraction and Class II malocclusion.

CONCLUSION

Based on the present findings, alveolar density in the apical region of upper incisors assessed by means of periapical radiographs is not predictive of root resorption 12 months after orthodontic treatment in cases without extraction.

REFERENCES

1. Mirabella AD, Årtun J. Risk factors for apical root resorption of maxillary anterior teeth in adult orthodontic patients. Am J Orthod Dentofacial Orthop. 1995;108(1):48-55.

2. Sameshima GT, Sinclair PM. Predicting and preventing root resorption: Part I. Treatment factors. Am J Orthod Dentofacial Orthop. 2001;119(5):505-10.

3. Smale I, Artun J, Behbehani F, Doppel D, Van't Hof M, Kuijpers-Jagtman AM. Apical root resorption 6 months after initiation of fixed orthodontic appliance therapy. Am J Orthod Dentofacial Orthop. 2005;128(1):57-67.

4. Taithongchai R, Sookkorn K, Killiany DM. Facial and dentoalveolar structure of apical root shortening and the prediction of apical root shortening. Am J Orthod Dentofacial Orthop. 1996;110(3):296-302.

5. Marques LS, Ramos-Jorge ML, Rey AC, Armond MC, Ruellase ACO. Severe root resorption in orthodontic patients treated with the edgewise method: prevalence and predictive factors. Am J Orthod Dentofacial Orthop. 2010;137(3):384-8.

6. Scheibel PC, Micheletti KR, Ramos AL. External apical root resorption after six and 12 months of non-extraction orthodontic treatment. Dentistry. 2011;1(1). doi:10.4172/2161-1122.1000102

7. Linge L, Linge BO. Patient characteristics and treatment variables associated with apical root resorption during orthodontic treatment. Am J Orthod Dentofacial Orthop. 1991;99(1):35-43.

8. Årtun J, Smale I, Behbehani F, Doppel D, Van't Hof M, Kuijpers-Jagtman AM. Apical root resorption six and 12 months after initiation of fixed orthodontic appliance therapy. Angle Orthod. 2005;75(6):919-26.

9. Årtun J, Van't Hullenaar R, Doppel D, Kuijpers-Jagtman AM. Identification of orthodontic patients at risk of severe apical root resorption. Am J Orthod Dentofacial Orthop. 2009;135(4):448-55.

10. Kaley J, Phillips C. Factors related to root resorption in edgewise practice. Angle Orthod. 1991;61(2):125-32.

11. Horiuchi A, Hotokezaka H, Kobayashi K. Correlation between cortical plate proximity and apical root resorption. Am J Orthod Dentofacial Orthop. 1998;114(3):311-8.

12. Goldie RS, King GJ. Root resorption and tooth movement in orthodontically treated, calcium-deficient, and lactating rats. Am J Orthod Dentofacial Orthop. 1984;85(5):424-30.

13. Otis LL, Hong JS, Tuncay OC. Bone structure effect on root resorption. Orthod Craniofac Res. 2004;7(3):165-77.

14. Scheibel PC, Iwaki LCV, Ramos AL. Is there correlation between alveolar and systemic bone density? Dental Press J Orthod. 2013;18(5):78-83.

15. Rosa JE. Considerations about radiographic processing. Rev Catar Odont. 1975;2:29-36.

16. Esteves T, Ramos AL, Pereira CM, Hidalgo MM. Orthodontic root resorption of endodontically treated teeth. J Endod. 2007;33(2):119-22.

17. Capelozza Filho L, Benicá NCM, Silva Filho OG, Cavassan AO. Root resorption in the orthodontic practice: application of a radiographic method for early diagnosis. Ortodontia. 2002;35(2):14-26.

18. Martins MM, Silva ACP, Mendes AM, Goldner MTA. External apical root resorption frequency and severity degree in cases treated with and without first-premolar extraction. Ortodon Gaúcha. 2003;7(2):121-8.

19. Spurrier SW, Hall SH, Joondeph DR, Shapiro PA, Riedel RA. A comparison of apical root resorption during orthodontic treatment in endodontically treated teeth and vital teeth. Am J Orthod Dentofacial Orthop. 1990;97(2):130-4.

20. Levander E, Malmgren O. Long-term follow-up of maxillary incisor with severe apical root resorption. Eur J Orthod. 2000;22(1):85-92.

21. Valladares Neto J, Albernaz PI, Almeida GA. Aproximation of palatal cortex versus external root resorption: is there a correlation during orthodontic treatment. ROBRAC. 2002;11(31):57-60.

22. Santos ECA, Lara TS, Arantes FM, Coclete GA, Silva RS. Computer-assisted radiographic evaluation of apical root resorption following orthodontic treatment with two different fixed appliance techniques. Rev Dental Press Ortod Ortop Facial. 2007;12(1):48-55.

23. Dudic A, Giannopoulou C, Leuzinger M, Kiliaridis S. Detection of apical root resorption after orthodontic treatment by using panoramic radiography and cone-beam computed tomography of super-high resolution. Am J Orthod Dentofacial Orthop. 2009;135(4):434-7.

24. Silveira HL, Silveira HE, Liedke GS, Lermen CA, Santos RB, Figueiredo JA. Diagnostic ability of computed tomography to evaluate external root resorption in vitro. Dentomaxillofac Radiol. 2007;36:393-6.

25. Scheibel PC, Albino CC, Matheus PD, Ramos AL. Correlation among mandibular, femoral, lumbar and cervical bone density. Dental Press J Ortod. 2009;14(4):111-22.

26. Southard KA, Southard TE, Schlechte JA, Meis PA. The relationship between the density of the alveolar processes and that of post-cranial bone. J Dent Res. 2000;79(4):964-9.

27. Jonasson G, Bankvall G, Kiliaridis S. Estimation of skeletal bone mineral density by means of the trabecular pattern of the alveolar bone, its interdental thickness, and the bone mass of the mandible. Oral Surg Oral Med Oral Pathol Oral Radiol Endod. 2001;92(3):346-52.

28. Jonasson G, Jonasson L, Kiliaridis S. Changes in radiographic characteristics of the mandibular alveolar process in dentate women with varying bone mineral density: a 5 year prospective study. Bone. 2006;38(5):714-21.

29. Jonasson G. Bone mass and trabecular pattern in the mandible as an indicator of skeletal osteopenia: a 10year follow up study. Oral Surg Oral Med Oral Pathol Oral Radiol Endod. 2009;108(2):284-91.

30. Lindh C, Obrant K, Petersson A. Maxillary bone mineral density and its relationship to the bone mineral density of the lumbar spine and hip. Oral Surg Oral Med Oral Pathol Oral Radiol Endod. 2004;98(1):102-9.

31. Oliveira RCG, Leles CR, Normanha MD, Lindh C, Ribeiro-Rotta RF. Assessments of trabecular bone density at implant sites on CT images. Oral Surg Oral Med Oral Pathol Oral Radiol Endod. 2008;105(2):231-8.

32. Choi J, Park C, Yi S, Lim H, Hwang H. Bone density measurement in interdental areas with simulated placement of orthodontic miniscrew implants. Am J Orthod Dentofacial Orthop. 2009;136(6):766.e1-12.

33. Wainwright WM. Facial lingual tooth movement: its influence on the root and cortical plate. Am J Orthod Dentofacial Orthop. 1973;64(3):278-302.

34. Mohandesan H, Ravanmehr H, Valei N. A radiographic analysis of external apical root resorption of maxillary incisors during active orthodontic treatment. Eur J Orthod. 2007;29(2):134-9.

35. Segal GR, Schiffman PH, Tuncay OC. Meta analysis of the treatment-related factors of external apical root resorption. Orthod Craniofac Res. 2004;7(2):71-8.

24

Lateral cephalometric radiograph *versus* lateral nasopharyngeal radiograph for quantitative evaluation of nasopharyngeal airway space

Suelen Cristina da Costa Pereira[1], Rejane Targino Soares Beltrão[2], Guilherme Janson[3], Daniela Gamba Garib[3]

Objective: This study compared lateral radiographs of the nasopharynx (LN) and lateral cephalometric radiographs (LC) used to assess nasopharyngeal airway space in children. **Material and Methods:** One examiner measured the nasopharyngeal space of 15 oral breathing patients aged between 5 and 11 years old by using LN and LC. Both assessments were made twice with a 15-day interval in between. Intergroup comparison was performed with t-tests (P < 0.05). **Results:** Comparison between LN and LC measurements showed no significant differences. **Conclusion:** Lateral cephalometric radiograph is an acceptable method used to assess nasopharyngeal airway space.

Keywords: Radiology. Nasopharynx. Orthodontics.

» The authors report no commercial, proprietary or financial interest in the products or companies described in this article.

[1] PhD Orthodontic Resident, School of Dentistry — University of São Paulo/Bauru.

[2] PhD in Orthodontics, School of Dentistry — University of São Paulo/Bauru.

[3] Full professor, Department of Orthodontics, School of Dentistry — University of São Paulo/Bauru.

Suelen Cristina da Costa Pereira
E-mail: sucristina@hotmail.com

INTRODUCTION

Two modalities of conventional and extraoral radiographs are used to assess nasopharyngeal airway space: lateral nasopharyngeal radiograph (LN), also known as cavum radiography, and lateral cephalometric radiograph (LC). The former is requested most frequently by physicians to assess the nasopharynx of patients with nasal obstruction, whereas the latter has been used for several years in Orthodontics to assess the morphology and development of dental occlusion, including soft and skeletal tissues of the face.[1,2] Moreover, several authors show that lateral cephalometric radiograph allows one to assess adenoid and dimension of nasopharynx.[1-11]

With the aim of establishing a baseline for measuring nasopharyngeal space on lateral radiographs, McNamara Jr[7] defined it as the shortest distance between the convex surface of the adenoid (or posterior wall of nasopharynx) and the dorsal surface of the soft palate. Patients with nasopharynx width less or equal to 5 mm reveal apparent airway obstruction. It is used only as an indicator of possible airway impairment. A more accurate diagnosis can be made only by an otorhinolaryngologist during clinical examination.

According to Kohler[12] and Almeida et al,[3] lateral cephalometric radiograph and lateral nasopharyngeal radiograph can be used by orthodontists and otorhinolaryngologists as integrated medical-dental examinations. Moreover, they can be obtained during the same procedure, which eliminates the need for additional radiographic exposure.

Ikino et al[2] assessed the degree of nasopharynx obstruction by means of applying Cohen and Konak[21] score to both lateral cephalometric radiograph and lateral nasopharyngeal radiograph. His results revealed that similar outcomes were produced by both radiographs in 73.1% of children. The author stated that lateral cephalometric radiograph yields better results in comparison to lateral nasopharyngeal radiograph, since patient's head positioning is standardized in the former. Head position is fixed in LC, which avoids variation in the sagittal and transverse planes and allows a more secure airway analysis without the artifacts produced by head rotation. This information is important since children hardly remain in the desired position. Based on these findings, the authors concluded that LC is the radiograph of choice for assessing nasal obstruction due to equally showing nasopharynx airway and minimizing changes in head positioning.

According to Almeida et al,[3] computed tomography (CT) is also used in diagnosis of nasopharyngeal obstruction; however, despite being more accurate, it is also more expensive. Montgomery et al[13] evaluated the results obtained by tomography and concluded that radiographic examination is poor in information. The authors suggest that CT should be used as the gold standard. Conversely, cephalometric radiography should be used to determine whether a more detailed tracking is necessary or not, bearing in mind that this is a two-dimensional and, therefore, limited examination.

No previous study compared lateral nasopharyngeal radiograph with lateral cephalometric radiograph used for quantitative evaluation of nasopharynx. For this reason, the objective of this study was to compare lateral cephalometric radiograph and lateral nasopharyngeal radiograph for a quantitative evaluation of nasopharyngeal airway space.

MATERIAL AND METHODS

This research was approved by the Federal University of Paraíba (UFPB) Institutional Review Board under protocol 574/06. All research subjects signed an informed consent form. This study assessed the orthodontic records of patients from the School of Dentistry of the University of São Paulo. In selecting the sample, the following inclusion criteria were applied: patients aged between 5 and 11 years old; recent lateral cephalometric radiograph of good quality (Fig 1A); signs of mouth breathing including open mouth posture, short upper lip and everted lower lip; large, varying degrees of narrow face; small nostrils, and poorly developed, deep, narrow palate which demonstrated the need for otorhinolaryngologist analysis.

The final sample comprised 15 patients who were referred to an otorhinolaryngologist for examination of the nasopharynx. A lateral nasopharyngeal radiograph (Fig 1B) was requested for all patients as a supplementary diagnostic tool. The interval between LC and LN was less than three months. Seven patients (46.7%) were males, whereas 8 (53.3%) were females. Patients had a mean age of 8.07 ± 1.58 years (varying from 5 to 11 years) as shown in Table.

Radiographs were manually traced by the same operator using Ultraphan sheets and a 0.35 mm mechanical pencil. Nasopharyngeal space was measured in millimeters with a ruler, from the point of the anterior half

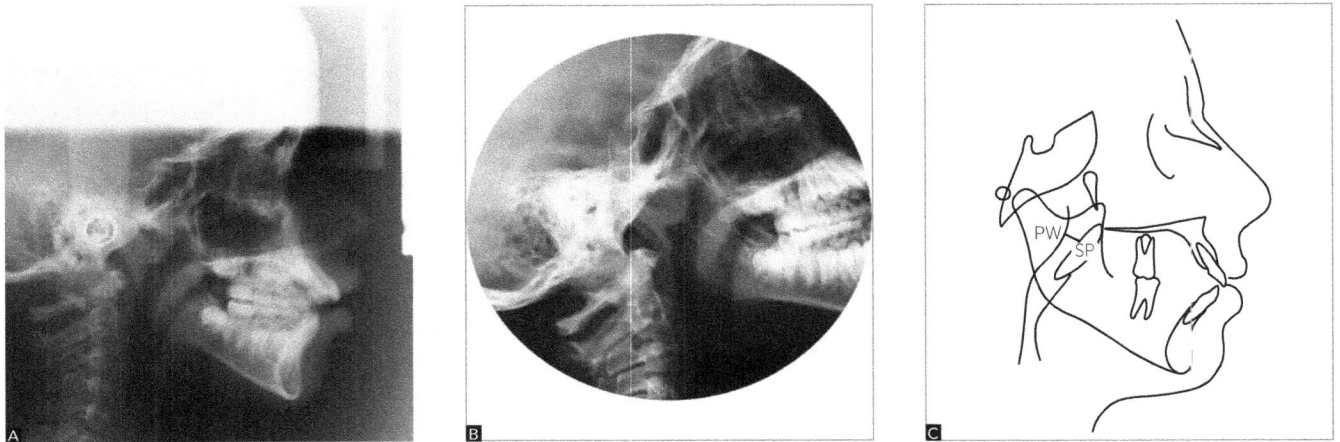

Figure 1 - A) Nasopharyngeal space measurement expressed in millimeters from the point of the anterior half of the contour of the soft palate (SP) to the nearest point of the pharyngeal wall (PW). **B)** Lateral nasopharyngeal radiograph (LN). **C)** Lateral cephalometric radiograph (LC).

of the contour of the soft palate to the nearest point of the nasopharyngeal posterior wall (Fig 1C).

Rotograph Plus (Villa Sistemi Medicali, Buccinasco, Italy) was used for lateral cephalometric radiograph, while Siemens (AG, Munich, Germany) was used for lateral nasopharyngeal radiograph under 10% and 20% image magnification, respectively. Magnification factors were corrected before comparison.

LC was obtained with the patient positioned in a cephalostat with the Frankfurt Horizontal Plane (FHP) parallel to the ground, lips at rest and in centric occlusion. Focus-sagittal midplane distance was 1.52 m and the exposure parameters were 85 KVp, 10 mA and 0.5 to 1 second of exposure time, depending on patient's age.

LN was performed with the child standing in profile with the head horizontally oriented and the mouth closed during inspiration. Focus-sagittal midplane distance was 1.42 m and the exposure parameters were 64 kV and 3.5 mA.

Data were processed in a statistical program (SPSS 11.0) for descriptive and inferential analyses. To calculate error of the method, all radiographs were remeasured after a 15-day interval. The formula proposed by Dahlberg[14] ($Se^2 = \Sigma d^2/2n$) was used to estimate the order of magnitude of casual errors, while systematic errors were analyzed by paired t-tests, as advocated by Houston.[15] Independent t-tests were used for intergroup comparison of nasopharynx width in LC and LN (significance level was set at 5%).

RESULTS

Casual errors were 0.56 and 0.07 for LN and LC, respectively. No statistically significant systematic errors were observed (Table 1).

There were no significant differences between nasopharynx measurements in LN and LC (Table 1).

DISCUSSION

Intragroup analyses showed no significant errors when the first and second measurements for lateral nasopharyngeal radiograph and lateral cephalometric radiograph were compared, thus demonstrating good precision and reproducibility of measurements.

Previous studies reported that nasopharynx evaluation is important to diagnose adenoid size and permeability of airway space.[16,17,18] This study aimed at comparing nasopharynx width in LC and LN. Correction of image magnification of both types of radiograph allowed comparison of nasopharynx measurements. No significant differences were observed between LC and LN (Table 1), corroborating the study by Ikino et al.[2] These authors conducted a qualitative analysis of nasopharynx and found an agreement in the degree of airway space obstruction for both types of radiographs, an important factor to consider when dealing with patients who will undergo orthodontic treatment and are likely to have lateral cephalometric radiograph requested for diagnosis, regardless of their respiratory condition. For these patients, evaluation of nasopharynx by means of LC can avoid unnecessary financial and biological costs of taking an extra radiographic exam.[1,19,20]

Table 1 - Patients' age, analysis of systemic and random errors and comparison between nasopharynx width in LC and LN.

Patients' age (years)			
Mean	Standard deviation	Minimum	Maximum
8.07	1.58	5	11

Analysis of systemic and random errors					
	First analysis		Second analysis			
	Mean	SD*	Mean	SD*	P**	Dahlberg
Lateral cephalometric radiograph	11.92	5.41	11.66	5.03	0.212	0.56
Lateral nasopharyngeal radiograph	11.47	3.16	11.49	3.17	0.427	0.07

Comparison between nasopharynx width in LC and LN				
Lateral cephalometric radiograph		Lateral nasopharyngeal radiograph		T-test
Mean	SD	Mean	SD	P
11.82	5.22	11.48	3.16	0.385

SD*= Standard deviation P** = 0.05.

The technique used to obtain LC yields better results in comparison to LN, since patient's head positioning is standardized in the former. For this reason, it avoids variations in the sagittal, frontal and transverse planes. Rotation of the head may produce undesired effects, especially in children who do not always remain in a desired position.[2] In addition, LC has the advantage of having a fixed distance between focal point and film.[21]

Major et al[22] assessed the capability of lateral cephalometric radiographs to diagnose hypertrophied adenoids and obstructed nasopharyngeal airway. They conducted a systematic literature review and concluded that LC performed reasonably well in evaluating adenoid size. Quantitative measures of adenoid area and subjective grading of adenoid size on LCs had reasonable correlations with actual adenoid size.

Barbosa et al[1] compared the use of LC and endoscopy of nasopharynx to evaluate nasopharynx obstruction. They concluded that LC allows visualization of soft and hard tissue structures , in addition to assessing location, configuration and growth of nasopharynx and adenoid tissue. Moreover, it allows structures closely related to oral cavity and nasopharynx to be visualized. Although this type of radiograph has greater limitations in comparison to two-dimensional interpretation of nasopharynx, it has proved to be effective as a diagnostic tool. This fact was evidenced by the strong correlation between LC results and nasal endoscopy.

CONCLUSION

No significant differences were found between measurements obtained with lateral nasopharyngeal radiograph and lateral cephalometric radiograph. Lateral cephalometric radiograph proved an acceptable method to evaluate nasopharyngeal airway space by both the orthodontist and the otorhinolaryngologist.

REFERENCES

1. Barbosa MC, Knop LAH, Lessa MM, Araujo TM. Avaliação da radiografia cefalométrica lateral como meio de diagnóstico da hipertrofia da adenoide. Rev Dental Press Ortod Ortop Facial. 2009;14(4):83-91.

2. Ikino CMY, D'Antonio WEPA, de la Cortina RAC, Lessa M, Castilho AM, Goto EY, et al. Tele-radiografia lateral de crânio e radiografia de cavum: estudo comparativo em crianças com obstrução nasal. Rev Bras Otorrinolaringol. 2000;66(6):592-6.

3. Almeida RCC, Artese F, Carvalho FAR, Cunha RD, Almeida MAO. Comparison between cavum and lateral cephalometric radiographs for the evaluation of the nasopharynx and adenoids by otorhinolaryngologists. Dental Press J Orthod. 2011;16(1):32-3.

4. David AF, Castilho JCM. Estudo comparativo entre os traçados manual e computadorizado da análise do espaço aéreo nasofaríngeo em radiografias

cefalométricas laterais. Ortodontia. 1999;32(2):88-93.

5. Chami FAI. Avaliação nasofibroscópica e radiológica de pacientes com hiperplasia da amígdala faríngea. Rev Bras Atual Otorrinolaringol. 1998;5(4):118-24.

6. Cohen LM, Koltai PJ, Scott JR. Lateral cervical radiographs and adenoid size: do they correlate? Ear Nose Throat J. 1992;71(12):638-42.

7. McNamara JA Jr. A method of cephalometric evaluation. Am J Orthod. 1984;86(6):449-69.

8. Poole MN, Engel GA, Chaconas SJ. Nasopharyngeal cephalometrics. Oral Surg Oral Med Oral Pathol. 1980;49(3):266-71.

9. Holmberg H, Linder-Aronson S. Cephalometric radiographs as a means of evaluating the capacity of the nasal and nasopharyngeal airway. Am J Orthod. 1979;76(5):479-90.

10. Fujioka M, Young LW, Girdany BR. Radiographic evaluation of adenoidal size in children: adenoidal-nasopharyngeal ratio. AJR Am J Roentgenol. 1979;133(3):401-4.

11. Pruzansky S. Roentgencephalometric studies of tonsils and adenoids in normal and pathologic states. Ann Otol Rhinol Laryngol. 1975;84(2 pt 2 Suppl 19):55-62.

12. Köhler GI. Mensuração dosimétrica e otimização imageológica de exames radiológicos na face infantil e adolescente. Departamento de Engenharia Biomédica [dissertação]. Curitiba (PR): Centro Federal de Educação Tecnológica do Paraná; 2005.

13. Montgomery WM, Vig PS, Staab EV, Matteson SR. Computed tomography: a three-dimensional study of the nasal air way. Am J Orthod. 1979;76(4):363-75.

14. Dahlberg G. Statistical methods for medical and biological students. New York: Interscience; 1940.

15. Houston WJB. The analysis of errors in orthodontic measurements. Am J Orthod. 1983;83(5):382-90.

16. Paradise JL, Bernard BS, Colborn DK, Janosky JE. Assessment of adenoidal obstruction in children: clinical signs versus roentgenographic findings. Pediatrics 1998;101(6):979-86.

17. Weimert TA. Evaluation of the upper airway in children. Ear Nose Throat J. 1987;66:196-200.

18. Jeans WD, Fernando DC, Maw AR. How should adenoidal enlargement be measured? A radiological study based on interobserver agreement. Clin Radiol. 1981;32(3):337-40.

19. Cassano P, Gelardi M, Cassano M, Fiorella ML, Fiorella R. Adenoid tissue rhinopharyngeal obstruction grading based on fiberendoscopic findings: a novel approach to therapeutic management. Int J Pediatr Otorhinolaryngol. 2003;67(12):1303-9.

20. Kubba H, Bingham BJ. Endoscopy in the assessment of children with nasal obstruction. J Laryngol Otol. 2001;115(5):380-4.

21. Cohen D, Konak S. The evaluation of radiographs of the nasopharynx. Clin Otolaryngol Allied Sci. 1985;10(2):73-8.

22. Major MP, Flores-Mir C, Major PW. Assessment of lateral cephalometric diagnosis of adenoid hypertrophy and posterior upper airway obstruction: a systematic review. Am J Orthod Dentofacial Orthop. 2006 ;130(6):700-8.

25

Reliability of CBCT in the diagnosis of dental asymmetry

Antônio Carlos de Oliveira Ruellas[1], Leonardo Koerich[2], Carolina Baratieri[3], Claudia Trindade Mattos[4], Matheus Alves Junior[5], Daniel Brunetto[5], Lindsey Eidson[6]

Objective: The aim of this study was to validate a method used to assess dental asymmetry, in relation to the skeletal midline, by means of CBCT. **Methods:** Ten patients who had CBCT scans taken were randomly selected for this study. Five different observers repeated 10 landmarks (x, y and z variables for each) and 12 linear measurements within 10 days. Measurements were taken in both arches to evaluate symmetry of first molars, canines and dental midline in relation to the skeletal midline. Intraclass correlation coefficient (ICC) was carried out to assess intra- and interobserver reliability for landmarks and distances. Average mean difference was also assessed to check measurement errors between observers. **Results:** ICC landmarks was ≥ 0.9 for 27 (90%) and 25 (83%) variables for intra- and interobserver, respectively. ICC for distances was ≥ 0.9 for 7 (58%) and 5 (42%), respectively. All ICC landmarks for distances were >0.75 for both intra- and interobserver. The mean difference between observers was ≤ 0.6 mm for all the distances. **Conclusion:** The method used to assess dental asymmetry by means of CBCT is valid. Measurements of molars, canines and dental midline symmetry with the skeletal midline are reproducible and reliable when taken by means of CBCT and by different operators.

Keywords: Cone-beam computed tomography. Imaging. Three-dimensional diagnosis. Dental arch.

» The authors report no commercial, proprietary or financial interest in the products or companies described in this article.

[1] Phd in Dentistry and Adjunct Professor, Federal University of Rio de Janeiro (UFRJ).
[2] MSc in Orthodontics, UFRJ.
[3] Phd in Orthodontics, UFRJ.
[4] Phd in Orthodontics, UFRJ. Adjunct Professor, UFF.
[5] Doctorate student in Orthodontics, UFRJ.
[6] MSc in Orthodontics, University of North Carolina.

Antônio Carlos de Oliveira Ruellas
Rua Professor Rodolpho Paulo Rocco, 325 – Rio de Janeiro/RJ — Brazil.
CEP: 21941-913 – E-mail: antonioruellas@yahoo.com.br

INTRODUCTION

Patients with malocclusion often present one or more characteristics related to asymmetry, for instance, Class II or III subdivision, dental midlines that are not coincident with each other, and/or dental midlines that are not coincident with the facial midline.[1] Proper orthodontic treatment planning requires a correct diagnosis. Dental arch rotation on the vertical axis, known as yaw, is often omitted in classifications and diagnosis. This important piece of information can determine the need for asymmetric mechanics or extractions to correct a dental midline shift or a unilateral Class II or III relationship, for example.[2]

Different methods can be used for diagnosis of patient's dental symmetry in relation to the skeletal midline (midsagittal plane). Burstone[1] has suggested, within a few limitations, the use of posteroanterior radiography to evaluate maxillary and mandibular discrepancies and the upper and lower dental midlines in relation to the skeletal midline. Another method suggests that the median raphe is the patient's skeletal midline.[3] In this method, the relationship between teeth and bone can be analyzed by means of dental casts. Furthermore, the methods described by Moyer[3] or Proffit[4] can help to identify asymmetry by means of a ruler and a bow divider or a symmetric grid, respectively. More recently, advances in technology have allowed the transfer of plaster models to a computer by using scanners.[5] They have also enabled three-dimensional models to be created on the basis of data obtained from Cone Beam Computed Tomography (CBCT), reproducing the patient's teeth and surrounding bone structures.[6] These models, however, are not linked to the patient's face anatomy; therefore, the advantages that a CBCT can provide, such as skeletal and dental diagnosis, are not used to their full potential. With a view to addressing such issue, some computer programs allow navigation in CBCT data through tomographic slices taken in the three planes of space and, with adjustment of the threshold, it is possible to visualize, at the same time, the teeth, bone and soft tissues.[7] Thus, the aim of this study was to validate a method used to evaluate, by means of CBCT, dental asymmetry (molars, canine and dental midline) in relation to the skeletal midline.

MATERIAL AND METHODS

Sample size calculation was carried out (α = 0.05; β = 0.2; ρ_0 = 0.45; ρ_1 = 0.90)[8] and revealed that ten patients would be enough for 10 observations (twice, 5 observers).

This study, approved by the Federal University of Rio de Janeiro Institutional Review Board, comprised ten patients who were being orthodontically treated and had CBCT taken. Patients were randomly selected. In selecting the sample, the following exclusion criteria were applied: absence of canines and incisors; presence of restorations at the evaluated sites; and syndromes, such as cleft lip and palate, by which maxillary bone formation could be affected.

The CBCT equipment used was an i-CAT (Imaging Sciences, Hatfield, PA), with a 13 x 17 cm field of view, voxel dimension of 0.4 mm and exposure time of 20 seconds. The images were obtained at 120 kVp and 5 mA. All patients were in maximum intercuspation during the scan.

After the images were taken, one operator imported all DICOM (Digital Images and Communication in Medicine) files into Dolphin 3D (Dolphin Imaging, version 11.0, Chatsworth, CA) software. For standardization purposes, the Frankfort Horizontal Plane was horizontally oriented for all patients. In addition, slice thickness was set to be equal to the voxel size. Patients' data were saved and all the observers started taking the measurements at this point. Each observer had to orient the patient's head (turning to left or right, only) and had to try to match the skeletal midline with the sagittal plane (Fig 1),

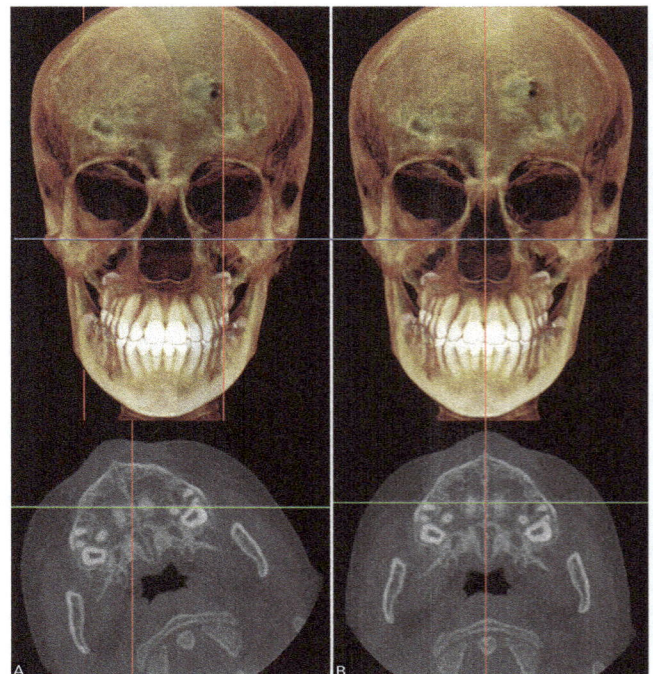

Figure 1 - **A)** Example of a patient with the Frankfort Horizontal Plane horizontally oriented. **B)** After one operator reoriented the skeletal midline with the sagittal plane (red).

using nasion, anterior nasal spine and posterior nasal spine as reference, before beginning the analyses.

Five different observers — all students of Orthodontics, with one to two years of experience working with CBCT — were asked to test the reproducibility of 10 landmarks and 12 distances using the CBCT scans, as shown in Tables 1 and 2. Calibration was done

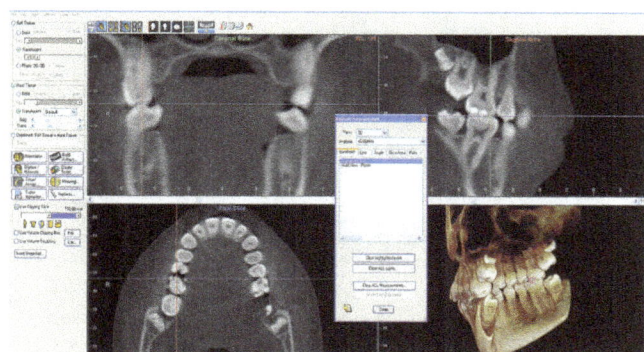

Figure 2 - Example of landmark positioning. After being identified in three different slices, the landmark was plotted in the axial view of the multiplanar reconstruction (lower left box).

with two scans that were not included in the sample. Evaluations were carried out independently and repeated within an interval of ten days. For more accuracy in the following step, the size of the landmarks was set at 0.01 mm. All four views (sagittal, axial, coronal and the rendered image) were used as reference to locate the landmarks. However, landmarks were only plotted in the axial slices of the multiplanar reconstruction (Fig 2). Figure 3 and 4 show the distances between the landmarks used in the study.

Landmarks and distances were obtained by means of the Digitize/Measurement tool available in the 3D view of the software. After all landmarks were plotted, the next step was to measure the distance between them. The software did not allow automatic connection between two landmarks. For this reason, this step had to be taken manually. To calculate the distance between two landmarks, the observer only connected the landmarks of interest. Both landmarks and distances were exported to Microsoft Excel (Microsoft Corporation, Redmond, WA).

STATISTICAL ANALYSES

Analyses were carried out with the Statistical Package for the Social Sciences 17.0 (Chicago, IL, USA). Intra-examiner and inter-examiner reliability values for both landmarks and distances were determined by using intraclass correlation coefficients (ICCs).

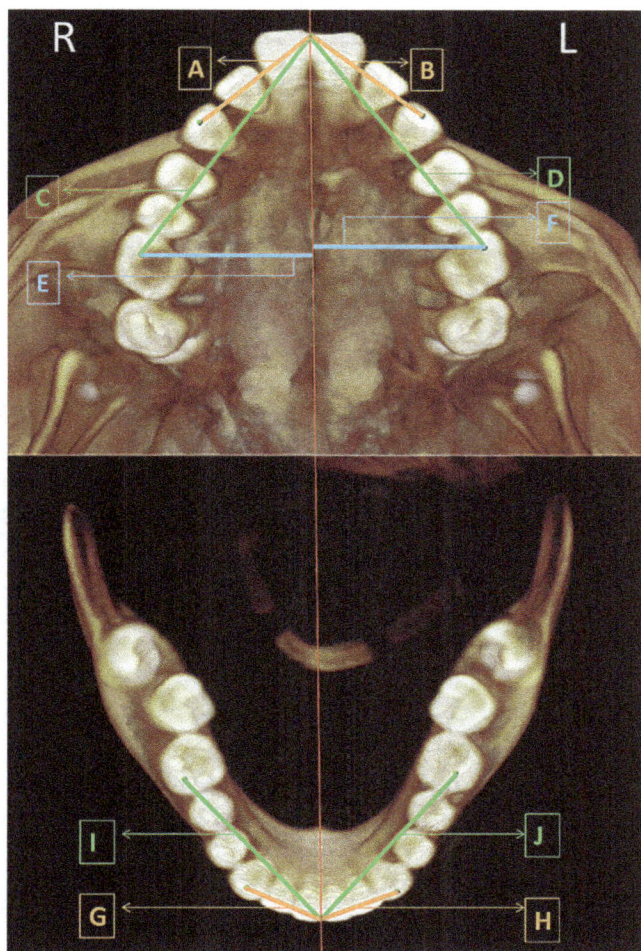

Figure 3 - Linear distances as shown in Table 2.

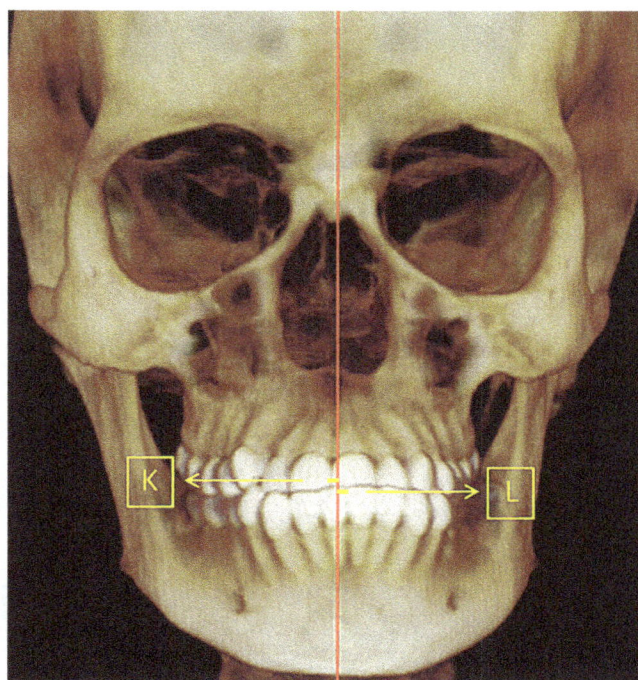

Figure 4 - Linear distances as shown in Table 2.

Table 1 - Localization of the landmarks used in the study.

Landmark	Anatomic region	Coronal slice	Axial slice	Sagittal slice
Maxilla				
UR6	Right molar mesiobuccal cusp tip	Middle-inferior-most point	Middle point	Middle-inferior-most point
UR3	Right canine cusp tip	Middle-inferior-most point	Middle point	Middle-inferior-most point
UML	Skeletal midline at upper incisors incisal edge	Middle-inferior-most point between incisors	Middle point between incisors	Anterior-inferior-most point
UL6	Left molar mesiobuccal cusp tip	Middle-inferior-most point	Middle point	Middle-inferior-most point
UL3	Left canine cusp tip	Middle-inferior-most point	Middle point	Middle-inferior-most point
Mandible				
LR6	Right molar mesiobuccal cusp tip	Middle-superior-most point	Middle point	Middle-superior-most point
LR3	Right canine cusp tip	Middle-superior-most point	Middle point	Middle-superior-most point
LML	Skeletal midline at lower incisors incisal edge	Middle-superior-most point between incisors	Middle point between incisors	Anterior-superior-most point
LL6	Left molar mesiobuccal cusp tip	Middle-superior-most point	Middle point	Middle-superior-most point
LL3	Left canine cusp tip	Middle-superior-most point	Middle point	Middle-superior-most point

Table 2 - Distance between landmarks.

Maxilla	
Distance A	Distance between UR3 and UML
Distance B	Distance between UL3 and UML
Distance C	Distance between UR6 and UML
Distance D	Distance between UL6 and UML
Distance E	Distance between UR6 90° to the skeletal midline
Distance F	Distance between UL6 90° to the skeletal midline
Mandible	
Distance G	Distance between LR3 and LML
Distance H	Distance between LL3 and LML
Distance I	Distance between LR6 and LML
Distance J	Distance between LL6 and LML
Midline	
Distance K	Distance between the skeletal midline and the midline of the upper teeth
Distance L	Distance between the skeletal midline and the midline of the lower teeth

Average mean differences for the distances measured by different examiners (measurement errors) were summarized, and descriptive statistics were applied. The paired t-test was also applied to detect significant mean differences. The level of significance was set at 0.05.

RESULTS

The reliability in defining the landmarks was estimated by ICC for each coordinate of each landmark. As a result, 30 variables (x, y and z for each landmark) were tested. The ICC was ≥ 0.9 for 27 (90%) of all intraobserver assessments, and the lowest intraobserver coefficient was 0.706. The ICC was ≥ 0.9 for 25 (83%) for all interobserver assessments, and the lowest interobserver coefficient was 0.591.

Table 3 shows the frequency of intraobserver and interobserver reliability estimated by ICC for the distances measured.

Table 4 shows the frequency of the mean difference for the distances measured by each observer. The mean difference was calculated using paired t-tests performed between every two observers for each distance. The results are summarized in Table 4 and illustrate that 10 (83%) measurements had a very small mean difference of less than 0.5 mm and no measurement had a mean difference greater than 1 mm.

Table 5 lists the reliability estimated by ICC and the interobserver mean difference for each distance.

DISCUSSION

Only skeletal structures were used to define the skeletal midline in this study. The references used were

Table 3 - Frequency of intra and interobserver reliability estimated by intraclass correlation coefficient (ICC) for the distances measured.

Values	Intraobserver		Interobserver	
	n	(%)	n	(%)
ICC ≥ 0.90	7	58	5	42
0.75 < ICC < 0.90	5	42	4	33
0.45 < ICC ≤ 0.75	0	0	3	25
ICC ≤ 0.45	0	0	0	0
Total	12	100	12	100

Table 4 - Frequency of the mean difference among observers on the distances measured.

Values (mm)	n	(%)
≥ 2	0	0
1 < x < 2	0	0
0.5 < x ≤ 1	2	17
≤ 0.5	10	83
Total	12	100

Table 5 - Reliability estimated by intraclass correlation coefficient (ICC) for each distance.

Distances	Intraobserver reliability	Interobserver reliability	Interobserver mean difference (mm)
A	0.932	0.920	0.31
B	0.883	0.859	0.34
C	0.959	0.934	0.35
D	0.969	0.900	0.54
E	0.886	0.916	0.60
F	0.949	0.867	0.41
G	0.813	0.862	0.23
H	0.917	0.741	0.26
I	0.893	0.866	0.50
J	0.963	0.946	0.22
K	0.781	0.591	0.35
L	0.958	0.740	0.38

landmarks such as anterior and posterior nasal spine and nasion. Differently from other studies using CBCT,[9,10] only the Frankfort Horizontal Plane was pre-oriented and each individual observer later established the skeletal midline. The reason was that if the head was already oriented with the skeletal midline in the sagittal plane, it would increase the likelihood for bias and make it easier for each observer to define the plane.

Head orientation does not influence linear measurements;[11] as long as the same landmarks were obtained, measurements should be the same.

Grauer et al[7] demonstrated that landmarks are better located when plotted in the stack of slices rather than in rendered images. This technique was employed by our study of which results corroborate the findings of other researches that showed high values for intraclass[9,10] and interclass[9,12] correlation for landmarks identified in dental structures.

Creed et al[6] showed that anteroposterior measurements for molars can be reliably taken using either digital models or surface models made on the basis of CBCT data. Asquith et al[13] investigated dental casts and 3D digital study models and found that intraexaminer mean differences for this variable were ≤0.05 mm and ≤0.32 mm, respectively. Our study had slightly higher mean differences; however, it was interexaminer instead of intraexaminer. In addition, the values were not clinically significant (all of them ≤ 0.54 mm). The present research also confirmed that the same type of anteroposterior evaluation can be applied for the canines.

Mean difference between observers for distances from skeletal to dental midlines were ≤ 0.4 mm. The other transversal measurement, molars perpendicular line to the skeletal midline, showed good reliability between observers. Other techniques have been applied for this evaluation. However, conventional or 3D digital models can use only the palatal rugae as reference, which is reliable for growing patients.[14] Nonetheless, using the raphe as the skeletal midline may not be the best option, as it has different shapes and curvatures.[1] Nevertheless, skeletal midline and raphe have been associated in the past.[15] With 3D surface models, one can obtain other structures that would likely provide a reliable skeletal midline. However, the production of these models involves either hiring a specialized company, which implies in higher costs,[6] or computer expertise, which is extremely time consuming.[9,16] To our view, the process involved in any of these options does not outweigh the benefits.

The advantages of the proposed method are as follows: the possibility of assessing and reproducing patients' skeletal midline and relating it to the teeth and soft tissues, and the possibility of directly taking measurements in the CBCT slices by means of simple techniques. Based on recent controversies, the main disadvantage is that not every patient needs a CBCT scan. Additionally, even though it is an important piece of data that can be obtained for cases of skeletal asymmetry, we do not recommend that CBCT scans be taken for this purpose only. In spite of being recommended for very specific cases, CBCT scans have lower radiation doses,[17,18] lower costs and good accuracy.[19] For this reason, the exam has been increasingly used, in addition to becoming more accepted.[20] The radiation doses involved in this type of exam are similar to those of a full-mouth series of radiographs. Furthermore, one single CBCT scan is able to provide data for airway, sinus and TMJ analyses.[21,22] On the other hand, another drawback is the potential presence of artifacts in the areas of interest and the need for specific software for evaluation.

Clinically determining dental midline shifts using the soft tissue as reference can be misleading when there are asymmetries in nose, chin or philtrum.[23] The proposed "imaginary plumb" method[24] as a true vertical line is affected by the patient and operator position as well as the parallax effect.

Anteroposterior dental asymmetry is often present in subdivision malocclusions. It can be corrected by means of minor dental movements or extractions depending on the degree of the discrepancy. It is necessary to diagnose in which arch and side the asymmetry is located to decide which mechanics will be applied. The evaluation on dental casts will use the raphe as the skeletal midline, but some degree of variation might occur between different operators due to the shape of the raphe. Therefore, evaluating dental asymmetry by means of CBCT images and having the skeletal midline as reference provides useful information for diagnosis.

CONCLUSION

Measurements for molars, canines and incisors in relation to the skeletal midline taken to assess dental asymmetry are reproducible and reliable when taken by means of CBCT.

REFERENCES

1. Burstone CJ. Diagnosis and treatment planning of patients with asymmetries. Semin Orthod. 1998;4(3):153-64.
2. Ackerman JL, Proffit WR, Sarver DM, Ackerman MB, Kean MR. Pitch, roll, and yaw: describing the spatial orientation of dentofacial traits. Am J Orthod Dentofacial Orthop. 2007;131(3):305-10.
3. Moyers RE. Handbook of orthodontics. Chicago: Year Book Medical Publishers; 1988.
4. Proffit WR, Fields HW, Sarver DM. Contemporary orthodontics. St. Louis: Mosby; 2007.
5. Boldt F, Weinzierl C, Hertrich K, Hirschfelder U. Comparison of the spatial landmark scatter of various 3D digitalization methods. J Orofac Orthop. 2009;70:247-63.
6. Creed B, Kau CH, English JD, Xia JJ, Lee RP. A comparison of the accuracy of linear measurements obtained from cone beam computerized tomography images and digital models. Semin Orthod. 2011;17:49-56.
7. Grauer D, Cevidanes LS, Proffit WR. Working with DICOM craniofacial images. Am J Orthod Dentofacial Orthop. 2009;136(3):460-70.
8. Walter SD, Eliasziw M, Donner A. Sample size and optimal designs for reliability studies. Stat Med. 1998;17(1):101-10.
9. Oliveira AE, Cevidanes LH, Phillips C, Motta A, Burke B, Tyndall D. Observer reliability of three-dimensional cephalometric landmark identification on cone-beam computerized tomography. Oral Surg Oral Med Oral Pathol Oral Radiol Endod. 2009;107(2):256-65.
10. Sanders DA, Rigali PH, Neace WP, Uribe F, Nanda R. Skeletal and dental asymmetries in Class II subdivision malocclusions using cone-beam computed tomography. Am J Orthod Dentofacial Orthop. 2010;138(5):542.e1-20; discussion 542-3.
11. El-Beialy AR, Fayed MS, El-Bialy AM, Mostafa YA. Accuracy and reliability of cone-beam computed tomography measurements: influence of head orientation. Am J Orthod Dentofacial Orthop. 2011;140(2):157-65.
12. Fuyamada M, Nawa H, Shibata M, Yoshida K, Kise Y, Katsumata A, et al. Reproducibility of landmark identification in the jaw and teeth on 3-dimensional cone-beam computed tomography images. Angle Orthod. 2011;81(5):843-9.
13. Asquith J, Gillgrass T, Mossey P. Three-dimensional imaging of orthodontic models: a pilot study. Eur J Orthod. 2007;29(5):517-22.
14. Almeida MA, Phillips C, Kula K, Tulloch C. Stability of the palatal rugae as landmarks for analysis of dental casts. Angle Orthod. 1995;65(1):43-8.
15. Harvold EP, Trugue M, Viloria JO. Establishing the median plane in posteroanterior cephalograms. In: Salzmann JA, editor. Roentgenographic cephalometrics. Philadelphia: J. B. Lippincott; 1961.
16. Cevidanes LH, Oliveira AE, Grauer D, Styner M, Proffit WR. Clinical application of 3D imaging for assessment of treatment outcomes. Semin Orthod. 2011;17:72-80.
17. Ludlow JB, Davies-Ludlow LE, Brooks SL. Dosimetry of two extraoral direct digital imaging devices: NewTom cone beam CT and Orthophos Plus DS panoramic unit. Dentomaxillofac Radiol. 2003;32:229-34.
18. Schulze D, Heiland M, Thurmann H, Adam G. Radiation exposure during midfacial imaging using 4- and 16-slice computed tomography, cone beam computed tomography systems and conventional radiography. Dentomaxillofac Radiol. 2004;33(2):83-6.
19. Mozzo P, Procacci C, Tacconi A, Martini PT, Andreis IA. A new volumetric CT machine for dental imaging based on the cone-beam technique: preliminary results. Eur Radiol. 1998;8(9):1558-64.
20. Kapila S, Conley RS, Harrell WE Jr. The current status of cone beam computed tomography imaging in orthodontics. Dentomaxillofac Radiol. 2011;40(1):24-34.
21. Cha JY, Mah J, Sinclair P. Incidental findings in the maxillofacial area with 3-dimensional cone-beam imaging. Am J Orthod Dentofacial Orthop. 2007;132(1):7-14.
22. Mah JK, Danforth RA, Bumann A, Hatcher D. Radiation absorbed in maxillofacial imaging with a new dental computed tomography device. Oral Surg Oral Med Oral Pathol Oral Radiol Endod. 2003;96(4):508-13.
23. Beyer JW, Lindauer SJ. Evaluation of dental midline position. Semin Orthod. 1998;4(3):146-52.
24. Jerrold L, Lowenstein LJ. The midline: diagnosis and treatment. Am J Orthod Dentofacial Orthop. 1990;97(6):453-62.

26

Comparative evaluation of cephalometric and occlusal characteristics between the Long Face pattern and Pattern I

Elisa Gurgel Simas de Oliveira[1], Célia Regina Maio Pinzan-Vercelino[2]

Objective: To compare the cephalometric and intraoral characteristics between Long Face pattern and Pattern I patients, besides evaluating associations between subjective facial patterns, cephalometric facial patterns and the intraoral characteristics. **Methods:** Through evaluation of frontal and right side extraoral photographs, three previously calibrated and experienced examiners selected 30 Long Face patients (Group 1) and 30 Pattern I patients (Group 2), aged between 9 and 19 years, of both genders. The cephalometric characteristics were assessed by the following variables: SN.GoGn, NS.Gn, AIFH, SNA, SNB, ANB, $1.\overline{1}$, 1.NA,1-NA, 1.NB, 1-NB, NA.Po, nasolabial angle and H-Nose. Clinical evaluations were also performed to determine the presence of posterior crossbite, anterior open bite and type of Angle's malocclusion. The cephalometric data were compared by independent t test. The chi-square test was used to evaluate the association between qualitative variables. **Results:** Significant differences were observed between groups regarding the variables SN.GoGn, NS.Gn, AIFH, ANB, NA.Pog, 1-NA, 1.NB and 1-NB, with an increase of these measures in Group 1. There were also significant differences between groups on variable $1.\overline{1}$, being lower in Group 1 than in Group 2. **Conclusions:** The Long Face was associated to Angle Class II malocclusion, to the presence of posterior crossbite and to anterior open bite. The Long Face subjective facial pattern was associated to dolichofacial cephalometric pattern.
Keywords: Cephalometry. Orthodontics. Diagnosis.

Elisa Gurgel Simas de Oliveira
Av. Dom Luís, 906/405 – Bairro Meireles – Brazil
CEP: 60.160-230 – Fortaleza/CE – E-mail: elisasimas@hotmail.com

[1] MSc in Orthodontics, UniCEUMA
[2] Professor, Post-Graduation Program – MSc in Orthodontics -UniCEUMA

INTRODUCTION

The long face is a deformity with skeletal implication and with unfavorable esthetics,[8,10] that can be observed in the three sagittal dental relations, being however, more associated to Class II sagittal discrepancies.[7,10]

The children, teenagers and adults that present this excessive vertical facial growth, have a peculiar characteristic, described in literature as "Long Face syndrome",[4,30] hyperdivergent facial type[16,24] and, recently, as Long Face pattern.[7-11]

The diagnosis of Long Face pattern is based in evaluations of the face morphology and cephalometry. The facial analysis allows to verify several characteristics common to these individuals such as: Absence of passive lip seal and contraction of mentalis muscles during labial closure,[1] besides a great exposure of upper incisors when lips are resting and great gingival exposure during smile,[1,4,30] the nose is generally long, with narrowing of the alar bases and the lower third of the face is increased, resulting in retrognathia appearance of the mandible.[1,26,30]

The cephalometry constitutes a necessary instrument to define, locate and quantify the skeletal disharmony present in patients with Long Face pattern, which can be associated to a horizontal growth of the condyle[6,26] and/or to an excessive posterior growth of the maxilla.[15,30]

Regarding the cephalometric characteristics, it is observed an increase on the total anterior height of the face and on the anterior and inferior facial height.[15,17] The anterior and superior facial height is generally normal,[1,4,30] but the proportion between medium and lower third is reduced.[3] The angle of the mandibular plane is increased,[4,8,11,15,28,29] as well as the gonial angle.[8,11] It is observed a mandibular repositioning in relation to the skull base.[1,11] The maxilla, however, is well positioned in relation to the skull base.[1,15]

Lately, it is observed in literature[13,21] that the cephalometric means, used in several cephalometric tracings, cannot be generically applied for diagnosis and treatment. Several researchers[5,20,23] concluded that most cephalometric standards varies significantly, when compared to several facial patterns. Before this, a more individualized interpretation of the cephalometry must become a rule, or rather, an association between the cephalometric analysis and the facial analysis must be standard for diagnosis, planning of treatment and orthodontic treatment. Therefore, the final decision of a planning must be taken based in cephalometric and facial findings. This way, this work had as objective to perform a comparative study of cephalometric and intraoral characteristics between Long Face patients and Pattern I, diagnosed by the subjective facial analysis, besides evaluating the associations between subjective facial patterns and cephalometric facial patterns.

MATERIAL AND METHODS
Material

The sample was selected according to the following criteria of inclusion:
- » Caucasians;
- » Long Face pattern or Pattern I;
- » Full orthodontic records;
- » Ages between 9 and 19 years;
- » No previous orthodontic treatment.

Methods
Orthodontic records

Extraoral, frontal and right side photographs from the orthodontic records belonging to patients registered for orthodontic treatment on the Specialization Course in Orthodontics, of the Odontology Academy of Ceará were used. The sample was selected by three experienced and previously calibrated examinators, in distinct moments and each one individually, to avoid that the evaluation of one examinator interfered on the others. Only the patients who had diagnostic concordance were selected.

All photographs were performed by the same radiology center (Prof. Perboyre Castelo), presenting a pattern. The patients during the photographs were in natural position of the head (NPH):[22] standing, with the feet 10 cm apart from each other, lips at rest, looking to an oval mirror located 1 meter before the patient and instructed to observe their own eyes reflection, keeping the pupils on the eye center.

The patients classified with Long Face pattern,[7-11] were on the frontal and right side photograph with excessive exposure of the resting teeth and gingiva when smiling, lower third of the face increased in relation to the medium third, difficulty of lip seal, resting upper lip with short appearance, everted lower lip, retruded mandible and short chin-neck line (Figs 1 and 2).

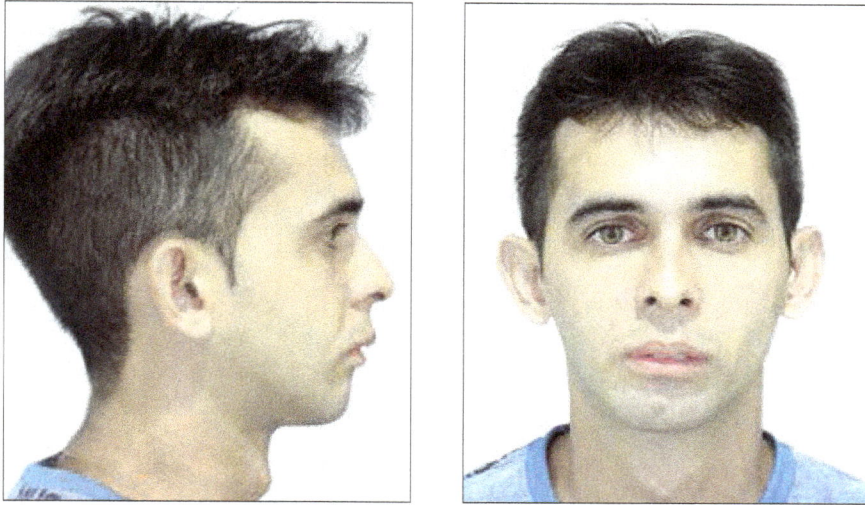

Figure 1 and 2 - Frontal and right side photograph of long face pattern patient.

The Pattern I patients[7-11,13] were identified by the facial normality and characterized by balanced vertical and skeletal sagittal relations on the front and profile evaluations. In frontal photograph they had apparent symmetry, proportion between the facial thirds, proportional volume of the lips vermilion and passive lip seal (Fig 3). On the evaluation of the right side photograph, Pattern I patients had mild facial convexity, expressive chin-neck line and parallel to Camper plane, and esthetically pleasant mentolabial sulcus, built with equal participation of the mentum and lower lip (Fig 4).

The patient's full name, gender and date of birth were obtained also from the orthodontic records. The date of birth allowed the accurate calculus of initial ages of the patients.

All patients that agreed to participate in the research filled out a form with their data, as well as signed a free informed term of consent (FITC), approved by the ethics committee in research (CER) of the University Center of Maranhão (UNICEUMA), protocol number 00469/08, according to standards of the resolution CNS 196/96.

Cephalometry

After evaluation of the photographs from orthodontic records for selection of the sample, the facial pattern was evaluated through cephalometry with variables that determined the facial growth pattern: SN.GoGn, NS.Gn (Axis Y) and AIFH (anterior inferior facial height).

Besides these variables, other measurements were performed of the skeletal components (SNA, SNB and ANB), dentoalveolar components ($1.\overline{1}$, 1.NA, 1-NA, 1.NB, 1-NB) and bone and tissue profiles (NAPog, nasolabial angle, H-Nose).

The radiographs were performed by the digital panoramic x-ray device (Orthopantomograph OP100-D, Instrumentarium, Palodex group, Tuusula, Finland, 2006). This digital device used a sensor that sent the images captured in the radiographic take to the computer screen. These images were saved in CD and printed in films by laser printer model Dryview 8150. The digital radiographic images were inserted on the program Cef X (CDT Software, Dourados, Mato Grosso, Brazil, version 2.1.24, 1995) and the reference points, lines and planes were demarcated.

The cephalometric facial pattern was determined when the patient showed at least two measures altered. It was considered: Dolichofacial the patient that showed SN.GoGn with values higher than 34 degrees,[19] NS.Gn (Axis Y) with values higher than 69.9 degrees[19] and AIFH with values higher than 71 mm;[27] mesofacial the patient that showed SN.GoGn with values within 30 and 34 degrees,[19] NS.Gn with values within 63.5 and 69.5 degrees[19] and AIFH with values within 63 and 71 mm[27] and brachyfacial the patient that showed SN.GoGn with values lower than 30 degrees,[19] NS.Gn with values lower than 63.5 degrees,[19] and AIFH with values lower than 63 mm.[27]

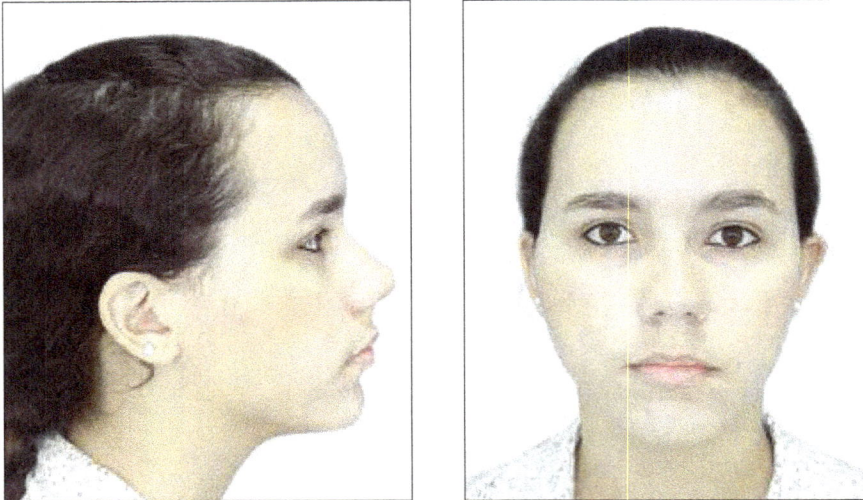

Figure 3 and 4 - Right side and frontal photograph of Pattern I patient.

Clinical assessment

It was filled out a clinical form for each patient containing data obtained from orthodontic records and observations such as: Initial age, presence of open bite and/or crossbite and classification of Angle's malocclusion.

The patients classified with presence of posterior crossbite, were those with abnormal buccolingual relation between superior and inferior teeth, of at least three teeth, when the dental arches were in centric relation, being uni or bilateral[25] and with presence of anterior open bite when showed a negative overbite between the edges of anterior, superior and inferior teeth, with measurement larger than 1 mm, obtained in millimetric ruler.[25]

On the investigation of the dental relation, it was observed a sagittal relation between the upper and lower permanent first molars.[2] The patients were classified as Class I, when presented a molar relation with the upper permanent first molar's mesiobuccal cusp occluding the lower permanent first molar's mesiobuccal sulcus,[2] as Class II when presented the lower permanent first molar positioned distally in relation to the upper permanent first molar and as Class III when presented the lower permanent first molars situated mesially to the upper permanent first molars.[2]

Statistical analysis
Method error

To determine the reliability of the obtained cephalometric results, after 15 days, it was randomly selected

a group of 20% of the radiographs, that were digitalized again and had their points demarcated by the same researcher. It was applied the dependent Student's t test in order to assess the systematic error.[18] For evaluation of the random error it was used the Dahlberg's formula.[12]

Statistical test

It was used the descriptive statistics (mean and standard deviation) for initial age and all cephalometric measures used.

The independent t test was applied to verify the compatibility between the initial ages of studied groups and to compare the cephalometric variables between groups.

It was applied the Chi-square test to evaluate the compatibility of groups regarding the proportion between genders, to verify the association between subjective facial pattern and cephalometric facial pattern and to evaluate the association of Long Face pattern and intraoral characteristics (posterior crossbite, anterior open bite and Angle's malocclusion).

Besides these tests, it was determined the prevalences of cephalometric facial patterns, posterior crossbite, anterior open bite and the type of Angle's malocclusion in relation to subjective facial pattern. Results with p < 0,05 were considered statistically significant. Tests were applied through BioEstat 5.0 (AYRES, Sociedade Civil Mamirauá, MCT-CNPq, Belém, PA, Brazil, 2005).

RESULTS

The sample consisted of photographs and teleradiographs of 60 patients, divided in two groups according to facial pattern (Table 1).

Regarding the method error, for the cephalometric variables it was not detected any random error and only one systematic error. For the variable NS.Gn, it was found, on the first measurement, a mean value of 72.62 degrees, and for the second measurement a mean value of 73.97 degrees. Considering that it occurred only one systematic error (7.15%) with variation of 1.35 degrees between the measurements, and none random error, the obtained results can be considered reliable.

The groups were compatible in relation to age and distribution of genders (Tables 2 and 3).

Regarding cephalometric variables, the studied groups presented statistically significant differences in: NS.GoGn, NS.Gn, AIFH, ANB, 1.1, 1-NA, 1.NB, 1-NB, NA.Pog (Table 2).

The Long Face pattern was associated to dolichofacial cephalometric facial pattern, and the Pattern I was associated to mesofacial cephalometric facial pattern (Table 3).

The Long Face pattern patients were associated to posterior crossbite, anterior open bite and Angle Class II malocclusion (Table 3).

Among the Long Face pattern patients 93.3% were dolichofacial patients, 43.3% with presence of posterior crossbite, 16.6% with presence of anterior open bite and 60% with Angle Class II malocclusion (Table 4).

Now, on the group of Pattern I patients 83.3% were mesofacial patients, 13.3% with presence of posterior

Table 2 - Comparative analysis of cephalometric variables and age between groups, according to independent t test.

Variables	GROUP 1 (n = 30) LONG FACE Mean ± SD	GROUP 2 (n= 30) PATTERN I Mean ± SD	p
Skeletal components			
SNA (degrees)	82.86 ± 4.29	82.59 ± 4.00	0.802
SNB (degrees)	78.00 ± 4.49	79.06 ± 3.92	0.333
ANB (degrees)	4.85 ± 2.22	3.57 ± 2.01	0.022*
Growth pattern			
SN.GoGn (degrees)	41.80 ± 6.78	34.37 ± 6.77	0.000*
NS.Gn (degrees)	70.90 ± 4.64	67.76 ± 4.03	0.006*
AIFH (mm)	77.49 ± 8.88	68.64 ± 6.23	0.000*
Dentoalveolar components			
$1.\overline{1}$ (degrees)	117.11 ± 14.56	124.79 ± 10.58	0.022*
1.NA (degrees)	26.27 ± 10.24	23.02 ± 7.26	0.161
1-NA (mm)	6.27 ± 3.91	4.45 ± 2.33	0.033*
1.NB (degrees)	31.80 ± 7.39	27.80 ± 6.13	0.026*
1-NB (mm)	8.32 ± 2.87	5.78 ± 2.42	0.000*
Osseous profile x tissue profile			
NA.Pog (degrees)	9.14 ± 4.91	6.07 ± 4.69	0.016*
ANL (degrees)	98.84 ± 13.54	101.24 ± 9.88	0.435
H-Nose (mm)	2.18 ± 4.62	2.99 ± 3.19	0.434
Compatibility between ages			
Age	13.43 ± 2.95	12.83 ± 3.02	0.444

*Statistically significant (p < 0.05).

Table 1 - Classification of the sample according to age and gender.

Variables	GROUP 1 (n = 30) LONG FACE	GROUP 2 (n= 30) PATTERN I
Age		
Mean ± SD	13.43 ± 2.95	12.83 ± 3.02
Maximum age	9	9
Minimum age	18	19
Gender		
Male	13	13
Female	17	17

Table 3 - Analysis of the compatibility of genders, facial pattern, cephalometric facial pattern, posterior crossbite, anterior open bite and classification of the Angle's malocclusions between the groups, according to Chi-square test.

Variables	GROUP 1 (n = 30) LONG FACE	GROUP 2 (n=30) PATTERN I	Total	χ²	P
Gender					
Female	17	17	34	0.00	
Male	13	13	26		1.00
Cephalometric facial pattern					
Brachyfacial	0	3	3	45.126	
Dolichofacial	28	2	30		0.000*
Mesofacial	2	25	27		
Posterior crossbite					
Absence	17	26	43	6.65	
Presence	13	4	17		0.010*
Anterior open bite					
Absence	25	30	55	5.45	
Presence	5	0	5		0.020*
Angle classification					
Class I	11	21	32	7.125	
Class II	18	9	27		0.028*
Class III	1	0	1		

*Statistically significant (p < 0.05).

Table 4 - Prevalence of cephalometric facial patterns, posterior crossbite, anterior open bite and type of Angle's malocclusion on the different groups.

Variables	GROUP 1 (n=30) LONG FACE	GROUP 2 (n=30) PATTERN I
Cephalometric facial pattern		
Brachyfacial	0%	10%
Dolichofacial	93.3%	6.6%
Mesofacial	6.6%	83.3%
Posterior crossbite		
Absence	56.6%	86.6%
Presence	43.3%	13.3%
Anterior open bite		
Absence	83.3%	100%
Presence	16.6%	0%
Angle classification		
Class I	36.6%	70%
Class II	60%	30%
Class III	3.3%	0%

crossbite, 70% with Angle Class I maloccusion and 30% with Angle Class II malocclusion. However, no Pattern I patient presented anterior open bite (Table 4).

DISCUSSION

The subjective facial analysis represents an important tool of orthodontic diagnosis,[13] that can be easily used for identification of Long Face pattern patients. These patients generally present several occlusal problems that may be associated to this facial growth pattern as: posterior crossbite, anterior open bite and Class II malocclusion. Many times, when the problem of vertical growth is identified through the face, the problem is also cephalometrically confirmed, however, when the problem is diagnosed cephalometrically first, it is not necessarily confirmed on the face, ie, the facial analysis allows a more accurate diagnosis of the Long Face pattern.

On the cephalometric assessment, the groups presented significative differences in relation to the following variables: SN.GoGn, NS.Gn, AIFH, ANB, 1.1, 1-NA, 1.NB, 1-NB and NA.Pog. The Long Face pattern patients presented increase on the angles: SN.GoGn (41.80±6.78), NS.Gn (70.90±4.64), indicating vertical growth pattern;

NA.Pog (9.14±4.91), showing increase of convexity of the bone profile; ANB (4.85±2.22), evidencing the increase on degree of sagittal discrepancy between maxilla and mandible and 1.NB (31.80±7.39) indicating vestibularization of lower incisors in relation to bone base. The linear measures 1-NA (26.27±10.24), 1-NB (8.32±2.87) and AIFH (77.49±8.88) were increased; indicating protrusion of upper and lower incisors and increase of the lower third of the face. The measure 1.1, that also presented significative difference between groups, showed decreased value for Long Face pattern patients, factor indicative of maxillomandibular retrusion.

Cardoso et al[11] also found significative differences in relation to the variables ANB, AIFH, SN.GoGn and NA.Pog when compared the cephalometric characteristics of Long Face pattern and of Pattern I.[11] They observed that Long Face patterr individuals presented increase of the cephalometric measures located below the palatal plane.[11]

Capelozza Filho et al[8] evaluating the cephalometric characteristics of Long Face pattern, did not observe significative differences in relation to sexual dimorphism and showed that male Long Face pattern patients, when compared to Pattern I patients, presented disparities in relation to magnitudes related to facial height, to growth pattern and to sagittal relation.

The assessment of maxillomandibular relation, based on value of angle ANB, was greater also in Long Face pattern individuals evaluated by Cardoso et al[9] and Capelozza Filho et al,[8] showing the tendency to Class II malocclusion that the carriers of this deformity present. The values for anterior and inferior facial height were higher for the Long Face pattern group with statistical significance, also observed in studies performed by Cardoso et al[9] and Capelozza Filho et al.[8] This result was also expected, since the increase on anterior inferior facial height constitutes the essence of the studied disease, being frequently found in literature.

Regarding the mandibular plane (SNGoGn), the mean values of this angle for Long Face pattern individuals were close to the maximum values of Pattern I individuals. This implies on the necessity of association of several cephalometric characteristics for definition of the Long Face pattern. Values above 37 degrees for the angle of the mandibular plane were reported in literature[4,14,15,16,20,28,29] as parameter to define Long Face pattern individuals. Although the values found in the studies performed by Capelozza Filho et al[8] and Cardoso et al[9] overcome this value, they cannot be used separately. In fact, the disease consists in an imbalance between the vertical components, and, therefore, a single parameter must not be used; therefore in this study it was associated to the mandibular plane (SN.GoGn), the measurement of the Y axis of growth (Ns.Gn) and the measurement of the anterior and inferior facial height for determination of cephalometric facial pattern.

The mandibular retrusion was emphasized with the assessment of NAP angle which was significantly different between Long Face pattern and Pattern I groups also in the study by Cardoso et al,[10] showing greater mandibular retrognathia and convexity of bone profile in Long Face pattern patients.

As for the cephalometric growth pattern, it was obtained 93,3% of dolichofacial patients on Group 1 (Long Face pattern) and 83.3% of mesofacial patients on Group 2 (Pattern I). The Chi-square test showed presence of association between the subjective facial pattern and the cephalometric facial pattern, which allows to conclude that the studied facial patterns, classified by the subjective analysis, are associated to cephalometric classification of the facial pattern, enabling the methodology used for identification of patients by subjective facial analysis, besides allowing the comparison between results from this study and other results from works in literature.

The patients on Group 1 presented a prevalence of 43.3% of posterior crossbite and the patients on Group 2 presented 13.3% of posterior crossbite. In relation to the Chi-square test it was observed an association between facial pattern and posterior crossbite. The prevalence of posterior crossbite in Long Face pattern patients is according to the observed in a study by Cardoso et al[10] in which the authors showed a prevalence of 34.2% of this malocclusion.

Regarding the presence of anterior open bite, the patients on Group 1 presented a prevalence of 16.6%, while on Group 2, no patients showed anterior open bite. In relation to the Chi-square test, it was observed an association between the Long Face pattern and the presence of anterior open bite.

About Angle's classification, the patients on Group 1 presented: 36.6% Class I, 60% Class II and 3.33% Class III; now the patients on Group 2 presented: 70% Class I and 30% Class II. As result of the Chi-square test, it was found an association between the facial pattern and Angle's classification. Patients on Group 1 were associated to Class II malocclusion and patients on Group 2 were associated to Class I malocclusion. This result agrees with the study performed by Cardoso et al[10] who found in Long Face pattern patients the following prevalences in relation to Angle malocclusions: 13.2% Class I, 71% Class II and 15.8% Class III. Probably, the Long Face pattern is associated to Class II malocclusion for these patients present a clockwise mandibular rotation, which facilitate a Class II sagittal relation.

CONCLUSIONS

The Long Face pattern was associated to Angle Class II malocclusion, to presence of posterior crossbite and to anterior open bite. The subjective Long Face pattern was associated to dolichofacial cephalometric facial pattern.

REFERENCES

1. Angelillo JC, Dolan EA. The surgical correction of vertical maxillary excess: long face syndrome. Ann Plast Surg. 1982;8(1):64-70.
2. Angle EH. Classification of malocclusion. Dent Cosmos. 1899;41(3):248-64.
3. Bell WH. Correction of skeletal type of anterior open bite. J Oral Surg. 1971;29(10):706-14.
4. Bell WH, Creekmore TD, Alexander RG. Surgical correction of the long face syndrome. Am J Orthod. 1977;71(1):40-67.
5. Bhat M, Enlow DH. Facial variations related to head form type. Angle Orthod. 1985;55(4):269-80.
6. Bjork A. Prediction of mandibular growth rotation. Am J Orthod. 1969;55(6):585-99.
7. Capelozza Filho L. Diagnóstico em Ortodontia. 1a ed. Maringá: Dental Press; 2004.
8. Capelozza Filho L, Cardoso MA, An TL, Bertoz FA. Características cefalométricas do padrão face longa: considerando o dimorfismo sexual. Rev Dental Press Ortod Ortop Facial. 2007;12(2):49-60.
9. Capelozza Filho L, Cardoso MA, An TL, Lauris JRP. Proposta para classificação, segundo a severidade, dos indivíduos portadores de más oclusões do padrão face longa. Rev Dental Press Ortod Ortop Facial. 2007;12(4):124-58.
10. Cardoso MA, Bertoz FA, Reis SAB, Capelozza Filho L. Estudo das características oclusais em portadores de padrão face longa com indicação de tratamento ortodôntico-cirúrgico. Rev Dental Press Ortod Ortop Facial. 2002;7(9):63-70.
11. Cardoso MA, Bertoz FA, Capelozza Filho L, Reis SAB. Características cefalométricas do padrão face longa. Rev Dental Press Ortod Ortop Facial. 2005;10(2):29-43.

12. Dahlberg G. Statistical methods for medical and biological students. New York: Interscience; 1940.

13. Feres R, Vasconcelos MHF. Estudo comparativo entre a análise facial subjetiva e a análise cefalométrica de tecidos moles no diagnóstico ortodôntico. Rev Dental Press Ortod Ortop Facial. 2009;14(2):81-9.

14. Fields HW, Proffit WR, Nixon WL, Phillips C, Stanek E. Facial pattern differences in long-faced children and adults. Am J Orthod. 1984;85(3):217-23.

15. Fish LC, Wolford LM, Epker BN. Surgical orthodontic correction of maxillary excess. Am J Orthod. 1978;73(3):241-57.

16. Fitzpatrick BN. The long face and V.M.E. Aust Orthod J. 1984;8:82-9.

17. Frost DE, Fonseca RJ, Turvey TA, Hall DJ. Cephalometric diagnosis and surgical-orthodontic correction of apertognathia. Am J Orthod. 1980;78(6):657-69.

18. Houston WJ. Analysis of errors in orthodontics measurements. Am J Orthod. 1983;83(5):382-90.

19. Interlandi S. Ortodontia bases para iniciação. 5ª ed. São Paulo: Artes Médicas; 2002.

20. Isaacson JR, Isaacson RJ, Speidel TM, Worms FW. Extreme variations in vertical face growth and associated variation in skeletal and dental relations. Angle Orthod. 1971;41(3):219-29.

21. Jacobson A. Planning for orthognatic surgery-art or science? Int J Adult Orthodon Orthognath Surg. 1990;5(4):217-24.

22. Lundström F, Lundström A. Natural head position as a basis for cephalometric analysis. Am J Orthod Dentofacial Orthop. 1992;101(3):244-7.

23. Metzdorf DW. A cephalometric study of cranial, mandibular and lower incisor morphology in adult face. Angle Orthod. 1977;47(4):288-92.

24. Moloney F, West RA, McNeill RW. Surgical correction of vertical maxillary excess: a re-evaluation. J Maxillofac Surg. 1982;10(2):84-91.

25. Moyers RE. Ortodontia. 4ª ed. Rio de Janeiro: Guanabara Koogan; 1991.

26. Nielsen IL. Vertical malocclusions: etiology, development, diagnosis and some aspects of treatment. Angle Orthod. 1991;61(4):247-60.

27. Pinzan A, Pinzan-Vercelino CRM, Martins DR, Janson G, Henriques JFC, Freitas MR, et al. Crescimento maxilomandibular no sentido antero-posterior e na altura anterior. In: Atlas de Crescimento Craniofacial. 10ª ed. São Paulo: Ed. Santos; 2006. p. 49-54.

28. Prittinen JR. Orthodontic diagnosis of long face syndrome. Gen Dent. 1996;44(4):348-51.

29. Schendel SA, Carlotti AE Jr. Variation of vertical maxillary excess. J Oral Maxillofac Surg. 1985;43(8):590-6.

30. Schendel SA, Eisenfeld J, Bell WH, Epker BN, Mishelevich DJ. The long face syndrome: vertical maxillary excess. Am J Orthod. 1976;70(4):398-408.

27

The use of three-dimensional cephalometric references in dentoskeletal symmetry diagnosis

Olavo Cesar Lyra Porto[1], Jairo Curado de Freitas[2], Ana Helena Gonçalves de Alencar[3], Carlos Estrela[4]

Objective: The aim of this study is to assess dentoskeletal symmetry in cone-beam computed tomography (CBCT) scans of Brazilian individuals with Angle Class I malocclusion. **Material:** A total of 47 patients (22 females and 25 males) aged between 11 and 16 years old (14 years) seen in a private radiology service (CIRO, Goiânia, GO, Brazil) were assessed. All CBCT scans were obtained from January, 2009 to December, 2010. Cephalometric measurements were taken by multiplanar reconstruction (axial, coronal and sagittal) using Vista Dent3DPro 2.0 (Dentsply GAC, New York, USA). Minimum, maximum, mean and standard deviation values were arranged in tables, and Student t-test was used to determine statistical significance (P < 0.05). **Results:** Data were homogeneous, and differences between the right and left sides were not significant. **Conclusions:** Cephalometric measurements of Brazilian individuals with Angle Class I malocclusion can be used to establish facial symmetry and three-dimensional standard references which might be useful for orthodontic and surgical planning.

Keywords: Facial asymmetry. Three-dimensional imaging. Cone-beam computed tomography.

» The authors report no commercial, proprietary or financial interest in the products or companies described in this article.

[1] PhD resident in Health Sciences, Federal University of Goiás (UFG).
[2] Professor, Department of Orthodontics, Brazilian Dental Association (ABOR).
[3] Professor, Department of Endodontics, UFG.
[4] Full professor, Department of Endodontics, UFG.

Carlos Estrela
Universidade Federal de Goiás, Departamento de Ciências Odontológicas, Praça Universitária, S/N – Setor Universitário
CEP: 74605-220 – Goiânia/GO — Brazil
E-mail: estrela3@terra.com.br

INTRODUCTION

Assessing skeletal asymmetry by means of cephalometric and panoramic radiograph of individuals in need of orthodontic treatment is an ongoing challenge that requires attention. Knowledge about craniofacial growth and growth direction, skeletal anatomy, tooth position, tooth relationship with bone structures, and facial profile is essential for accurate treatment planning.[1]

Cephalometry focuses on linear and angular dimensions established by bone, teeth and face measurements; and cephalometric findings aid diagnosis and help to establish treatment strategies.

Dentists use lateral cephalogram to establish the cephalometric references of normal individuals with a balanced face.[2,3] Despite potential limitations such as image distortion and superposition, posteroanterior radiograph is useful for other types of assessment. Nevertheless, it is considered reliable for surgical and orthodontic planning.[4]

Inaccurate image reading may be associated with superposition of anatomical structures and increased radiographic image distortion. Furthermore, correct management of patients during image acquisition is a risk factor that may affect quality. Two-dimensional radiographs are limited and might affect treatment planning and results negatively.[4,5,6]

The use of cone-beam computed tomography (CBCT) in Dentistry has raised several possibilities for planning, treatment and follow-up in a number of specialties.[7-21] Farman and Scarfe[16] reported that several CBCT systems may be used to obtain reconstructions similar to conventional cephalometric scans. According to these authors,[16] CBCT diagnostic precision and efficacy may be compared to conventional cephalometric imaging. Additionally, they also state that evidence-based selection criteria should be developed for CBCT use in Orthodontics.

Cephalometric analysis has been used to assess linear and angular measurements of hard and soft tissues of the craniofacial complex, while CBCT scans have been helpful in assessing facial asymmetry.[24] New facial examination models may be developed by combining the use of conventional cephalometric references and three-dimensional CBCT scans.[25,26] This study assessed dentoskeletal symmetry of Angle Class I patients by means of three-dimensional scans.

MATERIAL AND METHODS

Sample selection

Facial symmetry of a group of patients was determined and resulted in a clinically symmetrical sample. After that, three-dimensional scans of 47 patients (22 females and 25 males) aged between 11 and 16 years old (14 years) were retrieved and further assessed. The following inclusion criteria were applied: Angle Class I malocclusion, crowding, absence of dental caries and apical or marginal periodontitis. Exclusion criteria were: Angle Class II or III malocclusion, absence of teeth, traumatic bone and tooth injury, and previous orthodontic treatment. This study was approved by the local Institutional Review Board (Federal University of Goiás, Brazil, # 296/2011).

Method used to determine facial symmetry

Patients' digital frontal facial photographs were assessed by three specialists in Orthodontics. Facial symmetry was determined according to visual inspection and facial photographs. Clinically symmetrical patients were selected for cephalometric measurements.

Image acquisition method

CBCT scans were acquired in a private radiology clinic (CIRO, Goiânia, GO, Brazil) using an i-CAT scanner (Imaging Sciences International, Hatfield, PA, USA). Volumes were reconstructed according to the following exposure settings: 0.25-mm resolution, isometric voxel, 120 kVp, tube voltage, 3.8 mA current, exposure time of 40 seconds and field of view of 13 cm. Images were acquired at 14-bit grey scale at a focal distance of 0.5 mm and 360° rotation.

Images were assessed by Xoran 3.1.62 software (Xoran Technologies, Ann Arbor, USA) in a workstation Intel Core® 2 Duo 1.86 Ghz-6300 processor (Intel Corporation, Santa Clara, USA), NVIDIA GeForce 6200 turbo cache video card (NVIDIA Corporation, Santa Clara, USA), EIZO - S2000 FlexScan monitor (1600 x 1200 pixels resolution) and Microsoft Windows XP professional SP-2 operating system (Microsoft Corp, Redmond, USA). After reconstruction, data were stored in individual DICOM files according to each patient.

Cephalometric measurements

After three-dimensional measurements were obtained, the DICOM files were imported into VistaDent

3D Pro 2.00 (Dentsply GAC, New York, USA). A total of 17 cephalometric landmarks selected according to a specific protocol for dentoskeletal symmetry assessment were identified by a calibrated operator, who had more than five years experience, and plotted by means of axial, coronal and sagittal multiplanar reconstruction (Table 1; Figs 1 and 2). Subsequently, reference planes were determined (Tables 2 and 3) and the linear measurements were automatically calculated by the software (Table 3; Figs 4 and 5). Values were recorded in a Microsoft Office Excel® 2010 spreadsheet. Image upgrading and maximal magnification tools were used to ensure that all cephalometric landmarks were precisely plotted on each multiplanar reconstruction.

Table 1 - Cephalometric landmarks.

Cephalometric landmark	Cephalometric landmark description
Porion R (Po R)	The most superior point of the right auditory meatus
Porion L (Po L)	The most superior point of the left auditory meatus
Orbitale R (Or R)	The lowest point on the right inferior orbital margin
Orbitale L (Or L)	The lowest point on the left inferior orbital margin
Anterior nasal spine (ANS)	The lowest point of the maxillary anterior nasal spine
Posterior nasal spine (ENP)	The most posterior point of the maxillary posterior nasal spine
Capitulare R	Center of the head of right mandible
Capitulare L	Center of the head of left mandible
Condylion R (Co R)	The most superior posterior point of the right mandibular condyle
Condylion L (Co L)	The most superior posterior point of the left mandibular condyle
#16	The deepest point on the central fossa of right maxillary first molar
#26	The deepest point on the central fossa of left maxillary first molar
#36	Distobuccal cuspid tip of left mandibular first molar
#46	Distobuccal cuspid tip of right mandibular first molar
Gonion R (Go R)	The mid-point on the posterior outline of the angle of the mandible on the right side
Gonion L (Go L)	The mid-point on the posterior outline of the angle of the mandible on the left side
Gnathion (Gn)	The most anterior inferior point on the mandibular symphysis.

Table 2 - Cephalometric measurements reference planes

Reference plane	Plane description
Frankfort horizontal plane (FHP)	Line connecting right and left porion to left orbitale
Coronal plane (CP)	Line connecting right and left porion, perpendicular to the Frankfort horizontal plane
Midsagittal plane (MSP)	Line connecting anterior and posterior nasal spines, perpendicular to the Frankfort horizontal plane
Maxillary horizontal plane (MHP)	Line connecting anterior and posterior nasal spines, perpendicular to the midsagittal plane
Mandibular plane (MP)	Line connecting right and left gonion to gnathion

Table 3 - Cephalometric measurements.

Maxilla	Description
#16 - Coronal plane	From #16 central fossa to coronal plane
#26 - Coronal plane	From #26 central fossa to coronal plane
#16 - Sagittal plane	From #16 central fossa to sagittal plane
#26 - Sagittal plane	From #26 central fossa to sagittal plane
#16 - ANS	From #16 central fossa to anterior nasal spine
#26 - ANS	From #26 central fossa to anterior nasal spine
#16 - Maxillary Plane Height	From #16 central fossa to maxillary horizontal plane
#26 - Maxillary Plane Height	From #26 central fossa to maxillary horizontal plane
#16 - FHP height	From #16 central fossa to Frankfort horizontal plane
#26 - FHP height	From #26 central fossa to Frankfort horizontal plane
Mandible	**Description**
#36 - Coronal plane	From #36 distobuccal cuspid to coronal plane
#46 - Coronal plane	From #46 distobuccal cuspid to coronal plane
#36-Gn	From #36 distobuccal cuspid to gnation
#46-Gn	From #46 distobuccal cuspid to gnation
#36 - Mandibular Plane Height	From #36 distobuccal cuspid to mandibular plane on the left side
#46 - Mandibular Plane Height	From #46 distobuccal cuspid to mandibular plane on the right side
Condylion R-Gn	From condylion to gnation
Condylion L-Gn	From condylion to gnation
Condylion R-GoR	From right condylion to right gonion
Condylion L-GoL	From left condylion to left gonion
Go R-Gn	From right gonion to gnation
Go L-Gn	From left gonion to gnation
FHP-Go R	From Frankfort horizontal plane to right gonion
FHP-Go L	From Frankfort horizontal plane to left gonion
TJD	**Description**
R Capitulare - sagittal plane	From R Capitulare to midsagittal plane
L Capitulare - sagittal plane	From L Capitulare to midsagittal plane
R Capitulare - coronal plane	From R Capitulare to coronal plane
L Capitulare - coronal plane	From L Capitulare to coronal plane
R Capitulare – FHP	From R Capitulare to Frankfort horizontal plane
L Capitulare – FHP	From L Capitulare to Frankfort horizontal plane

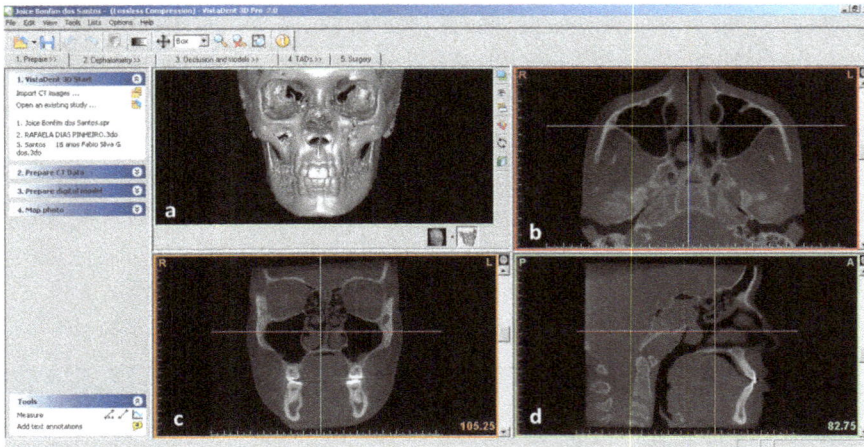

Figure 1 - 3D cephalometric module of VistaDent 3D Pro 2.00 software (Dentsply GAC, New York, USA). 3D reconstructions (**A**), Axial (**B**), coronal (**C**) and sagittal slices (**D**).

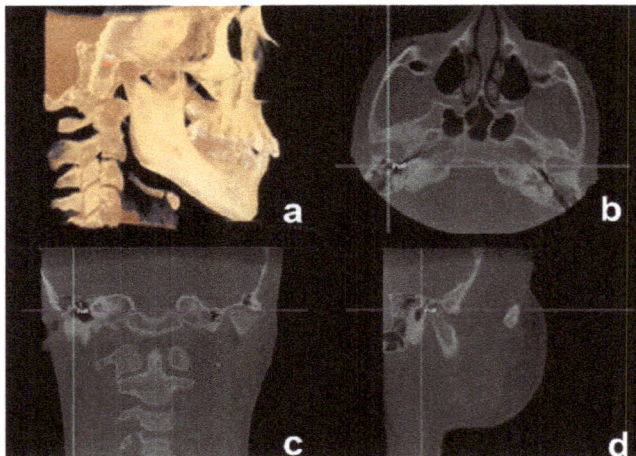

Figure 2 - Right porion cephalometric landmark (PoR) identified in the 3D (**A**), axial (**B**), coronal (**C**) and sagittal (**D**) multiplanar reconstructions.

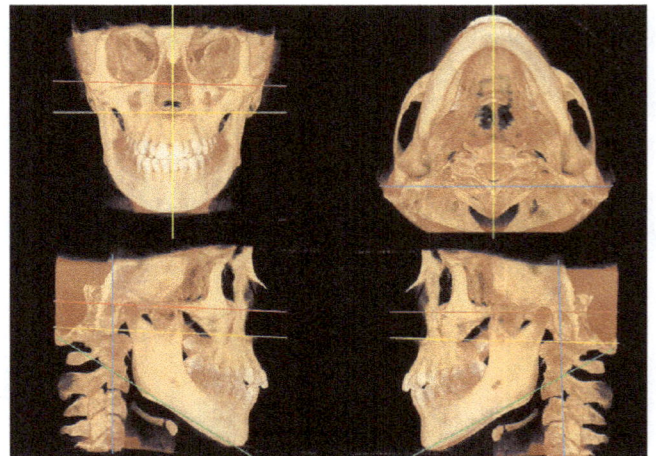

Figure 3 - Three-dimensional reconstructions of the reference planes: Frankfort Horizontal Plane (red), Coronal Plane (blue), Midsagittal Plane (yellow), Maxillary Plane (orange) and Mandibular (green).

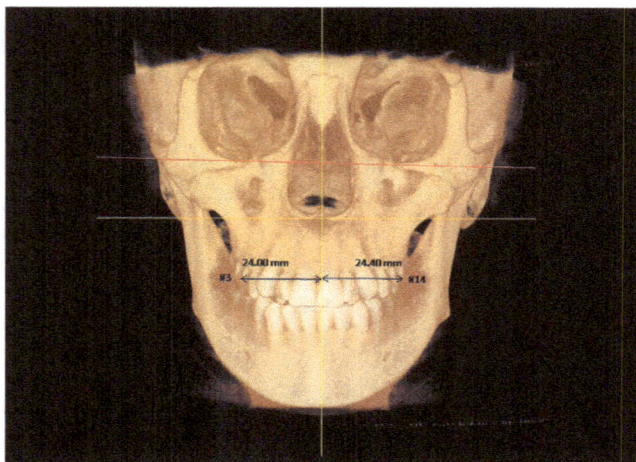

Figure 4 - Three-dimensional image of cephalometric measurements between #16, #26 and the midsagittal plane.

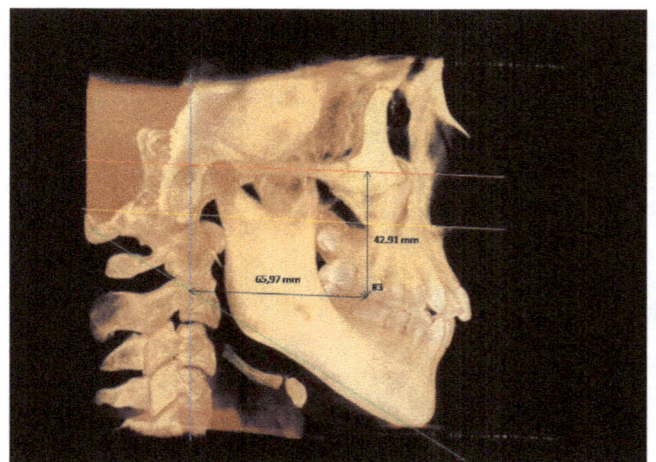

Figure 5 - Three-dimensional image of cephalometric measurements from #16 landmark to the Frankfort Horizontal and Coronal Planes.

Table 4 - Means and standard deviation of cephalometric measurements obtained from Angle Class I patients (n = 47).

Cephalometric measurements	Minimal and maximum values (mm)				Mean and standard deviation		
	Minimal	Maximum	Minimal	Maximum			
Maxilla	**#16**		**#26**		**#16**	**#26**	**p**
#16/26 - Coronal Plane	51.30	71.11	52.63	70.35	61.56 ± 4.47	61.22 ± 4.12	0.073
#16/26 - Sagittal Plane	19.96	26.47	19.56	26.51	23.33 ± 1.45	23.48 ± 1.51	0.453
#16/26 - ANS	38.60	51.74	38.36	51.37	44.75 ± 2.85	44.94 ± 2.91	0.240
#16/26 - MHP	15.10	25.69	14.61	27.44	20.56 ± 2.85	20.54 ± 2.79	0.348
#16/26 - FHP	31.97	49.21	31.32	47.82	40.36 ± 3.48	40.27 ± 3.45	0.610
Mandible	**#46**		**#36**		**#36**	**#46**	**p**
#16/26 - Coronal Plane	50.72	71.27	52.21	69.05	61.62 ± 4.33	61.60 ± 4.59	0.964
#16/26 - Gn	45.24	59.05	44.79	57.05	49.68 ± 2.50	49.74 ± 2.85	0.716
#16/26 - Height-GoGn	22.12	30.77	21.84	31.40	25.81 ± 2.19	25.92 ± 1.99	0.587
Mandible	**Right**		**Left**		**Left**	**Right**	**p**
Condylion-Gn	101.24	127.48	100.27	126.6	117.11 ± 4.74	117.42 ± 4.71	0.230
Condylion-Go	42.18	59.12	43.58	60.20	49.42 ± 3.33	49.84 ± 3.50	0.087
Go-Gn	76.45	92.85	77.61	90.4	84.51 ± 3.37	84.66 ± 3.44	0.569
FHP-Go	43.12	62.98	41.94	63.94	51.42 ± 4.23	51.88 ± 4.28	0.100
TMJ	**Right**		**Left**		**Left**	**Right**	**p**
Capitulare - MSP	43.83	51.43	42.55	51.25	47.84 ± 1.90	47.29 ± 2.17	0.036
Capitulare - Coronal Plane	6.66	12.96	5.93	13.18	10.18 ± 1.37	9.45 ± 1.32	0.000
Capitulare - FHP	3.27	11.61	3.40	11.65	7.33 ± 1.99	7.31 ± 1.79	0.894

Table 5 - Means and standard deviation (SD) of differences between right and left sides in Angle Class I patients (n = 47).

Maxilla	Minimal	Maximum	SD
#16/26 - Coronal Plane	0.05	3.02	1.07 ± 0.76
#16/26 - Sagittal Plane	0.02	3.07	1.13 ± 0.68
#6 - ANS	0.06	2.19	0.93 ± 0.64
#6 - MHP	0.01	5.43	1.50 ± 1.38
#6 - FHP	0.05	2.52	0.87 ± 0.68
Mandible			
Coronal Plane	0.06	3.65	1.15 ± 0.81
Condylion - Gn	0	4.33	1.37 ± 1.11
Condylion - Go	0.01	4.01	1.38 ± 0.95
Go-Gn	0.02	4.53	1.38 ± 1.14
FHP - Go	0.01	5.35	1.55 ± 1.14
#6 - Gn	0.01	3.43	0.83 ± 0.77
Height - GoGn	0.05	5.33	0.98 ± 0.90
TMJ			
Capitulare - MSP	0.10	4.31	1.43 ± 1.13
Capitulare - Coronal Plane	0.04	2.45	0.90 ± 0.54
Capitulare - Frankfort	0.15	2.12	0.99 ± 0.56

Statistical analysis

Mean and standard deviation of all cephalometric measurements were obtained. Cephalometric measurements from both left and right sides and the differences between them were recorded in two subsequent tables. Those differences were assessed by t-test for paired samples and Wilcoxon test. Data normality was assessed by Kolmogorov-Smirnov test. Values were significant at $P < 0.05$.

Differences between measurements obtained on the left and right sides were recorded by descriptive statistics in Table 5 which shows minimal, maximum, mean and standard deviation values. All statistical analyses were performed by means of SPSS (20.0, SPSS Inc, Chicago, USA).

RESULTS

Results are summarized in Tables 4 and 5. Table 4 shows minimal, maximum, mean and standard deviation values of cephalometric measurements obtained from the maxilla, mandible and temporomandibular joint (TMJ). Table 5 shows the differences between left and right measurements.

DISCUSSION

Facial harmony, an ancient esthetic concern of human beings, was confirmed by facial photographs of Angle Class I Brazilian patients, despite differences between right and left cephalometric measurements.

Orthodontic treatment is planned based on the linear and angular measurements of the craniofacial complex. For decades, measurements were taken on the basis of two-dimensional images. Lateral and posteroanterior cephalograms as well as panoramic radiographs were often used as complementary examination by specialized dentists, mainly in Orthodontics.[26,31-38] Measurements are usually obtained on the basis of two-dimensional scans of three-dimensional structures.

CBCT has redefined cephalometric analysis.[27-30,39] Methods may have to be adapted to CBCT risks and benefits, as well as to its three-dimensional scans so as to increase the accuracy of cephalometric measurements.

This study used VistaDent 3D Pro 2.00 (Dentsply GAC, Nova York, USA) which enables navigation in the axial, sagittal and coronal planes so as to take cephalometric measurements. Measurements taken on the basis of CBCT scans are more accurate and reliable due to better magnification and less distortion than two-dimensional images.[26,27,40-43]

Three-dimensional cephalometric analyses were carried out to establish reference values. Sievers et al.[44] assessed 70 patients and used the index by Katsumata et al[24] to measure asymmetry in Class I and II patients. The index was calculated based on the distances from the craniometric landmarks to the midsagittal, coronal and axial planes. The midsagittal plane was established by sella, nasio and dent landmarks; whereas the axial plane was established by the sella and nasio landmarks and was perpendicular to the midsagittal plane. Dent landmark was used to determine the coronal plane which was perpendicular to the other two planes. Angle Class II patients were not more asymmetrical than Class I patients.

In this study, landmarks and measurements were used to assess symmetry according to five planes: midsagittal, coronal, Frankfort horizontal, maxillary and mandibular. These planes were used as reference for cephalometric measurements. The midsagittal plane was established by the anterior and posterior nasal spines and was perpendicular to the Frankfort horizontal plane according to a model, which differs Katsumata et al.[24] The coronal plane connected the right and left porion and was perpendicular to the Frankfort horizontal plane. There were significant differences in Capitulare-MSP and Capitulare Coronal-Plane cephalometric measurements.

Using different methods to locate craniometric landmarks and three-dimensional cephalometric measurements affects the process of establishing reference values, which hinders comparison with results yielded by previous studies.[24,27,44,45] Some studies have used algorithms to demonstrate the use of three-dimensional cephalometry and to derive two-dimensional cephalometric references for three-dimensional evaluations.[26,41,46] New cephalometric methods using three-dimensional scans have been suggested.[27,28,29] Cheung et al[29] developed a model of cephalometric analysis of dentofacial abnormalities and established new cephalometric reference values for Chinese adult patients. Cavalcanti et al[30] assessed the accuracy of craniofacial bone and tissue measurements obtained by means of 3D computed tomography (CT) and a volume technique using an independent workstation with graphic tools. The 3D-CT measurements proved accurate in assessing growth and developmental changes. Takahashi et al[3] assessed facial skeletal structures using the vertical view of cephalometric lateral radiographs not only to establish the mean normality values for young Brazilians whose ancestors were white or Asian with normal occlusion, but also to assess the differences between males and females and ethnic groups under study. Their results suggested that males and females from both ethnic groups presented differences in some of the cephalometric measurements. Additionally, differences between the two ethnic groups under study were also observed.

The reference values obtained in this study are complementary to other dentoskeletal symmetry findings, such as those provided by clinical and model analyses. Tooth size discrepancies may result in midline deviation which also leads to asymmetry. The Bolton discrepancy analysis of digital CBCT models has been used to assess the effect of teeth on asymmetry. Tarazona et al[47] assessed the reproducibility and reliability of the Bolton index when using digital CBCT models and digitized images of conventional models. Although both methods proved clinically acceptable, CBCT results were accurate and reproducible. Sanders et al[48] compared the degree of dentoskeletal asymmetry in Class II patients and subjects with normal occlusion by means of CBCT. A total of 34 landmarks were used to assess dental, dentoalveolar, bone and condyle asymmetries. The distances from the contact points of maxillary and mandibular central incisors to the midsagittal plane were measured together with linear and angular measurements so as to establish dentoskeletal asymmetry. These measurements were essential for the precise diagnosis of dentoskeletal symmetry.

Asymmetries may result in esthetic and functional deviations of variable intensity. Thus, using cephalometry to determine the severity of asymmetry is an essential tool in orthodontic planning. CBCT may be used for cephalometric analysis, but this three-dimensional tool exposes patients to radiation. Therefore, care should be taken to ensure the best cost-benefit relationship between information and radiation dose,[22,23] and decisions should respect the ALARA principle (as-low-as-reasonably-achievable).

Further studies should be conducted to determine the clinical significance of differences and standard deviations. The faces of subjects included in our study were symmetrical, but cephalometric measurements revealed differences between the left and right sides as well as statistical differences in two cephalometric measurements of TMJ. Despite this discrepancy, CBCT scans may function as a three-dimensional guide to identify and measure dentoskeletal asymmetries during orthodontic and surgical planning.

CONCLUSION

The faces of Angle Class I subjects included in our study were symmetrical, but cephalometric measurements revealed differences between the left and right sides.

REFERENCES

1. Broadbent HB. A new x-ray technique and its application to orthodontia. Angle Orthod. 1931;1:45-66.
2. Graber TM. Orthodontics principles and practice. 2nd ed. Philadelphia: Saunders; 1966.
3. Takahashi R, Pinzan A, Henriques JFC, Freitas MR, Janson GRP, Almeida RR. Análise cefalométrica comparativa das alturas faciais, anterior e posterior, em jovens brasileiros, descendentes de xantodermas e leucodermas, com oclusão normal. Rev Dental Press Ortod Ortop Facial. 2005;10(6):42-58.
4. Kau CH, Bozic M, English J, Lee R, Bussa H, Ellis RK. Cone-beam computed tomography of the maxillofacial region: an update. Int J Med Robotics Comput Assist Surg. 2009;5:366-80.
5. Farman AG, Scarfe WC. Development of imaging selection criteria and procedures should precede cephalometric assessment with cone-beam computed tomography. Am J Orthod Dentofacial Orthop. 2006;130(2):257-65.
6. Castro IO, Alencar AH, Valladares-Neto J, Estrela C. Apical root resorption due to orthodontic treatment detected by cone beam computed tomography. Angle Orthod. 2013;83(2):196-203.
7. Angle EH. Classification of malocclusion. Dent Cosmos. 1899;41:248-64,350-7.
8. Arai Y, Tammisalo E, Hashimoto K, Shinoda K. Development of a compact computed apparatus for dental use. Dentomaxillfac Radiol. 1999;28:245-8.
9. Estrela C, Bueno MR, Alencar AHG, Mattar R, Valladares-Neto J, Azevedo BC, et al. Method to evaluate inflammatory root resorption by using cone beam computed tomography. J Endod. 2009;35(11):1491-7.
10. Dreiseidler T, Mischkowski RA, Neugebauer J, Ritter L, Zöller JE. Comparison of Cone-Beam Imaging with orthopantomography and computerized tomography for assessment in presurgical implant dentistry. Int J Oral Maxillofac Implants. 2009;24(2):216-25.
11. Lund H, Gröndahl K, Gröndahl H. Cone beam computed tomography for assessment of root length and marginal bone level during orthodontic treatment. Angle Orthod. 2010;80(3):466-73.
12. Kau CH, Richmond S, Palomo JM, Hans MG. Three-dimensional cone beam computerized tomography in orthodontics. J Orthod. 2005;32(4):282-93.

13. Mozzo P, Procacci C, Tacconi A, Martini PT, Andreis IA. A new volumetric CT machine for dental imaging based on the cone-beam technique: preliminary results. Eur Radiol. 1998;8(9):1558-64.
14. Capelozza Filho L, Fattori L, Matagliatti L. Um novo método para avaliar as inclinações dentárias utilizando a tomografia computadorizada. Rev Dental Press Ortod Ortop Facial. 2005;10(5):23-9.
15. Cattaneo PM, Bloch CB, Calmar D, Hjortshøj M, Melsen B. Comparison between conventional and cone-beam computed tomography-generated cephalograms. Am J Orthod Dentofacial Orthop. 2008;134(6):798-802.
16. Farman AG, Scarfe WC. Development of imaging selection criteria and procedures should precede cephalometric assessment with cone-beam computed tomography. Am J Orthod Dentofacial Orthop. 2006;130(2):257-65.
17. Oliveira AE, Cevidanes LH, Phillips C, Motta A, Burke B, Tyndall D. Observer reliability of three-dimensional cephalometric landmark identification on cone-beam computerized tomography. Oral Surg Oral Med Oral Pathol Oral Radiol Endod. 2009;107(2):256-65.
18. Cavalcanti MGP, Sales MAO. Tomografia computadorizada. In: Cavalcanti MGP. Diagnostico por Imagem da Face. São Paulo: Ed. Santos; 2008. p. 245-72.
19. Dudic A, Giannopoulou C, Leuzinger M, Kiliaridis S. Detection of apical root resorption after orthodontic treatment by using panoramic radiography and cone-beam computed tomography of super-high resolution. Am J Orthod Dentofacial Orthop. 2009;135(4):434-7.
20. You KH, Lee KJ, Lee SH, Baik HS. Three-dimensional computed tomography analysis of mandibular morphology in patients with facial asymmetry and mandibular prognathism. Am J Orthod Dentofacial Orthop. 2010;138(5):540.e1-8.
21. Freitas JC, Alencar AHG, Estrela C. Long-term evaluation of apical root resorption after orthodontic treatment using periapical radiography and cone beam computed tomography. Dental Press J Orthod. 2013;18(4):104-12.
22. Garcia Silva MA, Wolf U, Heinicke F, Gründler K, Visser H, Hirsch E. M. Effective dosages for recording Veraviewepocs dental panoramic images: analog film, digital, and panoramic scout for CBCT. Oral Surg Oral Med Oral Pathol Oral Radiol Endod. 2008;106(4):571-7.

23. Silva MA, Wolf U, Heinicke F, Bumann A, Visser H, Hirsch E. Cone-beam computed tomography for routine orthodontic treatment planning: a radiation dose evaluation. Am J Orthod Dentofacial Orthop. 2008;133(5):640.e1-5.

24. Katsumata A, Fujishita M, Maeda M, Ariji Y, Ariji E, Langlais RP. 3D-CT evaluation of facial asymmetry. Oral Surg Oral Med Oral Pathol Oral Radiol Endod. 2005;99(2):212-20.

25. Gribel BF, Gribel MN, Frazão DC, McNamara JA Jr, Manzi FR. Accuracy and reliability of craniometric measurements on lateral cephalometry and 3D measurements on CBCT scans. Angle Orthod. 2011;81(1):26-35.

26. Gribel BF, Gribel MN, Manzi FR, Brooks SL, McNamara JA Jr. From 2D to 3D: an algorithm to derive normal values for 3-dimensional computerized assessment. Angle Orthod. 2011;81(1):3-10.

27. Swennen GR, Schutyser F, Barth EL, De Groeve P, De Mey A. A new method of 3-D cephalometry part I: The anatomic Cartesian 3-D reference system. J Craniofac Surg. 2006;17(2):314-25.

28. Swennen GR, Schutyser F. Three-dimensional cephalometry: spiral multislicevs cone-beam computed tomography. Am J Orthod Dentofacial Orthop. 2006;130(3):410-6.

29. Cheung LK, Chan YM, Jayaratne YS, Lo J. Three-dimensional cephalometric norms of Chinese adults in Hong Kong with balanced facial profile. Oral Surg Oral Med Oral Pathol Oral Radiol Endod. 2011;112(2):e56-73.

30. Cavalcanti M, Rocha S, Vannier MW. Craniofacial measurements based on 3D-CT volume rendering: implications for clinical applications. Dentomaxillofac Radiol. 2004;33(3):170-6.

31. Chidiac JJ, Shofer FS, Al-Kutoub A, Laster LL, Ghafari J. Comparison of CT scanograms and cephalometric radiographs in craniofacial imaging. Orthod Craniofac Res. 2002;5(2):104-13.

32. Cevidanes LHS, Styner MA, Profit WR. Image analysis and superimposition of 3-Dimensional cone-beam computed tomography models. Am J Orthod Dentofacial Orthop. 2006;129(5):611-8.

33. Moraes ME, Hollender LG, Chen CS, Moraes LC, Balducci I. Evaluating craniofacial asymmetry with digital cephalometric images and cone-beam computed tomography. Am J Orthod Dentofacial Orthop. 2011;139(6):e523-31.

34. Janson GR, Metaxas A, Woodside DG, Freitas MR, Pinzan A. Threedimensional evaluation of skeletal and dental asymmetries in Class II subdivision malocclusions. Am J Orthod Dentofacial Orthop. 2001;119(4):406-18.

35. Rose JM, Sadowsky C, BeGole EA, Moles R. Mandibular skeletal and dental asymmetry in Class II subdivision malocclusions. Am J Orthod Dentofacial Orthop. 1994;105(5):489-95.

36. Bruntz LQ, Palomo JM, Baden S, Hans MG. A comparison of scanned lateral cephalograms with corresponding original radiographs. Am J Orthod Dentofacial Orthop. 2006;130(3):340-8.

37. Isik F, Nalbantgil D, Sayinsu K, Arun T. A comparative study of cephalometric and arch width characteristics of Class II division 1 and division 2 malocclusions. Eur J Orthod. 2006;28(2):179-83.

38. Sayinsu K, Isik F, Trakyali G, Arun T. An evaluation of the errors in cephalometric measurements on scanned cephalometric images and conventional tracings. Eur J Orthod. 2007;29(1):105-8.

39. Hajeer MY, Millett DT, Ayoub AF, Siebert JP. Applications of 3D imaging in orthodontics: part I. J Orthod. 2004;31(1):62-70.

40. Adams GL, Gansky SA, Miller AJ, Harrell WE, Hatcher DC. Comparison between traditional 2-dimensional cephalometry and a 3-dimensional approach on human dry skulls. Am J Orthod Dentofacial Orthop. 2004;126(4):397-409.

41. Cho Y, Moseley DJ, Siewerdsen JH, Jaffray DA. Accurate technique for complete geometric calibration of cone-beam computed tomography systems. Med Phys. 2005;32(4):968-83.

42. Hilgers ML, Scarfe WC, Scheetz JP, Farman AG. Accuracy of linear temporomandibular joint measurements with cone-beam computed tomography and digital cephalometric radiography. Am J Orthod Dentofacial Orthop. 2005;128(6):803-11.

43. Santoro M, Jarjoura K, Cangialosi TJ. Accuracy of digital and analogue cephalometric measurements assessed with the sandwich technique. Am J Orthod Dentofacial Orthop. 2006;129(3):345-51.

44. Sievers MM, Larson BE, Gaillard PR, Wey A. Asymmetry assessment using cone beam CT A Class I and Class II patient comparison. Angle Orthod. 2012;82(3):410-7.

45. Peck JL, Sameshima GT, Miller A, Worth P, Hatcher DC. Mesiodistal root angulation using panoramic and Cone Beam CT. Angle Orthod. 2007;77(2):206-13.

46. Halazonetis DJ. From 2-dimensional cephalograms to 3-dimensional computed tomography scans. Am J Orthod Dentofacial Orthop. 2005;127(5):627-37.

47. Tarazona B, Llamas JM, Cibrián R, Gandía JL, Paredes V. Evaluation of the validity of the Bolton Index using cone-beam computed tomography (CBCT). Med Oral Patol Oral Cir Bucal. 2012;17(5):e878-83.

48. Sanders DA, Rigali PH, Neace WP, Uribe F, Nanda R. Skeletal and dental asymmetries in Class II subdivision malocclusions using cone-beam computed tomography. Am J Orthod Dentofacial Orthop. 2010;138(5):542.e1-20.

Permissions

All chapters in this book were first published in DPJO, by Dental Press International; hereby published with permission under the Creative Commons Attribution License or equivalent. Every chapter published in this book has been scrutinized by our experts. Their significance has been extensively debated. The topics covered herein carry significant findings which will fuel the growth of the discipline. They may even be implemented as practical applications or may be referred to as a beginning point for another development.

The contributors of this book come from diverse backgrounds, making this book a truly international effort. This book will bring forth new frontiers with its revolutionizing research information and detailed analysis of the nascent developments around the world.

We would like to thank all the contributing authors for lending their expertise to make the book truly unique. They have played a crucial role in the development of this book. Without their invaluable contributions this book wouldn't have been possible. They have made vital efforts to compile up to date information on the varied aspects of this subject to make this book a valuable addition to the collection of many professionals and students.

This book was conceptualized with the vision of imparting up-to-date information and advanced data in this field. To ensure the same, a matchless editorial board was set up. Every individual on the board went through rigorous rounds of assessment to prove their worth. After which they invested a large part of their time researching and compiling the most relevant data for our readers.

The editorial board has been involved in producing this book since its inception. They have spent rigorous hours researching and exploring the diverse topics which have resulted in the successful publishing of this book. They have passed on their knowledge of decades through this book. To expedite this challenging task, the publisher supported the team at every step. A small team of assistant editors was also appointed to further simplify the editing procedure and attain best results for the readers.

Apart from the editorial board, the designing team has also invested a significant amount of their time in understanding the subject and creating the most relevant covers. They scrutinized every image to scout for the most suitable representation of the subject and create an appropriate cover for the book.

The publishing team has been an ardent support to the editorial, designing and production team. Their endless efforts to recruit the best for this project, has resulted in the accomplishment of this book. They are a veteran in the field of academics and their pool of knowledge is as vast as their experience in printing. Their expertise and guidance has proved useful at every step. Their uncompromising quality standards have made this book an exceptional effort. Their encouragement from time to time has been an inspiration for everyone.

The publisher and the editorial board hope that this book will prove to be a valuable piece of knowledge for researchers, students, practitioners and scholars across the globe.

List of Contributors

Daniel Santos Fonseca Figueiredo, Lucas Cardinal and Flávia Uchôa Costa Bartolomeo
Former Orthodontic residents, Pontifícia Universidade Católica de Minas Gerais (PUC-MG), Belo Horizonte, Brazil

Juan Martin Palomo
Associate Professor and Program Director, Case Western Reserve University, Department of Orthodontics, and Director of the Craniofacial Imaging Center, School of Dental Medicine, Cleveland, Ohio, USA

Martinho Campolina Rebello Horta
Associate Professor and Dean of Graduate Studies, Pontifícia Universidade Católica de Minas Gerais (PUC-MG), Belo Horizonte, Brazil

Ildeu Andrade Jr
Associate Professor of Orthodontics, Pontifícia Universidade Católica de Minas Gerais (PUC-MG), Belo Horizonte, Brazil

Dauro Douglas Oliveira
Associate Professor and Program Director of Orthodontics, Pontifícia Universidade Católica de Minas Gerais (PUC-MG), Belo Horizonte, Brazil

Antônio Carlos de Oliveira Ruellas
Phd in Dentistry and Adjunct Professor, Federal University of Rio de Janeiro (UFRJ)

Leonardo Koerich
MSc in Orthodontics, UFRJ

Carolina Baratieri
Phd in Orthodontics, UFRJ

Claudia Trindade Mattos
Phd in Orthodontics, UFRJ. Adjunct Professor, UFF

Matheus Alves Junior and Daniel Brunetto
Doctorate student in Orthodontics, UFRJ

Suelen Cristina da Costa Pereira
PhD Orthodontic Resident, School of Dentistry — University of São Paulo/Bauru

Elisa Gurgel Simas de Oliveira
MSc in Orthodontics, UniCEUMA

Célia Regina Maio Pinzan-Vercelino
Professor, Post-Graduation Program – MSc in Orthodontics -UniCEUMA

Adilson Luiz Ramos
Adjunct professor, Department of Dentistry, State University of Maringá, UEM

Lilian Cristina Vessoni Iwaki
Associate professor of Dental radiology and Stomatology, Department of Dentistry, State University of Maringá, UEM

Kelly Regina Micheletti
PhD resident in Orthodontics, State University of São Paulo, UNESP

Patrícia Superbi Lemos Maschtakow
Doctorate Student of the Program of Oral Biopathology at FOSJC-UNESP

Jefferson Luis Oshiro Tanaka
Professor of the Specialization Course in Orthodontics APCD

João Carlos da Rocha
Assistant Professor of Pediatric Dentistry at FOSJC-UNESP

Lílian Chrystiane Giannasi
Adjunct Professor, UNINOVE

Mari Eli Leonelli de Moraes and Julio Cezar de Melo Castilho
Assistant Professor of Dental Radiology at FOSJC-UNESP

Carolina Bacci Costa
Doctorate Student of the Program of Oral Biopathology at FOSJC-UNESP

Luiz Cesar de Moraes
Full Professor, Dental Radiology at FOSJC-UNESP

Mahtab Nouri
Associate professor, Dentofacial Deformities Research Center of Shahid Beheshti University of Medical Sciences, Iran

Arash Farzan
Postgraduate student of Orthodontics, Research Center of Shahid Beheshti University of Medical Sciences, Iran

Lindsey Eidson
MSc in Orthodontics, University of North Carolina

Ana Cláudia de Castro Ferreira Conti
Professor of Orthodontics, Universidade do Sagrado Coração (USC), Bauru, São Paulo, Brazil

Ali Reza Akbarzadeh Baghban
Assistant professor of Biostatistics, Faculty of Paramedicine, Shahid Beheshti, University of Medical Sciences, Iran

Reza Massudi
Professor, Laser and Plasma Research Institute, Shahid Beheshti University, Iran

Fabiano Paiva Vieira
Professor, Federal Institute of Paraná

Arnaldo Pinzan
Associate professor, Department of Pediatric Dentistry, Orthodontics and Collective Health, School of Dentistry — University of São Paulo/Bauru

Guilherme Janson
Full professor, Department of Pediatric Dentistry, Orthodontics and Collective Health, School of Dentistry — University of São Paulo/Bauru

Thais Maria Freire Fernandes
Professor, University of Northern Paraná (UNOPAR)

Renata Carvalho Sathler
Professor, Hospital for Rehabilitation of Craniofacial Anomalies/USP

Rafael Pinelli Henriques
Professor, Central-West College Pinelli Henriques

Mayur S. Bhattad
Senior lecturer, Sharad Pawar Dental College and Hospital, Department of Pedodontics and Preventive Dentistry, Sawangi, Wardha, Maharashtra, India

Sudhindra Baliga
Professor, Sharad Pawar Dental College and Hospital, Department of Pedodontics and Preventive Dentistry, Sawangi, Wardha, Maharashtra, India

Pavan Vibhute
Associate professor, Sharad Pawar Dental College and Hospital, Department of Orthodontics, Sawangi, Wardha, Maharashtra, India

Daniela Gamba Garib
Full professor, School of Dentistry — University of São Paulo/Bauru.(FOBUSP)

Maria Helena Ocké Menezes
MSc in Orthodontics, University São Paulo, UNICID

Omar Gabriel da Silva Filho
MSc in Orthodontics, São Paulo State University (UNESP)

Patricia Bittencourt Dutra dos Santos
PhD resident in Applied Dental Sciences (FOB-USP)

Paulo Roberto Barroso Picanço and Gracemia Vasconcelos Picanço
MSc in Orthodontics, Uningá. Professor, Paulo Picanço Center of Orthodontics

Fabricio Pinelli Valarelli and Rodrigo Hermont Cançado
Adjunct Professor, Uningá

Karina Maria Salvatore de Freitas
Post-Doc in Orthodontics, University of Toronto. Professora, Uningá

Michele Machado Vidor
Masters student in Clinical Dentistry, Radiology, Universidade Federal do Rio Grande do Sul (UFRGS), Santa Cecília, Rio Grande do Sul, Brazil

Rafael Perdomo Felix
Masters student in Dental Prosthesis, Pontifícia Universidade Católica do Rio Grande do Sul (PUCRS), Porto Alegre, Rio Grande do Sul, Brazil

Ernani Menezes Marchioro
Adjunct professor, Pontifícia Universidade Católica do Rio Grande do Sul (PUCRS), Department of Dentistry, Porto Alegre, Rio Grande do Sul, Brazil

Luciane Hahn
Professor, São Leopoldo Mandic, School of Dentistry, Postgraduate program in Orthodontics, Porto Alegre, Rio Grande do Sul, Brazil

Alexandre Durval Lemos
Professor, Department of Dentistry, State University of Paraíba, UEPB

Cintia Regina Tornisiello Katz and Mônica Vilela Heimer
Assistant professor, Department of Social Dentistry, Federal University of Pernambuco, UFPE

Aronita Rosenblatt
Full professor, Department of Social Dentistry, University of Pernambuco, UPE

João Paulo Schwartz, Daniele Salazar Somensi, Priscila Yoshizaki and Luciana Laís Savero Reis
Specialist in Orthodontics, Hospital for Rehabilitation of Craniofacial Anomalies – São Paulo University (HRAC-USP)

Rita de Cássia Moura Carvalho Lauris and Omar Gabriel da Silva Filho
MSc in Orthodontics, HRAC-USP

Gisele Dalbén
PhD in Pediatric Dentistry, HRAC-USP

Daniela Gamba Garib
Professor and assistant professor of Orthodontics, School of Dentistry — University of São Paulo/Bauru

Yalil Augusto Rodriguez-Cardenas
Specialist in Orthodontics, National University of Colombia. Specialist in Oral and Maxillofacial Radiology, Universidad Peruana Cayetano Heredia

Luis Ernesto Arriola-Guillen
Associate Professor, Department of Orthodontics, School of Dentistry, Universidad Científica del Sur-UCSUR and Universidad Nacional Mayor de San Marcos, UNMSM

Carlos Flores-Mir
Associate Professor and Head of the Department of Orthodontics, University of Alberta
Professor, University of Alberta, Department of Dentistry, Edmonton, Alberta, Canada

Jordana Rodrigues Amorim
Student at the specialization course in Preventive Orthodontics, Hospital for Rehabilitation of Craniofacial Anomalies/USP

Diogo de Vasconcelos Macedo
Degree in Dentistry, Federal University of Pará (UFPA)

David Normando
Adjunct professor, Federal University of Pará (UFPA)

Ana Cláudia Laureano Navarro
Specialist in Orthodontics, Londrina State University

Luiz Sérgio Carreiro, Ricardo Takahashi, Carlos Eduardo de Oliveira Lima and Claudenir Rossato
Associate Professor, Londrina State University

Tehnia Aziz
Private practice, Edmonton, Alberta, Canada

Francis Carter Wheatley
Graduate student in Computer Sciences, Boston University, Boston, Massachusetts, USA

Kal Ansari
Assistant professor, University of Alberta, Department of Surgery, Edmonton, Alberta, Canada

Manuel Lagravere
Assistant professor, University of Alberta, Department of Dentistry, Edmonton, Alberta, Canada

Michael Major
Clinical assistant professor, University of Alberta, Department of Dentistry, Edmonton, Alberta, Canada

Rejane Targino Soares Beltrão
PhD in Orthodontics, School of Dentistry — University of São Paulo/Bauru

Guilherme Janson and Daniela Gamba Garib
Full professor, Department of Orthodontics, School of Dentistry — University of São Paulo/Bauru

Paula Cabrini Scheibel
MSc in Integrated Dentistry, State University of Maringá, UEM

Pimchanok Foosiri and Korapin Mahatumarat
Chulalongkorn University, Department of Orthodontics (Bangkok, Thailand)

Soontra Panmekiate
Chulalongkorn University, Department of Radiology (Bangkok, Thailand)

Caroline Nemetz Bronfman
PhD resident in Orthodontics, Universidade de São Paulo (USP), School of Dentistry, Bauru, São Paulo, Brazil

Guilherme Janson
Full professor, Universidade de São Paulo (USP), School of Dentistry, Department of Orthodontics, Bauru, São Paulo, Brazil

Arnaldo Pinzan
Associate professor, Universidade de São Paulo (USP), School of Dentistry, Department of Orthodontics, Bauru, São Paulo, Brazil

Thais Lima Rocha
PhD resident in Orthodontics, Universidade de São Paulo (USP), School of Dentistry, Bauru, São Paulo, Brazil

Maurício Barbosa Guerra da Silva
MSc in Orthodontics

Bruno Cabús Gois
Specialist in Radiology, APCD. MSc in Dentistry, UNESP

Eduardo Franzotti Sant'Anna
Assistant Professor of Orthodontics, Federal University of Rio de Janeiro (UFRJ)

Henrique M. Villela, Mario Vedovello Filho, Heloísa C. Valdrighi, Milton Santamaria-Jr, Carolina Carmo de Menezes and Silvia A. S. Vedovello
Uniararas, Fundação Hermínio Ometto, Programa de Pós-graduação em Ortodontia (Araras/SP, Brazil)

João Paulo Schwartz and Taisa Boamorte Raveli
PhD resident, Universidade Estadual Paulista (UNESP), Department of Orthodontics, Araraquara, São Paulo, Brazil

Humberto Osvaldo Schwartz-Filho
Adjunct Professor, Universidade Federal do Paraná (UFPR), Department of Stomatology, Curitiba, Paraná, Brazil

Dirceu Barnabé Raveli
Professor, Universidade Estadual Paulista (UNESP), Department of Orthodontics, Araraquara, São Paulo, Brazil

Marcio Rodrigues de Almeida and Paula Vanessa Pedron Oltramari-Navarro
Full professor of Orthodontics, Universidade Norte do Paraná (UNOPAR), Londrina, Paraná, Brazil

Cristina Futagami
MSc in Orthodontics, Universidade Norte do Paraná (UNOPAR), Londrina, Paraná, Brazil

Ricardo de Lima Navarro
PhD in Orthodontics, Universidade de São Paulo (USP), São Paulo, São Paulo, Brazil

Luciana Flaquer Martins
Visiting professor, Ciodonto College

Julio Wilson Vigorito
Full professor of Orthodontics, University of São Paulo (USP)

Olavo Cesar Lyra Porto
PhD resident in Health Sciences, Federal University of Goiás (UFG)
MSc in Health Sciences, UFG

Jairo Curado de Freitas
Professor, Department of Orthodontics, Brazilian Dental Association (ABOR)
PhD in Health Sciences, UFG

Ana Helena Gonçalves de Alencar
Post-doc in Endodontics, Cardiff University. Professor of Endodontics, School of Dentistry, UFG

Carlos Estrela
Full Professor in Endodontics, USP. Professor of Endodontics, School of Dentistry, UFG

Index

www.ingramcontent.com/pod-product-compliance
Lightning Source LLC
Chambersburg PA
CBHW080644200326
41458CB00013B/4724